Perioperative Care of the Child

A Nursing Manual

Edited by

Linda Shields

PhD, MMedSci, BAppSci (Nursing), FRCNA, FRSM

WILEY-BLACKWELL

A John Wiley & Sons, Ltd., Publication

This edition first published 2010
© 2010 Blackwell Publishing Ltd

Blackwell Publishing was acquired by John Wiley & Sons in February 2007. Blackwell's publishing programme has been merged with Wiley's global Scientific, Technical, and Medical business to form Wiley-Blackwell.

Registered offices
John Wiley & Sons Ltd, The Atrium, Southern Gate, Chichester, West Sussex, PO19 8SQ, United Kingdom

Editorial offices
9600 Garsington Road, Oxford, OX4 2DQ, United Kingdon
2121 State Avenue, Ames, Iowa 50014-8300, USA

For details of our global editorial offices, for customer services and for information about how to apply for permission to reuse the copyright material in this book please see our website at www.wiley.com/wiley-blackwell.

Library of Congress Cataloging-in-Publication Data
Perioperative care of the child : a nursing manual / edited by Linda Shields.
　　p. ; cm.
　Includes bibliographical references and index.
　ISBN 978-1-4051-5595-3 (pbk. : alk. paper) 1. Children—Surgery—Nursing—Handbooks, manuals, etc.
2. Operating room nursing—Handbooks, manuals, etc. I. Shields, Linda.
　　[DNLM: 1. Perioperative Nursing—methods. 2. Adolescent. 3. Child. 4. Pediatric Nursing—methods. WY 161 P4445 2010]
RD137.P47 2010
617.9′8—dc22

2009021834

A catalogue record for this book is available from the British Library.

Set in 9.5/12 pt Palatino by Macmillan Publishing Solutions, Chennai, India
Printed and bound in Malaysia by KHL Printing Co Sdn Bhd

1   2010

Contents

Contributors

Bernie Carter *PhD, PGCE, PGCE, BSc, RSCN, SRN, FRCN*
Bernie Carter is currently Professor of Children's Nursing at the University of Central Lancashire and at Alder Hey Children's NHS Foundation Trust. Bernie has been involved in researching and writing about children's pain for many years. Her particular interests lie in pain assessment and especially the assessment, care and pain management of children with severe cognitive impairment. She is currently involved in researching the pain experiences of boys and young men with Duchenne Muscular Dystrophy.

Julie Grasso *(nee Mill) RN*
Julie Grasso is the Clinical Nurse Consultant at The Stuart Pegg Paediatric Burns Centre at the Royal Children's Hospital, Brisbane. Her special interests include distraction therapy for children and burn assessment.

Eunice Hanisch *BSc (Nursing), BSocComm, PR*
Eunice has been working at the Mater Children's Hospital in Brisbane, Australia, since 1995. Eunice joined the Mater Children's Paediatric Postoperative Anaesthetic Care Unit in 2005, and before that worked in the surgical/orthopaedic ward.

Jeremy Jolley *PhD, MA, BN, PGCEA, PGCTheol, SRN, RSCN*
Jeremy Jolley is a Senior Lecturer – Paediatric Nursing at the University of Hull, East Yorkshire in the UK. He initially worked in general paediatric nursing before becoming a nurse teacher in 1989. Since then, he has managed pre- and post-registration programmes in paediatric nursing at the undergraduate and postgraduate levels. His research interests centre around the history of paediatric nursing, and his publishing has focussed on the individual needs of the child and the ways in which nursing can provide a service that is properly orientated to the needs of each child rather than to the needs of the hospital or community nursing team. Jeremy argues that each child should be seen as a 'person' and as a member of a family, that the child has a right, not just to be respected but to be regarded with affection.

Denise Jonas *RSCN, RGN, MSc, BSc (Hons), PGCHEPR, RNT*
Denise Jonas is currently a lecturer/practitioner in children's pain management and child health at University of Salford and Royal Manchester Children's Hospital. Denise has specialised for many years in the field of children's pain management. Her interests include the management of pain following day surgery and chronic pain in children.

Roy Kimble *MD (Qld), MBChB (Glas), FRCS, FRACS (Paed Surg)*
Professor Kimble is a Paediatric Surgeon and Director of Burns & Trauma in the Combined Department of Paediatric Surgery at The Royal Children's and Mater Children's Hospitals, Brisbane, Australia. His special areas of interest include paediatric burns and antenatal

diagnosis and treatment of fetal anomalies. He is Professor of Paediatrics at the University of Queensland Department of Paediatrics and Child Health.

Wendy McAlister *BN, RN*
Wendy holds a Bachelor of Nursing and works at the Mater Children's Hospital, Brisbane, Queensland, Australia, as a Registered Nurse. She has been a paediatric nurse for 12 years, worked as a paediatric recovery nurse for 5 years and an anaesthetic nurse for 4 years.

Janet Roper *BN, GradDip Perioperative Nursing, PGC Anaesthetic Nursing, RN*
Janet's interests in paediatric perioperative nursing began in her early training days at the Royal Children's Hospital in Brisbane, Australia. After various positions in Australia, Janet moved to the UK where she worked as practice educator in the Operating Department of the John Radcliffe Hospital in Oxford. Janet has now returned to her home town of Brisbane and is a perioperative nurse at the Redcliffe Hospital.

Linda Shields *PhD, MMedSci, BAppSci (Nursing), FRCNA, FRSM*
Linda Shields is Professor of Paediatric and Child Health Nursing and the Child and Adolescent Health Service and Curtin Health Innovation Research Institute, Curtin University of Technology, Perth, Western Australia, Australia, and is an Honorary Professor in the Department of Paediatrics and Child Health, The University of Queensland, Brisbane, Queensland, Australia. She maintains a small clinical load in post-operative recovery, and her research interests include family-centred care across health services, health of children in developing countries and the history of nursing.

Rebecca Smith *MA, BA (Hons), RN*
Rebecca is an In-House Donor Transplant Co-ordinator for the Hull and East Yorkshire Hospitals NHS Trust in the UK and a regional Transplant Co-ordinator for St James University Hospital in Leeds. She worked for many years on a General Intensive Care Unit that nursed both adults and children. She is also a lecturer at the University of Hull, specialising in health care ethics.

Susan Louise Tame *MSc (Dist), PGDip, BSc (Hons), PGCE (FE), RN (Adult)*
Susan began working in theatres at Hull and East Yorkshire Hospitals NHS Trust, England, in 1999 and worked in a number of specialities as a scrub practitioner before becoming a senior nurse and then sister in maxillofacial and ENT theatres. Susan currently works as a training advisor, providing advice and support to pre- and post-registered operating department practitioners and nurses working within theatres across the Trust. She is also a clinical practice educator for student operating department practitioners.

Ann Lesley Tanner *RN, MHlthSc (HlthProm)*
Ann Lesley Tanner became a Registered General Nurse at the Royal Adelaide Hospital, Adelaide, South Australia, in 1984, and gained a Master's degree in Health Science, majoring in Health Promotion in 1998 from Queensland University of Technology, Brisbane, Australia. She works as a Registered Nurse at the Royal Children's Hospital, Brisbane, Queensland, in the day procedure centre, PACU (post-anaesthetic care unit) and a major surgical/burns ward. She has been working in paediatric surgical wards and operating suites for the past 15 years.

Introduction

Operating theatres are frightening places, a foreign environment where highly specialized techniques that involve opening and invading a human body take place. As such, they present unique challenges for both those who use them, and those who work there. For children who require surgery and their families, the surgical environment is potentially one in which consideration must be given to the whole psychosocial aspect of care, even more so than in any other hospital environment. This is the 50th anniversary of publication of the Platt Report, a policy document that saw, around the world, the protection of the psychological state of children during hospital admission. This book about the care of children in the perioperative area celebrates the benefits brought about by the changes implemented in the paediatric surgical area since. While we have covered many topics surrounding different areas of paediatric surgical practice, there are some we may have missed, and would welcome suggestions from your readers for future editions.

In this book, we aim to provide the reader with a range of information about the specialised care of children (and their families) who are having a surgical procedure in a perioperative area. However, we have not included detailed accounts of standard perioperative practice, e.g. sterilising techniques, as this book is about children and their families. For standard perioperative practice, many large and detailed books exist. The authors of this book are all experienced clinicians, who have highly specialised skills in particular areas. While we all live in different countries, we all care for children and their families when they come into a health service for a surgical procedure of some kind.

A note on terminology. We often refer to parents. For our purposes, 'parent' means any person who has primary responsibility to care for a child. This can mean the natural parents, any extended family member, foster parents and carers or anyone in whose charge the child is deemed to be at the time. However, for brevity, we use the word 'parent/s'. We use the term 'child' to mean child in the legal sense, i.e. a minor in legal terms (in many countries, someone under the age of 18 years). However, we recognise that adolescents, young people or any other term considered politically correct could be used for those in their teenage years, whom we include in this book. We also include people who may be older than 18 years, but who still use paediatric operating theatres for any reason whatsoever. For ease of use, all will be referred to as 'child' or 'children'. We use the terms 'operating theatre' and 'operating room' interchangeably, and often use the abbreviation 'OR' for operating room. The paediatric postanaesthetic care unit, or post-operative recovery room, is denoted as 'PPACU'. Induction rooms are part of many paediatric ORs, and are the rooms adjoining the operating theatre itself where the anaesthetic is induced before the child is wheeled into the theatre and placed on the operating table. Induction rooms are often colourful places with pictures on the wall and a range of distraction tools such as music and puppets to relax the child and his or her parents. This precludes a range of people having to enter the theatre itself, thereby preventing possible spread of microorganisms.

We hope that you enjoy reading this book, and that it is useful to anyone who is caring for children and families.

Linda Shields

Acknowledgements

This book is dedicated to the memory of Mary Ann Doslick (1953–1999), a committed and caring children's nurse who worked at the Mater Children's Hospital in Brisbane, Queensland, Australia, for many years. Some of us who have written this book knew Mary well, and miss her very much.

My personal thanks must go to the contributors, many of whom had serious family events occur during the time they wrote their chapters. I applaud their persistence and commitment, and for sticking with what must have become onerous tasks at times. Ms Canay Brown Coghill and Master Alfred Jack Coghill helped enormously with their patience and willingness to be photographed in many different situations.

I also want to thank Ms Vicki Adams from the Medical Graphics Department at the Mater Hospitals in Brisbane, Australia, who helped provide many of the images in the book. Ms Jenny Hall and staff of the University of Queensland Mater Library also helped with searches. A special thanks to Ms Jeanette Gilchrist from the Faculty of Health and Social Care at the University of Hull, who did much of the administration and co-ordination of authors, chapters etc. I thank my husband, Allan Shields, who put up with the late nights, stress and confusion that writing any book causes in a household.

And last but not least, I wish to thank Ms Magenta Lampson and her team at Wiley-Blackwell in Oxford for their support, encouragement and editorial eyes.

Abbreviations

<	less than
>	greater than
ABC	airway, breathing and circulation
ABG	arterial blood gasses
ACORN	Australian College of Operating Room Nurses
ANZCA	Australia & New Zealand College of Anaesthesists
AORN	Association of Operating Room Nurses
ASPAN	American Society of PeriAnaesthesia Nurses
BP	blood pressure
BSD	brainstem death
BTS	British Transplant Society
C	centigrade
Ca^+	calcium
CAAS	Cardiac Analgesia Assessment Scale
CCAM	congenital cystic adenomatoid malformation
CDH	congenital diaphragmatic hernia
CIT	cautery inferior turbinates
CJD	Creutzfeld–Jakob disease
cm	centimetre
CMI	continuous morphine infusions
CMV	cytomegalovirus
CNS	central nervous system
CO_2	carbon dioxide
CSF	cerebrospinal fluid
CT	computerised tomography
CVP	central venous pressure
DIC	disseminated intravascular coagulation
ECG	electrocardiogram
ENT	ear, nose and throat
ETT	endotracheal tube
EUA	examination under anaesthetic
EXIT	*ex utero* intrapartum treatment
FCC	family-centred care
FiO_2	fraction of inspired oxygen
FLACC	Faces, Legs, Activity, Cry and Consolability pain assessment tool
FPS-R	Revised Faces Pain Scale
GA	general anaesthetic
GMC	General Medical Council (UK)
GP	general practitioner

H_2O	water
HIV	human immunodeficiency virus
HLA	human leukocyte antigen
hr	hour
ICP	intracranial pressure
ICU	intensive care unit
IDC	indwelling catheter
IM	intramuscular
IPPV	Intermittent Positive Pressure Ventilation
IV	intravenous
kg	kilogramme
LMA	laryngeal mask airway
LWI	local wound infiltration
MAC	minimum alveolar concentration
mEq	milli-equivalents
MH	malignant hyperthermia
mins	minutes
MIS	minimally invasive surgery
mls	millilitres
mm	millimetre
mmHg	millimetres of mercury
MRI	magnetic resonance imaging
MSPCT	Multiple Size Poker Chip Tool
NB	*nota bene* (note well)
NCA	nurse-controlled analgesia
NCCPC-PV	Non-Communicating Children's Pain Checklist-Post-operative Version
NCCPC-R	Non-Communicating Children's Pain Checklist
NEC	necrotising enterocolitis
NG	nasogastric
NHBD	non–heart beating donation
NIBP	non-invasive blood pressure
NSAID	non-steroidal anti-inflammatory drugs
O_2	oxygen
OA	oesophageal atresia
ODP	operating department practitioner
ODR	National Organ Donor Register (UK)
OR	operating room (or operating theatre)
OSA	obstructive sleep apnoea
PARS	post-anaesthesia recovery score
PAS	post-anaesthesia shivering
PCA	patient-controlled analgesia
PEG	percutaneous enteric gastrostomy
PIPP	Premature Infant Pain Profile
PO_2	oxygen pressure
PONV	post-operative nausea and vomiting
PPACU	paediatric post-operative care unit

PPP	Paediatric Pain Profile
PPPM	Parents Post-operative Pain Measure
RN	registered nurse
SaO$_2$	oxygen saturation
SCAN	suspected child abuse and neglect
secs	seconds
T3	tri-iodothyronine
T4	thyroxine
TBI	total body irradiation
TBSA	total body surface area
TDC	thyroglossal duct cyst
TIVA	total intravenous anaesthesia
TOF	tracheo-oesophageal fistula
TPN	total parenteral nutrition
TTTS	twin–twin transfusion syndrome
U&E	urea and electrolytes
UK	United Kingdom
USA, US	United States of America
WHO	World Health Organization

1 The history of children's perioperative care

Jeremy Jolley

Why history is important

We may question what place history has in perioperative care today, care that is, by definition, modern, technical and advanced. There are several reasons why it can be useful to pause for a while and consider what history has to offer. We can learn from what has gone before, from the mistakes that have been made and also from the way that practitioners have managed to advance the discipline and improve the care that can be provided to the surgical child. History also gives our discipline a depth that it would not otherwise have. Perioperative nursing is not just a discipline that is going places, it has a past, too, and a history that is rich and fascinating.

The written history of perioperative nursing as a speciality of nursing, rather than surgery, is difficult to find, and needs rigorous research and examination. Most of the written history is about the development of operating theatre nursing during times of war (Holder, 2003a,b, 2004a–c; Rae, 2004a,b), or about its development as an adjunct to the surgeon (Cumber, 2006; Nelson, 2007). A critical history of the speciality is badly needed.

What is perioperative nursing?

The lack of a single and inclusive definition of the speciality makes historical investigation difficult. The term 'perioperative nursing' emerged in the 1970s (McGarvey *et al.*, 2000), and in 1978, the Association of Operating Room Nurses in the USA defined it as encompassing engagement with the patient from the initial decision to undertake surgery to the final discharge of the patient from the outpatient clinic. By 2006, this had changed little, with the following definition on the website of the Association of Operating Room Nurses (USA). However, a search in 2008 showed it is not possible to find this definition again:

AORN defines the term "perioperative nursing" as the practice of nursing directed toward patients undergoing operative and other invasive procedures. AORN recognizes the "perioperative nurse" as one who provides, manages, teaches, and/or studies the care of patients undergoing operative or other invasive procedures, in the preoperative, intraoperative, and postoperative phases of the patient's surgical experience. Perioperative nurses work on the surgical front lines, so no one is better qualified or has the capacity to advocate for and ensure patient safety in the surgical setting. Association of Operating Room Nurses (2006)

Other definitions are scarce. Nursing within the perioperative environment is implied in the definition of the Association for Perioperative Practice in the UK, but there is no definition of the perioperative nurse: 'the area utilised immediately before, during and after the performance of a clinical intervention or clinically invasive procedure' (Association for Perioperative Practice, 2005). The Australian College of Operating Room Nurses Standards for Perioperative Nursing contain the following definitions:

Perioperative: The period before, during and after an anaesthetic, surgical or other procedure.
Perioperative Environment: The service area where the provision of an anaesthetic, surgical or other procedure may be undertaken.
Perioperative nurse: A nurse who provides patient care during the perioperative period.

Australian College of Operating Theatre Nurses (2006).

While the American and Australian definitions are for and about nurses, the shortage of nurses in the UK and the governmental financial restrictions placed on the National Health Service have led to the emergence of other practitioners such as 'operating department practitioners'. These technicians are being educated by nurses (Shields & Watson, 2007) without a realisation of the effects of such roles on the nursing profession.

In 1999, at the Association of Operating Room Nurses (AORN) national conference in the USA, members decided to change the organisation's name to the Association for PeriOperative Registered Nurses (Editorial, 1999) and in so doing ensured that the term 'perioperative' nursing became part of modern language. It is probably the case that such broad definitions of perioperative nursing are not yet universally accepted. Most practitioners would confine the term 'perioperative nursing' to that care which is given in and around the theatre suite (Association for Perioperative Practice, 2005).

While the discipline's focus is still on the patient in the operating theatre, paediatric perioperative nurses are beginning to see their role as something broader, as child patients cannot be properly understood by their need for surgery alone. Their proper care requires an understanding of the child as a child, as a member of a family and as a person with a life outside the theatre suite.

A brief history of perioperative nursing

War is always good for the development of health sciences, in particular, those related to surgery, and perioperative nursing is no exception. The Crimean War (1853–1856) and the American Civil War (1861–1965) saw the emergence of nurses who assisted with surgery (Holder, 2003a; Schultz, 2004). During First World War, technology and machines became the cornerstone of armed conflict, and surgery developed exponentially, as did operating theatre nursing (Holder, 2004a–c; Rae, 2004a,b). Similar rates of advances in knowledge occurred during Second World War, the Korean War and the Vietnam War, and in all armed conflicts since then (Bassett, 1992; Biedermann, 2002). Much of the development of surgery took place on the battlefield, and throughout history we see both women and men providing nursing care (Holder, 2003b; Schultz, 2004).

However, it is necessary to note that for the most part, the individuals concerned were not members of any discipline of nursing and would not have regarded themselves as professional nurses. Furthermore, there was a lack of organisation to the often *ad hoc* services that were provided. It was this deficiency that brought Florence Nightingale to fame. While the existence of nursing during ancient battles is interesting, it is only from the time of Florence Nightingale and perhaps the mid-19th century when we can say that the history of perioperative nursing begins. This should not be surprising, for nursing as a discipline, that is, an organised body of people who saw themselves as nurses, did not exist much before this time. In fact, both paediatric nursing and perioperative nursing came about because of the growth of the hospital as a means of providing health care. By the mid-19th century, most large towns in Britain and Western Europe possessed a general hospital and by the end of that century, most large towns also had a children's hospital (Lomax, 1996).

For paediatric perioperative nursing to exist on any scale, there first needed to be hospitals for children and surgeons working within those hospitals. Such history does not begin much before the middle of the 19th century (the first children's hospital in Britain opened in 1852). At that time, almost all surgery were orthopaedic or associated with the repair of wounds. Additionally, children's hospitals often provided only medical care; surgery was hardly considered part of the medical profession and most children's hospitals did not possess an operating theatre. Over the next 100 years, paediatric surgery tended to develop more from adult surgery in the general hospitals than it did from the activities of the medically orientated children's hospitals. This slowed its development and resulted in paediatric surgery and paediatric perioperative care being largely a 20th century invention. In other words, there were about 50 years (between about 1850 and 1900) when paediatric perioperative care developed especially slowly. However, paediatric surgery and perioperative nursing did benefit from the fact that practitioners came to work with children, already having experience of adult surgery. Children's hospitals, on the other hand, with their focus on medical care, were often ill prepared to develop surgical services for children. Well into the 20th century, this schism between the general and children's hospitals affected perioperative paediatric nursing to a degree that was both deep and dysfunctional. Even today, perioperative paediatric nurses can sometimes align themselves more to theatre nursing than to paediatric nursing. We can learn from the mistakes of the past and ensure that perioperative and paediatric nurses work together to progress their mutual interest for the benefit of children having surgery.

An overview of the history of surgery

Historically, there are two forms of surgery, 'external' and 'deep'. External surgery avoids the opening of body cavities and is concerned with skin wounds, fractured bones, etc. Deep surgery involves the opening of body cavities such as the peritoneum and the thorax. The history of deep surgery is relatively recent. Although external surgery was practiced in ancient Egypt, Rome, Greece and Arabia, deep surgery was considered too risky, especially in children (Figure 1.1). Even relatively simple procedures such as appendicectomy appeared only in the last 150 years. However, external surgery, involving the skin, associated tissue and bones, has been practiced

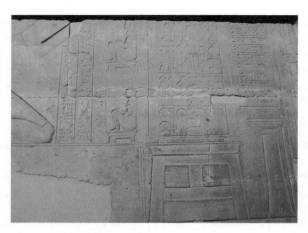

Fig. 1.1   Hieroglyphs of surgical instruments, Kom Ombo Temple, Aswan, Egypt, 2nd century BC.

for at least as long as historical records exist. Cranial surgery and cutting for (bladder) stone are exceptions to this rule and were carried out in ancient times (Mariani-Costantini *et al.*, 2000).

In 1755, Samuel Johnson defined chirurgery (surgery) as 'the art of curing by external applications' (Johnson, 1755). This shows that at this time, deep surgery did not exist and that almost by definition, surgeons did not give medicine or open body cavities. The prescription of medicine was the province of the physician; however, the labels for medical and nursing trades-people were often confused, especially in the provinces where multi-tasking was much more in evidence. Wyman (1984) points out that the labels 'surgeon' and 'apothecary', which should have been quite distinct, were in fact often confused. The label 'surgeon' has at times been taken to mean a 'general practitioner', inferring that surgeons were less well qualified than physicians, and tended to have a broad field of practice. It is largely for this reason that general practitioners are said to work from 'surgeries'. 'Surgery' was a label for the practice of someone qualified in only the cruder aspects of medicine.

We have noted two exceptions to the historical division of external and deep surgery: the procedures cutting for stone (lithotomy) and trephination of the skull that have been practiced for hundreds of years. These procedures were not at all safe, especially when practiced on children, but were measures of last resort. Trephination was carried out to relieve intracranial pressure, much as it might be practiced today. Cutting for stone, too, is, more or less, a procedure that we would see practiced on adults today. However, in the past and for reasons that are quite unclear (Ellis, 2001), children commonly suffered from bladder stones and so lithotomy was a procedure of paediatric surgery.

Deep surgery depended on the advent of anaesthesia and of antibiotics. By the time these developments were available in the late 19th century, surgery was becoming an educated and professionalised discipline. So it is that we see two almost separate surgical histories. There is an ancient history of the management of wounds and fractures. Here, surgeons were a wide range of individuals, perhaps best understood by the archetypal barber-surgeon of the 16th to 19th centuries, whose practices could be identified by a white pole on which bloody rags were hung to dry in the wind. The red-and-white pole, still seen outside the barber's shop, is what remains today of this once more varied craft.

Surgery's reputation as being an educated, professional occupation is a relatively new invention. Even 100 years ago, surgeons were widely considered to be a lower class of medic; they were often poorly educated and were considered trades-people. Prior to the mid 19th century, surgeons were not considered to be professionals but would have received on-the-job training of one sort or another. The surgeon's practice was thought crude, even barbaric in an age when practical work was not a proper activity for the well-heeled and well-educated classes. If we go back further, to the medieval period, we find that surgery was a dangerous occupation for if the patient died, the surgeon could forfeit his or her own life (Rawcliffe, 1997; Editorial, 2003). In a sense, surgery has often been a courageous activity. The early cardiac surgeons (20th century) were not at risk of losing their own lives even where their developing practices had fatal consequences for the patient. Even so, their reputation and their careers were often very much at risk (Waldhausen, 1997). The history of child surgery seems fashioned by courage, individuality and brave-endeavour. Children's perioperative nurses were part of the courage that was played out time and time again as endeavour upon endeavour turned once-hazardous procedures into operative events that were both safe and routine. Paediatric perioperative nursing is still developing as a discipline, despite a long and interesting history. Like any developing discipline, its practitioners also require a degree of courage. Frontiers of practice were never pushed forward by a rigid adherence to rules.

The development of perioperative nursing

Both barber-surgeons and bonesetters were largely trades-people who learned their craft from being apprenticed to a surgeon or from being born into a family of barber-surgeons or bonesetters (Adams, 1997). Before the migration of surgical education into universities, it was not at all uncommon for a surgeon to be female (Jonson, 1950; Talbot & Hammon, 1965; Clark, 1968). In 1563, a certain Mother Edwin was called in to St. Thomas' Hospital, London to treat a boy's hernia (Wyman, 1984). The division between surgeons and nurses was once very blurred. Wyman (1984, p. 32) offers the example of Margaret Colfe (1564–1643) who was the wife of the vicar of Lewisham. Her memorial stone reads 'having bene above 40 yeares a willing wife, nurse, mid-wife, surgeon, and in part physitian to all both rich and poore … [*sic*]'. However, male surgeons often sought to exclude female practitioners (Clark, 1968). From the mid-19th century males have dominated medicine. Even within the 20th century Gellis (1998) recalls working in a leading American children's hospital on the day that the first female doctor was employed, when the whole medical staff wore black arm-bands in protest.

The dominance of medicine today makes it all too easy to view children's surgery from a medical perspective. In fact, the roles of surgeon, nurse and paramedic have changed constantly through the years and are changing even today. History shows us that in the past nurses have performed surgery (Wyman, 1984; Wolff & Wolff, 1999). Robinson (1972) reports that between 1923 and 1948, an outpatient sister at a Scottish hospital routinely performed minor operations, often administering the anaesthetic herself. Similarly, surgeons have been active in caring for the child patient both before and after the operation. Wolff and Wolff (1999) note the existence of sub-surgeons (*subchirurgen*) between 1750 and 1850 in Germany and Austria. These individuals were trained in medical or surgical schools and taught by qualified doctors rather than surgical trades-people. The curriculum included wound care (debridement, etc.) and nursing. Some of the graduates worked as nurses, supervisors of nursing and some as country doctors. These sub-surgeons belonged to a sub-professional class. The sub-surgeons died out in the mid-19th century, the result of the professionalisation of medicine and the newly created profession of nursing. Nurses were then available to manage the patient's perioperative care, making the *subchirurgens* unnecessary.

We understand perioperative care as an activity that has been, and still is, performed by a variety of people. Today, it is often assumed that surgery is the province of the surgeon, a registered medical practitioner. However, history would beg to differ and even today English law does not confine the practice of surgery to medical surgeons; indeed chiropodists, nurses, acupuncturists and others, all perform techniques that are surgical in that they are invasive.

Key discoveries in perioperative care

Much of the history of surgery is directly related to a number of key discoveries. One of the most important was the discovery by Lister of antisepsis in ca. 1870. Lister's work, however, took some time to be accepted (Porter, 2003). Florence Nightingale energetically adopted the principles of antisepsis, despite her initial rejection of germ theory. Much of Nightingale's ideology was based on accepted methods of managing a large household with their heavy emphasis on discipline and cleanliness (Nightingale, 1860). While Lister's work on antisepsis struggled to be accepted by an inflexible medical brotherhood, Nightingale's influential work became widely accepted and gave credence to it (Larson, 1989). This is one example of the way in which the development of surgery has been dependant on nurses. However, nursing's important role in the development of surgery has often been hidden. This is the result, in part, of nurses failing to write about their endeavours (Nightingale being an exception) and of the subjugation of nurses by a male-dominated medical hierarchy.

The first effective anaesthetic (chloroform) was introduced around 1847 and it is this single discovery that marks the effective beginning of deep surgery (Porter, 2003). Chloroform and the anaesthetics that were developed after it, freed the surgeon from being confined to the treatment of superficial wounds, dental disease and fractures. Radiography was discovered in 1895 and unlike Lister's work on antisepsis, the use of x-rays quickly became an important tool to aid diagnosis. More complicated surgery and more complex procedures were at the forefront of scientific discoveries and became associated with surgeons who were increasingly well educated. This, in time, would enable surgery to be considered properly part of the medical profession.

The change of direction brought about by advances in surgery, secondary to the introduction of anaesthetic and antisepsis, is illustrated in an excerpt from an article by E.P.:

> *I have often heard my mother describe an incident in her early life; it would be between the years 1828 and 1832. She was the youngest daughter, and had much of the care of two brothers, both younger. The one next to her in age developed, when about two years' old,*

a small lump on the temple. He was a very bright, lively child. The lump was first like a smooth pea, and slowly grew on and on. The doctor attending said he could do nothing as it was too near the brain. As the lump grew the child did not lose intelligence, but merely became an invalid, as the head was too heavy to hold up, and at the last could only lie down, with the huge mass resting on the shoulder. The doctor had a picture painted of the child, but the artist represented him as sitting up playing with a whip, a vein stretched over the tumour. One night it burst, the blood spurting to the ceiling, and before morning the child died. The doctor asked permission to hold an autopsy, which was granted, as my grandfather was a man who desired to do everything to help on science. Seven doctors came to the little old-world Devonshire cottage. I have heard the younger brother say how pleased he was to see the seven doctors' horses at the cottage door, but my mother's recollection was very different. She stifled her sobs and crept upstairs, silently and gently raised the old latch and through the round latch-hole, saw her father standing looking on whilst the doctors worked. She saw the large growth removed, the skull under it smooth and thin; the skull was opened, showing the one half of the brain well developed for a child, the half under the growth shrivelled and compressed, and she heard the doctor's words to her father: "If we had only had the courage to try, this could have been removed, like a lump of fat; but, thanks to you, sir, the next patient we have may live." The child was carried to his grave by his sisters in white, the coffin suspended by white ropes. His picture is in some museum, I do not know where. Old surgery was conservative and death dealing; the new is daring and life saving. (E.P., 1905, p. 399)

Early beginnings of surgery for children

Radical approaches became characteristic of surgery in the late 19th and 20th centuries. History is often changed by just a few individuals who stand out, not so much for their chances in life or for their education but for their individuality, determination and courage. So it is with paediatric surgery. William Ladd became a full-time surgeon in the USA in 1936. Ladd was ahead of his time in appreciating that if paediatric surgery was to develop, it would need to be recognised as a separate speciality with special training for those involved and specialised nurses to provide the required care. The recognition he called for did not come until 1974 (in the USA), after 33 years of frustrated effort. By the development of techniques to deal with oesophageal atresia, malrotation of the gut (Ladd's procedure), extrophy of the bladder and cleft lip, Ladd proved that children's congenital conditions were amenable to surgery (Hendren, 1998).

In the UK, Denis Browne (Williams, 1999) was perhaps Britain's first full-time paediatric surgeon. In 1954 he helped found the British Association of Paediatric Surgeons and became its first president (Dunn, 2006). He did much to develop children's surgery, and without the professional infrastructure that exists today. All this was achieved in the early and middle years of the 20th century and against a backdrop of hostility towards children's medicine and especially toward children's surgery. Denis Brown was a fighter, a characteristic perhaps strengthened by his service in Gallipoli and France during the First World War (Smith, 2000).

It was due to the endeavours of Ladd, Browne and those they influenced and encouraged that by 1950 all had changed; surgery was then a heroic activity.

Paediatric surgery possessed new confidence, experimentation was expected and (Figure 1.2) new techniques thrived:

> *In September 1946, Barbara was born with a cleft soft palate, and owing to the professional observation of the nurse, consultations took place, when it was decided that before reaching the age of one year, plastic surgery should be performed. When a month or two old, this child was attacked by bronchitis, but by careful nursing, was able to be taken to the famous Plastic Surgery Centre at East Grinstead on the appointed date. An operation on this minute mouth was performed, and after a few weeks in hospital the child was returned to her parents with some simple directions for the care of her mouth. Before she was two years of age, she was gaily chattering away in "Harry Hemsley's Horace" dialect, but within another year she was able to compete in conversation with any normal child of her own age. Now, at four years old, thanks to the devoted services of the eminent Surgeons practising at the Plastic Surgery Centre at East Grinstead, she is the possessor of a full set of baby teeth, if slightly uneven, and is a most intelligent child, with a delightful sunny disposition. Mankind in general, and our heroic servicemen in particular ... owe much to the miraculous performance of Plastic Surgery.* (Anonymous, 1950, p. 118)

In more recent years, neonatal surgery has been an important development (Adzick & Nance, 2000a,b). By the 1970s, sufficient work had been done in this field for texts on baby surgery to be produced for nurses (Young & Martin, 1979). This area of work is almost impossible to visualise outside a construct of experimentation and endeavour. Perioperative nurses had to become more knowledgeable. At the same time, nurse education was rapidly becoming more academic with nursing's migration into the university sector. Developing in the last 15 years, prenatal surgery will probably become another milestone in the history of paediatric surgery (Koop, 1997; MacKenzie & Adzick, 2001) (see Chapter 9). These advances confront nursing with important challenges and an increasing need both for professional organisation and education.

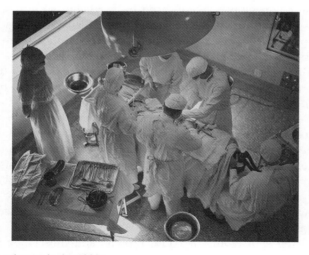

Fig. 1.2   Operating theatre in the 1960s.

Surgeons and children's perioperative nurses work collaboratively in the interest of the child. Both disciplines have contributed to the development of children's surgery and neither could have existed independently of the other. It is probably the case, however, that the role of the perioperative nurse in history has not been given the prominence that it deserves. The challenges faced by perioperative nurses today are not as new as we may have assumed. In truth, perioperative nurses have been involved in the development of children's surgery from its very beginning.

The growth of paediatric surgery

One of the earliest paediatric hospitals in Europe was the *l'hôpital des enfants malade* in Paris, which existed as a hospital from 1802. There were one or two general hospitals (which were in existence prior to the children's hospitals) which opened children's wards. For example, Guy's Hospital in London opened a children's ward in 1848 and the London Hospital opened one in 1840 (Lomax, 1996). However, these were short-lived, and on the whole, children were admitted to adult wards, something of which Florence Nightingale approved. It was not until ca. 1920 that most general hospitals possessed children's wards and performed paediatric surgery (Lomax, 1996). By this time, the specialist children's hospitals mostly practiced only medicine. Physicians and surgeons distrusted each other, with physicians regarding their practice as essentially more intellectual. Charles West, the founder of The Hospital for Sick Children, Great Ormond Street, London, is known to have had a poor view of surgery and saw no need for the hospital to employ a surgeon (Twistington-Higgins, 1952). However, some surgery must have been practiced in the early days of Great Ormond Street because the surgeon Timothy Holmes was working there when he published his text 'Treatise on the surgical treatment of the diseases of infancy and children' in 1868 (Lomax, 1996). He moved to St. George's Hospital in London that same year, indicating perhaps that surgery at Great Ormond Street was a less than consistent service. Timothy Holmes' surgery would have been limited to the treatment of wounds and of bone and joint disease.

Children's surgery for bladder stones seems to have been fairly commonplace until the beginning of the 20th century, when for reasons that remain unclear (Ellis, 2001), the condition became uncommon. It was not until the 20th century that surgery for congenital conditions such as cleft lip and club foot became relatively commonplace, as did tonsillectomy and adenoidectomy, and the first closed repair of intussusception, performed by Jonathan Hutchinson, took place at the London Hospital (Lomax, 1996). However, the specialist children's hospitals were still doing mainly minor and more specialist surgery. Even by 1900 most major and trauma surgery was being undertaken in general hospitals where children's services were often poorly developed. There was competition between the children's and general hospitals which resulted in a lack of cooperation. The general hospital's insistence on being general prevented specialist services from developing. At the same time, the children's hospital's emphasis on medical treatment and more specialist surgery meant that the general hospitals were still performing an essential role by providing major and trauma surgery. Professional rivalry has often been dysfunctional in the development of specialist services.

Before the speciality of paediatric surgery began to develop, what surgery did take place was performed by general and anatomically specialist surgeons. From these early years in the mid-20th century, medicine and nursing were both institutional in delaying the progress of paediatric surgery. Paediatric surgery and the specialist paediatric nursing upon which it so depended were subjected to resentment and antipathy from general surgery and general nursing. It took 25 years for paediatric surgery to be recognised as a separate discipline in the USA in 1970 (Koop, 1993). Koop set up the first neonatal intensive care unit in the USA (Pennsylvania Children's Hospital) with a grant from the US Children's Bureau. Previous attempts to set up the unit had been thwarted by the hospital's failure to acknowledge that neonatal intensive care required specialist nurses. In Britain, the same antagonism to the development of paediatric surgery can be discerned. The British Association of Paediatric Surgeons did not come about until 1954, 26 years after the establishment of the British Paediatric Association (Forfar *et al.*, 1989), the forerunner of the Royal College of Paediatric and Child Health. In his review of a lifetime of work in paediatric surgery, Koop (1993) recalls that paediatricians would allow children to die of correctable surgical pathology rather than suffer the ignominy of making a referral to a paediatric surgeon. This seems all the more strange because medical paediatrics was itself a small and poorly recognised discipline. Gellis (1998) recalls working as a paediatrician in the mid-20th century and of not being allowed to go to the neonatal unit without a specific invitation.

The lack of acceptance of paediatric surgery in the wider world of medicine and nursing meant that surgeons were working with few resources and almost always with no specialist nurses. As the head of paediatric surgery in a major US children's hospital, Koop recalls spending the night before surgery fashioning endotracheal tubes from urinary catheters because it was not possible to purchase endotracheal tubes small enough for babies. In this same way, Koop also recalls of the 1950s 'Rigid brass scopes were used to do laryngoscopy, oesophagoscopy and bronchoscopy because there were no flexible scopes. Patients (children) were never anaesthetised … visibility was hampered by poor lighting and by the constant explosive splattering of saliva and other secretions over one's face and glasses' (Koop, 1993, p. 619). Gellis (1998) recalls wards full of children with outstretched arms receiving subcutaneous infusions because there were no paediatric-sized cannulae for intravenous infusions.

Conclusion: perioperative nursing of children

The struggle for the recognition of paediatric perioperative nursing still continues. Fotheringham (1994) notes that education programmes for adult anaesthetic and recovery nurses did not commence until the mid 1980s; today, similar programmes for paediatric perioperative nurses are rare. It is problematic for the small and under-represented speciality of perioperative children's nurses to organise and achieve recognition for the very specialist service they provide. It is easy for loyalties to be divided between theatre and paediatric nursing. However, history teaches us that divided loyalties and professional rivalry achieve nothing but failure. Perioperative paediatric nurses (whatever their qualification) have one thing in common, an overriding concern for the welfare of the surgical child. In this, they share their orientation with paediatric surgeons, paediatric anaesthetists and children's nurses. Just as in days of old, those (whatever their qualification) prepared to place children in their role title are in an important sense, part of one single profession.

References

Adams, J. (1997). From crippledom to orthopaedic nursing: Pyrford, Surrey 1908–1945. *International History of Nursing Journal*, 2: 23–37.

Adzick, N.S., Nance, M.L. (2000a). Pediatric surgery: First of two parts. *New England Journal of Medicine*, 342: 1651–1657.

Adzick, N.S., Nance, M.L. (2000b). Pediatric surgery: Second of two parts. *New England Journal of Medicine*, 342: 1726–1732.

Anonymous (1950). A little child with a laughing look. *British Journal of Nursing*, 98: 118.

Association for Perioperative Practice (Incorporating NATN). (2005). *Definition of a perioperative environment*. Available at http://www.afpp.org.uk/document_downloads/position_statements/NATN%20definition%20of%20a%20perioperative%20environment.pdf (accessed 19 January 2008).

Association of Operating Room Nurses. (2009). About AORN. Available at: **http://www.aorn.org/AboutAORN/ (accessed 23 June 2009).**

Australian College of Operating Theatre Nurses. (2006). *ACORN Standards 2006*. Personal communication, 13 September 2006, ACORN Secretariat.

Bassett, J. (1992). *Guns and brooches: Australian Army nursing from the Boer War to the Gulf War*. Oxford University Press, Melbourne.

Biedermann, N. (2002). Experiences of Australian Army theatre nurses. *Association of Operating Room Nurses Journal*, 75: 337–340.

Clark, A. (1968). *Working life of women in the seventeenth century*. Frank Cass, London.

Cumber, K. (2006). Perioperative nursing: From handmaiden to nursing professional: A brief history of professional evolution. *DNA Reporter*, 31: 3–4.

Dunn, P.M. (2006). Sir Denis Browne (1892–1927): The father of paediatric surgery in Britain. *Archives of Diseases in Childhood*, 89(Suppl 1): A54–A55.

Editorial. (1999). AORN changes. *Nursing*, 29: 62–63.

Editorial. (2003). The responsibility of surgeons and their fees B.C. 2300. *British Medical Journal*, 327(7424): 1143.

Ellis, H. (2001). *A history of surgery*. Greenwich Medical Media Limited, London.

E.P. (1905). Surgery, old and new. *British Journal of Nursing*, 35: 399.

Forfar, J.O., Jackson, A.D.M., Laurance, B.M. (1989). *The British Paediatric Association 1928–1988*. The Royal College of Child Health and Paediatrics, London.

Fotheringham, D. (1994). The development of anaesthetic and recovery nurse education. *British Journal of Theatre Nursing*, 3: 7–8.

Gellis, S.S. (1998). General pediatrics. *Pediatrics*, 102: 286.

Hendren, W.H. (1998). Pediatric surgery. *Pediatrics*, 102: 275.

Holder, V.L. (2003a). From handmaiden to right hand – the Civil War – first in an ongoing series about the history of perioperative nursing. *Association of Operating Room Nurses Journal*, 78: 448, 450, 453.

Holder, V.L. (2003b). From handmaiden to right hand – the birth of nursing in America … Second in an ongoing series about the history of perioperative nursing in the United States. *Association of Operating Room Nurses Journal*, 78: 618–620, 622–624, 626.

Holder, V.L. (2004a). From handmaiden to right hand – World War I – the mud and the blood … fourth in an ongoing series about the history of perioperative nursing. *Association of Operating Room Nurses Journal*, 80: 527–528, 530, 533–536.

Holder, V.L. (2004b). From handmaiden to right hand – World War I – the mud and the blood … fifth in an ongoing series about the history of perioperative nursing. *Association of Operating Room Nurses Journal*, 80: 652–660, 663–665.

Holder, V.L. (2004c). From handmaiden to right hand – World War I and advancements in medicine … sixth in an ongoing series about the history of perioperative nursing. *Association of Operating Room Nurses Journal*, 80: 911–919, 921–923.

Johnson, S. (1755). *A dictionary of the English language*. W. Pickering, London.

Jonson, B. (1950). *The alchemist*. Librairie Universitaire, Louvain.

Koop, C.E. (1993). Pediatric surgery: The long road to recognition. *Pediatrics*, 92: 618–622.

Koop, C.E. (1997). The tiniest patients. *Newsweek*, 129: 51.

Larson, E. (1989). Innovations in health care: Antisepsis as a case study. *American Journal of Public Health*, 79: 92–99.

Lomax, E.M.R. (1996). Small and special: The development of hospitals for children in Victorian Britain. Wellcome Institute for the History of Medicine, London.

MacKenzie, T.C., Adzick, N.S. (2001). Advances in fetal surgery. *Journal of Intensive Care Medicine (Blackwell Publishing Limited)*, 16: 251–262.

Mariani-Costantini, R., Catalano, P., di Gennaro, F., di Tota, G., Angletti, L.R. (2000). New light on cranial surgery in ancient Rome. *Lancet*, 355(9200): 305–308.

McGarvey, H.E., Chambers, M.G.A., Boore, J.R.P. (2000). Development and definition of the role of the operating department nurse: A review. *Journal of Advanced Nursing*, 32: 1092–1100.

Nelson, D. (2007). Perioperative nursing and its history. *Dissector*, 35: 19–23.

Nightingale, F. (1860). *Notes on nursing: What it is, and what it is not*. D. Appleton and Company, New York.

Porter, R. (2003). *Blood and guts: A short history of medicine*. W.W. Norton, New York.

Rae, R. (2004a). Operating in the theatre of World War I: France. *ACORN: The Journal of Perioperative Nursing in Australia*, 17: 10–13.

Rae, R. (2004b). Operating in the theatre of World War I: Egypt. *ACORN: The Journal of Perioperative Nursing in Australia*, 17: 14–16.

Rawcliffe, C. (1997). Medieval surgery. *British Journal of Theatre Nursing*, 6: 8–10.

Robinson, E. (1972). *The Yorkhill story: The history of the Royal Hospital for Sick Children, Glasgow*. The Board of Management for Yorkhill and Associated Hospitals, Glasgow.

Schultz, J.E. (2004). *Women at the front: Hospital workers in Civil War America*. The University of North Carolina Press, Chapel Hill.

Shields, L., Watson, R. (2007). The demise of nursing in the United Kingdom: A warning for medicine. *Journal of the Royal Society of Medicine*, 100, 70–74.

Smith, A. (2000). Denis Browne: Maverick or master surgeon? *Australian & New Zealand Journal of Surgery*, 70: 770–777.

Talbot, C., Hammon, E.A. (1965). *The medical practitioners in medieval England*. Wellcome Historical Medical Library, London.

Twistington-Higgins, T. (1952). *Great Ormond Street 1852–1952*. Odhams Press, London.

Waldhausen, J. (1997). The early history of congenital heart surgery: Closed heart operations. *Annals of Thoracic Surgery*, 64: 1533–1539.

Williams, D.I. (1999). Denis Browne and the specialization of paediatric surgery. *Journal of Medical Biography*, 7: 145–150.

Wolff, H., Wolff, J. (1999). Nursing in the profession of the "sub surgeons" between 1750 and 1850. *Pflege*, 12: 347–351.

Wyman, A.L. (1984). The surgeoness: The female practitioner of surgery 1400–1800. *Medical History*, 28: 22–41.

Young, D.G., Martin, E.J. (1979). *Young and Weller's baby surgery*. HM and M Publishers, Aylesbury.

2 The psychosocial care of children in the perioperative area

Linda Shields

Children's perceptions of the operating theatre

Children see things differently to adults. While this seems self-evident, a visit to a hospital where children receive care demonstrates that, for example, this is not always well understood. Look around any children's ward and find where the pictures or wall paintings are placed. Are they at a level children will be able to see, or are they too high? Adults can rationalise what they are seeing, but often children, especially little ones, cannot. To demonstrate how a child sees things, Figure 2.1 shows a child's view from the operating table, while Figure 2.2 shows what an

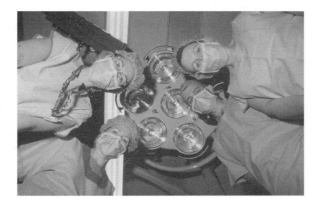

Fig. 2.1 A child's view from the operating table. *Source*: Photograph courtesy of Mater Health Services.

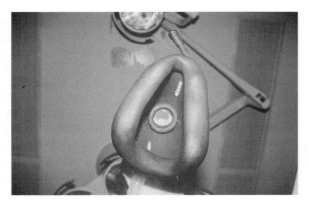

Fig. 2.2 A child's view of an anaesthetic mask. *Source*: Photograph courtesy of Mater Health Services.

anaesthetic mask looks like when it is coming towards a child's face. Necessary pieces of equipment can look very frightening to small children.

The paediatric operating room (OR) must reflect this idea. When a child enters the OR reception it should be 'child-friendly'. Pictures and cartoons on the walls, bright curtains and hangings, colourful mobiles and full toyboxes will make a child feel comfortable in what is, in reality, a very strange environment. In the OR, pictures on walls need to be at heights children can see – low down on walls for children who walk into the OR, and higher up for children who come on a trolley. Toys, books, television and videotapes make waiting time pass, and the children, who often do not have premedication, play on the floor until taken into the theatre. Parents should stay with their child until the child is anaesthetised if at all possible, either in induction rooms or in the OR itself. Instead of trolleys, some hospitals have toy cars for children to ride in from the ward to the OR, others have trolleys dressed up as boats or other 'fun' vehicles. Unless there are very good reasons to clothe children in OR gowns or hospital pyjamas, it is important that children be allowed to come to the OR in their own pyjamas or clothes (Figure 2.3).

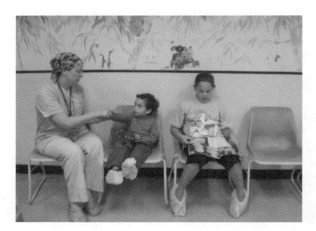

Fig. 2.3   Children coming to theatre in their own pyjamas.

The effect of hospitalisation on children

The emotional and psychological effect of surgery and operative procedures on children, and the effect of hospitalisation have been studied extensively. Historically, admission to hospital has been portrayed as a character-forming experience for children, something necessary for optimum growth and development (Jessner *et al.*, 1952; Blom, 1958; Oremland & Oremland, 1973). As late as 1992, Lansdown suggested that children could gain psychologically from a hospital admission (Lansdown, 1992). However, in what we would now consider a more enlightened approach, many investigators (Strachan, 1993) have studied psychological trauma encountered by children due to hospital admission, and often, similar investigations have studied parents. It is known that duration of hospital stay for children is shortened if their parents stay with them (Taylor & O'Connor, 1989) but several factors have all been shown to have a detrimental effect on the child's emotional experience of hospital admission, including the child's age and variations in personality. Others include admission for longer than 2 weeks, if the child is undergoing painful and/or traumatic illnesses or injuries, if there has been inadequate preparation for a routine admission, if any previous admission experiences were traumatic or upsetting, if at least one parent is not present, and if there is a lack of paediatric training for staff. In addition, highly anxious parents might impart a degree of anxiety to the child, and unconsciously add to a child's emotional upset, while a punishing style used by parents can be disastrous.

It is well recognised that children have needs different to adults (Price, 1994). In any of the specialities of health care, and most importantly in perioperative care, it is important to know that children's metabolism, development and physiological functioning is different to that of adults, and children can never be regarded as 'little adults'. All care for children has to recognise that these physical differences make it imperative that care delivery is different to models of care used for adults, and should be planned so. In fact, the most important factor differentiating the needs of children from those of adults is their level of physical and psychological development (Table 2.1).

Table 2.1 Developmental stages of children and perioperative nursing considerations

Age	Developmental Issues	Children's Fears	Coping Methods	Techniques/Interventions
Infant (birth to 11 months)	Close bond to parents Sensitivity to environment Minimal language	Distrust	Stranger Anxiety Withdrawal Crying	Encourage parent contact Warm hands, equipment Avoid patient hunger
Toddler (1–3 years)	Becoming an individual Assertiveness Limited language	Pain Short separation from parents	Loss of control Anger/aggression Hyperactivity	Allow choices if possible Encourage parent contact Use verbal communication
Preschool child (4–5 years)	Rich fantasy life Magical thinking Good expressive and receptive language Independence/strong sense of self	Pain Disfigurement Long separation from parents Frustration	Withdrawal Fantasy Anger/guilt Regression	Use puppets for expression Encourage fantasy or play Allow care participation Explain procedures with puppets
School-age child (6–12 years)	Well-developed language Some understanding of bodily functions Ability to reason Better self-control Incomplete idea of death	Death Disfigurement Being punished/hurt	Withdrawal Regression Demanding behaviour	Respect child's modesty Explain procedures with puppets or play Be positive about outcomes Encourage child to master situation, socialise with peers and maintain schoolwork
Adolescent (13–18 years)	Independence Self-determination Realistic view of death Importance of peers	Loss of autonomy Humiliation Entrapment Death Loss of peer acceptance	Depression Independence Helplessness Tough attitude Anger	Encourage adolescent to express concerns and fears Stress peer acceptance Allow control and choice when appropriate Encourage adult contact

Source: Davis & Klein (1994, p. 569).

Consequently, the models of care used with children in the perioperative environment (as in all branches of health care) must be cognizant of children's needs.

Models of care

Various models and theories have been tried in paediatrics. A series of educational case study papers used an example of a case study of an 8-year-old boy with leukaemia to describe how the theories of Neumann (Piazza *et al.*, 1992), Orem (Foote *et al.*, 1993) and Roy (Wright *et al.*, 1993) could be used to organise delivery of care. They were all found to be applicable to paediatrics, although they focused on the child and did not necessarily include parents, and did not mention perioperative care. With a recognition that most nursing models were not relevant to children, some paediatric nurses devised their own; for example, a model that linked activities of daily living with developmental stages (Clarke, 1988; MacDonald, 1988; Smith, 1995). No specific models of paediatric perioperative care have come to light (and this absence provides wonderful opportunities for a large research project), so a brief explanation of paediatric models of care is given here. All of these could equally well be applied in perioperative practice, except for care-by-parent, which is a structural model requiring physical and environmental facilities for its implementation.

Care-by-parent model

In USA in the 1960s, care-by-parent units, in which the parents (and family) live in with the sick child, were first introduced (Goodband & Jennings, 1992). A care-by-parent unit has rooms with a bed for the parent and *en suite* facilities, furnished in a comfortable, home-like style (Editorial, 1986). There are tea and coffee making and laundry facilities, dining and play areas and a treatment room. Parents live with the children and provide care in conjunction with the nurses. The role of the parent is outlined and expectations negotiated on admission. Although care-by-parent is not something that would be applicable in an operating theatre, children cared for in this manner could be surgical patients.

Partnership in care

A scenario about Tamar, who has broken her arm, illustrates how partnership in care can be given in the OR (Scenario 2.1). Partnership in care, which can work well in the perioperative arena, was first devised in 1988 by Anne Casey. Its main principles are that nursing care for a child in hospital can be given by the child's parents with support and education from the nurse, and that family or parental care can be given by the nurse if the family is absent (Casey, 1995). The role of the family, or parent, is to take on everyday care of the child, while the role of the paediatric nurse is to teach, support, and if necessary, refer the family to others. In 1995, Coyne examined parents' views of partnership in care, in a phenomenological study of 18 parents (Coyne, 1995). All viewed their participation as necessary for the child's well-being, a non-negotiable part of parenthood while nurses were seen as too busy to provide consistent care. Parents were prepared to learn more complex care, but only when

Scenario 2.1   Partnership in care

Tamar broke her arm when she fell off her bike, and needs it pinned under anaesthetic. She is in the surgical ward and will have to stay overnight.

Tamar is very worried about going to theatre. She had had her tonsils out 6 months before, and she remembered the sore throat, the smell of the anaesthetic gasses and the way the theatre looked – a strange, frightening place. When Tamar had her tonsillectomy, her father, Peter, had taken her into theatre and held her until she became unconscious. This time, though, Peter is away, and Donna, her mother, can't stay, as she has no one who can mind the other children.

The nurses in the ward realise that this could be a frightening time for 5-year-old Tamar, and so ask one of the nurses who will be on duty when Tamar goes to theatre to come to the ward and meet her. They work in partnership with Donna, Tamar and the other children (who have also come to the hospital) to try to negotiate the best possible experience for them all. Adam, the nurse in charge of the surgical ward, Ellen, the perioperative nurse, Donna and Tamar sit down and plan a pathway for Tamar's care. Adam tells Donna that the ward nurses will make sure Tamar is not left alone when she returns from theatre, while Ellen talks with Tamar and explains what is going to happen when she goes into theatre, and tells Tamar that she will meet her at the theatre reception and stay with her until she is asleep. Also, Ellen will see Tamar in the recovery room, though she tells Tamar that she will be cared for by another nurse there. Donna is confident that Tamar will be well cared for, Tamar feels safe even though her mother can't stay, and Donna and the other children go home, while Tamar goes to the operating theatre.

necessary, preferring to leave it to the nurses because of the anxiety it caused. Information, communication and negotiation were the most important part of ensuring successful partnerships with the nurses, and these are particularly important if a child is having an operation. Again, we have found no research that specifically examines partnership in care in the perioperative setting.

Family-centred care

The most commonly cited paediatric model of care now is family-centred care (FCC), and this is a very effective model of care in the operating theatre. Tomas's story provides us with an example of this (Scenario 2.2). FCC is 'a way of caring for children and their families within health services which ensures that care is planned around the whole family, not just the individual child/person, and in which all the family members are recognised as care recipients' (Shields *et al.*, 2006). The Institute for Family-Centered Care in the United States (USA) lists several core concepts which make up the model (Institute for Family-Centered Care, 2007) (Box 2.1). The term 'FCC' is widely used in paediatrics, though it is known that it is difficult to implement in any setting (Darbyshire, 1994; Coyne, 2003), and its effectiveness has never been properly tested (Shields *et al.*, 2007). However, it is, at this stage, the model most widely used around the world, and, as we can see from Tomas's story, it can be done. However, cases like Tomas's will work only in a health system which is very well funded, where the success and efficiency of the system is not based on numbers – surgeons whose income depends on the number of cases they do in a session may not be able to wait for the amount of negotiation and time it took Tomas to agree to the anaesthetic. In other words, it will be very difficult to implement in a health service which is not well funded or cannot find adequate staff.

Scenario 2.2 Family-centred care

Tomas is an 8-year-old boy who has come to theatre for his fifth operation for re-implantation of ureters. George, his father, accompanies him. Because he has had multiple admissions and much experience of surgery, Tomas knew he wanted an intravenous rather than a gaseous induction, but the doctors and nurses could not access a vein. Rather than force Tomas to have a gaseous induction, the nurses and doctors spent a great deal of time negotiating with him. The remaining children on the list stayed in the wards and the operating teams were delayed until this child was anaesthetised. Team members accepted this as good practice, and families whose children's surgery was delayed were equally tolerant, as they knew that if this happened during their turn the same consideration would be shown. In addition, George was considered and included at every stage. As Tomas persistently refused the gas mask, his father became agitated and began to speak roughly to him. The nurses and doctors communicated with George in such a way that he felt less frightened, explaining why they were happy to wait till the boy was ready, and in this way calmed him, thereby minimising Tomas's upset. Eventually, after about 2 hours, the boy had a successful and stress-free anaesthetic.

Box 2.1 Core concepts of FCC

Dignity and Respect: Health care practitioners listen to and honour patient and family perspectives and choices. Patient and family knowledge, values, beliefs, and cultural backgrounds are incorporated into the planning and delivery of care.

Information Sharing: Health care practitioners communicate and share complete and unbiased information with patients and families in ways that are affirming and useful. Patients and families receive timely, complete, and accurate information in order to effectively participate in care and decision-making.

Participation: Patients and families are encouraged and supported in participating in care and decision-making at the level they choose.

Collaboration: Patients, families, health care practitioners and leaders collaborate in policy and programme development, implementation, and evaluation; in health care facility design; and in professional education as well as the delivery of care.

Source: Institute for Family-Centered Care (2007).

In FCC, the child is central, because anything that happens to this child affects all members of the family; the care the child receives in relation to his or her illness or condition for which he or she has entered the health service must at all times be planned around the whole family, and whoever that family sees as an integral part of its family group. This calls for all health professionals who deal with the family to have exceptional communication and negotiation skills, and for recognition by health service managers that such a model of care calls for increased staff-to-patient ratios. These requirements are necessary because the 'unit' to whom care is delivered is never a single individual (Shields *et al.*, 2006).

It is important that all health care is supported by rigorous evidence. To that end, we must critically examine FCC and how it is delivered. While we can intuitively think that FCC is the best for all, we must question if that is so. A Cochrane systematic review of FCC (Shields *et al.*, 2007) has shown that despite a very large literature on the topic, it has not been effectively evaluated. In other words, while it sounds good, we really do not know if it either works or makes any difference to the emotional well-being of children and their families. This fits with the works of Darbyshire (1994) and Coyne (1996, 2003), who have found that FCC is a wonderful ideal, but difficult to implement effectively. However, in the perioperative field, where emotional stress for both parents and children is heightened, it may be that FCC is the best way of delivering care. At least, it ensures that the whole family's needs are recognised, and again, research is needed to determine if FCC is a model which works in perioperative care of children.

The presence of parents

As described in Chapter 1, until the 1960s, parents were often excluded from a hospital during a child's admission (Shields & Nixon, 1998), and while this has changed so that parents are now encouraged and often expected to stay for the duration of the child's admission, parental presence in the OR is a more contentious issue. There is good evidence that parental presence during anaesthetic induction (PPI) is beneficial to the child (Association for the Welfare of Children in Hospital, 1989; Burns, 1997) and anxiety is lessened for both children and parents (Schulman, 1967; Landers, 1994; LaRosa-Nash & Murphy, 1996, 1997; Astuto *et al.*, 2006). Many hospitals and anaesthetists now encourage parents to accompany their children into theatre, at least until the child is anaesthetised. However, it is of supreme importance that parents are well prepared for what they will see happening to their child; for example, they know what their child will look like as he or she becomes unconscious, they are told everything that will happen, and they be escorted out of the theatre and assured that everything went well. Some paediatric postoperative anaesthetic care units (PPACUs) allow parents to be with their child, but there is little published about the presence of parents in the PPACU. In some countries, parents are expected to remain with their recovering child. There are several reasons for this. In some Nordic countries (Shields, 2001), children are given heavy sedation as a premedication and, as a consequence, have a postoperative recovery period of several hours (as opposed to the practice of giving little or no premedication and where the child wakes up rapidly and the recovery period is short). In these countries, parents receive financial compensation if they stay home from work to care for sick children, and so are expected to accompany their child to hospital, and this includes the PPACU, where the child may stay for at least 2 hours, and where the nursing staff care for several postoperative patients at once. In some developing countries, parents stay in PPACU with their child because of the lack of available nursing staff. Whatever the reason or scenario, more research is needed in this area.

At this point in history, and in these stages of nursing and medical science and knowledge, it is unnecessary for parents to accompany their child into the OR itself. Infection control demands that as few people as possible enter an OR; seeing a child cut may be traumatic for a parent, and they could suffer emotional trauma from seeing their child in such a foreign environment. However, it is a wise clinician who learns to assess and balance the accepted knowledge of the day with possible benefits (psychosocial or emotional) for their patients and act in the patient's best interests, even if this goes against accepted practice. It is only 20 years ago that parents were excluded from resuscitation attempts on their children, and yet today, in many hospitals it is normal practice, as evidence showed that parents (and children) benefitted from this rather than waiting outside not knowing what was happening to their child (Dingeman *et al.*, 2007). Some time in the future it may be possible for parents to watch their children having surgery.

Play in the operating theatre suite

Play is often used to alleviate a child's fears about impending surgery. Play is commonly used as an important therapeutic tool for hospitalised children, either through formal play sessions with a trained play therapist, or in an informal situation with other children and staff. Through play a child maintains a normal perspective on living, thus reducing anxiety, and is part of hospital routine in many hospitals (Woon, 2004). The child can communicate ideas, cope with new perceptions, recognise feelings, decrease fear, clarify distortions and comprehend threatening occurrences. Children develop mastery over adverse situations by playing. Through play, teachers, nurses and other health staff can handle a child's aggressive and hostile behaviour, and help children prepare for impending situations such as operations (Li, 2007). In many paediatric hospitals, the play leader/therapist is an important part of the OR team.

In some hospitals and ORs, clowns (Spitzer, 2006; Li, 2007), puppet shows (McCormack, 1998) and theatre entertainers (Martin, 1995) are used to make the hospital experience relatively enjoyable for children and they are particularly useful in the OR, as is music therapy, which offers opportunities for structured social interaction, enhancement of education, decreasing fear and anxiety, distraction for painful procedures, relaxation and pain control (Avers *et al.*, 2007).

Emotional, social and spiritual needs of the patient

Having an operation can be particularly traumatic for children, and they, and their parents, have the right to know that they are in competent hands and will be treated in a dignified, respectful manner, and that they will be informed, in ways they can understand, of what is going to happen to the child. Training in communication skills is vitally important for perioperative nurses to ensure they are able to assess the child's and parent's ability to understand, and their comprehension of what they are being told. Children and parents whose first language is different to the prevailing language of the dominant culture must be provided with translators and written information in their own language.

Many families find the need to reinforce their spiritual beliefs before impending surgery. Part of good perioperative care is to include the people involved in the family's spiritual well-being as part of the team. They may require a priest, Imam, minister of religion or may require counselling from a professional counsellor to help them through this difficult phase. They may require members of their own family or friends to support them. The nurses' duty is to ascertain the family' needs and ensure they are satisfactorily met before surgery and in the immediate postoperative period, if required.

Conclusion

When a child comes to the OR, their psychosocial care is every bit as important as their surgical care. The presence of their parents is probably the most important contributing factor to their emotional safety, and their presence for induction of a child's anaesthetic is widely used. There are many other things that must be considered and techniques to be used that protect the child's well-being. Different models of care are used in the OR, but (like most paediatric areas) the one that is most common now is FCC.

References

Association for the Welfare of Children in Hospital. (1989). *A recommended policy relating to the provision of care for children undergoing anaesthesia.* Association for the Welfare of Children in Hospital, Sydney.

Astuto, M., Rosano, G., Rizzo, G., Disma, N., Raciti, L., Sciuto, O. (2006). Preoperative parental information and parents' presence at induction of anaesthesia. *Minerva Anestesiologica*, 72: 461–465.

Avers, L., Mathur, A., Kamat, D. (2007). Music therapy in pediatrics. *Clinical Pediatrics*, 46: 575–579.

Blom, G.E. (1958). The reactions of hospitalized children to illness. *Pediatrics*, 22: 590–600.

Burns, L.S. (1997). Advances in pediatric anesthesia. *Nursing Clinics of North America*, 32: 45–71.

Casey, A. (1995). Partnership nursing: Influences on involvement of informal carers. *Journal of Advanced Nursing*, 22: 1058–1062.

Casey, A.A. (1988). Partnership with child and family. *Senior Nurse*, 8: 8–9.

Clarke, D. (1988). Framework for care. *Nursing Times*, 84: 33–35.

Coyne, I.T. (1995). Partnership in care: Parents' views of participation in their hospitalized children's care. *Journal of Clinical Nursing*, 4: 71–79.

Coyne, I.T. (1996). Parent participation: A concept analysis. *Journal of Advanced Nursing*, 23: 733–740.

Coyne, I.T. (2003). *A grounded theory of disrupted lives: Children, parents and nurses in the children's ward.* Unpublished PhD thesis. King's College University of London, London.

Darbyshire, P. (1994). *Living with a sick child in hospital: The experiences of parents and nurses.* Chapman & Hall, London.

Davis, J.L., Klein, R.W. (1994). Perioperative care of the pediatric trauma patient. *AORN Journal*, 60(4): 561–570.

Dingeman, R.S., Mitchell, E.A., Meyer, E.C., Curley, M.A. (2007). Parent presence during complex invasive procedures and cardiopulmonary resuscitation: A systematic review of the literature. *Pediatrics*, 120: 842–854.

Editorial. (1986). Care-by-parent in a Canadian hospital. *Pediatric Mental Health*, 5: 3.

Foote, A., Holcombe, J., Piazza, D., Wright, P. (1993). Orem's theory used as a guide for the nursing care of an eight-year-old child with leukemia. *Journal of Pediatric Oncology Nursing*, 10: 26–32.

Goodband, S., Jennings, K. (1992). Parent care: A US experience in Indianapolis. In: Cleary J. (ed.). *Caring for children in hospital: Parents and nurses in partnership.* Scutari Press, London.

Institute for Family-Centered Care. (2007). *Patient- and family-centered care.* Maryland Institute for Family-Centered Care, Bethesda, MD. Available at: http://www.familycenteredcare.org/pdf/CoreConcepts.pdf (accessed 8 January 2008).

Jessner, L., Blom, G.E., Waldfogel, S. (1952). Emotional implications of tonsillectomy and adenoidectomy on children. *Psychoanalytic Study of the Child*, 7: 126–169.

Landers, H. (1994). Anaesthesia induction: Should parents be present? *Info Nursing*, 25: 10–12.

Lansdown, R. (1992). The psychological health status of children in hospital. *Journal of the Royal Society of Medicine*, 85: 125–126.

LaRosa-Nash, P.A., Murphy, J.M. (1996). A clinical case study: Parent-present induction of anesthesia in children. *Pediatric Nursing*, 22: 109–111.

LaRosa-Nash, P.A., Murphy, J.M. (1997). An approach to pediatric perioperative care: Parent-present induction. *Nursing Clinics of North America*, 32: 183–199.

Li, H.C. (2007). Evaluating the effectiveness of preoperative interventions: The appropriateness of using the Children's Emotional Manifestation Scale. *Journal of Clinical Nursing*, 16: 1919–1926.

MacDonald, A. (1988). A model for children's nursing. *Nursing Times*, 84: 52–55.

Martin, G. (1995). Once upon a time: The story of the All sports Hospital Entertainers. *Children in Hospital*, 21: 1–2.

McCormack, M. (1998). Have puppets, will travel. How a magical puppet theater cheers young patients. *The Volunteer Leader*, 39: 6.

Oremland, E.K., Oremland J.D. (1973). *The effects of hospitalization on children: Models for their care*. Charles C. Thomas, Springfield, IL.

Piazza, D., Foote, A., Wright, P., Holcombe, J. (1992). Neumann systems model for the nursing care of an 8-year-old child with leukemia. *Journal of Pediatric Oncology Nursing*, 9: 17–24.

Price, S. (1994). The special needs of children. *Journal of Advanced Nursing*, 20: 227–232.

Schulman, J.L., Foley, J.M., Vernon, M.A., Allan, D. (1967). A study of the effect of the mother's presence during anaesthesia induction. *Pediatrics*, 39: 111–114.

Shields, L. (2001). The delivery of family-centred care in hospitals in Iceland, Sweden and England: A report for The Winston Churchill Memorial Trust 2001. Available from: URL http://www.churchilltrust.com.au/res/File/Fellow_Reports/Shields%20Linda%202000.pdf (accessed 10 January 2008).

Shields, L., Nixon, J. (1998). I want my mummy – changes in the care of children in hospital. *Collegian*, 5: 16–19.

Shields, L., Pratt, J., Hunter, J. (2006). Family-centred care: A review of qualitative studies. *Journal of Clinical Nursing*, 15: 1317–1323.

Shields, L., Pratt, J., Davis, L.M., Hunter, J. (2007). Family-centred care for children in hospital. Cochrane Database of Systematic Reviews 2007, Issue 1. Art. No.: CD004811. DOI: 10.1002/14651858.CD004811.pub2.

Smith, F. (1995). *Children's nursing in practice: The Nottingham model*. Blackwell Science, Oxford.

Spitzer, P. (2006). Hospital clowns-modern-day court jesters at work. *Lancet*, 368: 34–35.

Strachan, R.G. (1993). Emotional responses to paediatric hospitalization. *Nursing Times*, 89: 45–49.

Taylor, M.R.H., O'Connor, P. (1989). Resident parents and shorter hospital stay. *Archives Diseases in Childhood*, 64: 274–276.

Woon, R. (2004). Hospital play therapy: Helping children cope with hospitalisation through therapeutic play. *Singapore Nursing Journal*, 31: 16–19.

Wright, P.S., Holcombe, J., Foote, A., Piazza, D. (1993). The Roy adaptation model used as a guide for the nursing care of an 8-year-old child with leukemia. *Journal of Pediatric Oncology Nursing*, 10: 68–74.

3 Care of the child in the operating room

Linda Shields and Ann Tanner

Preparation of children for theatre

Children and their parents going into theatre are often anxious about their surgery and many have little idea of the actual procedure. The nurse who admits the family to hospital must establish their needs, and it is the responsibility of the surgeon to adequately inform them of the type and extent of surgery required and the associated risks. Pre-operative education is of paramount importance, and the admitting nurse can educate children and parents on expected events when they return from theatre. Pain is often one of the most frequent concerns of patients who are about to undergo surgery, and the anaesthetist can alleviate these anxieties by explaining in detail the type of analgesia they can expect to receive in surgery and post-operatively. The admitting nurse can reinforce this information as well as give the child and parents information about the expected post-operative interventions such as intravenous lines, drains, indwelling catheters, and intravenous or epidural infusions for analgesia. For some procedures in older children and young people who may be having major surgery, it may be necessary for them to be reviewed and educated by a physiotherapist prior to surgery to teach them safe methods of turning in bed, and for the importance of deep breathing exercises for those who may need prolonged bed rest following surgery.

While preparing a child for theatre, family members must be afforded an opportunity to express anxieties and concerns on an individual basis and to determine how they can be most supportive to the child during the perioperative period (Kristensson-Hallström, 2000). The perioperative nurse requires an awareness of the psychosocial needs of children and good communication skills to recognise the importance of input from family members. Communication among the individuals caring for the child is paramount. Established lines of communication permit the efficient and meaningful transfer of information and provide the most efficient means of informing the patient about necessary procedures. Familiarity with operating room and day surgery unit policies helps alleviate patient and parent anxieties.

Evidence about the importance of effective preparation of children for hospital admission abounds in the nursing and early childhood studies literature. No-where is it more important than for OR. America saw the first pre-admission programmes in hospitals in the 1970s (Johnson, 1974). They provide the opportunity to prepare children for surgery, explain the reason for the operation, interview the family, give written information and facilitate discussions between nurses, doctors and parents. Because of the range of ages of children who have operations, written and oral information should be age-appropriate, and it is important that operations are never suggested as a threat or punishment. Storybooks, video games, board games, puppets of children having surgery and various other techniques can be used to prepare a child (Eckhardt & Prugh, 1978). Written material and discussions must be in the language of the patient. In Britain, the Action for Sick Children, and in Australia, The Association for the Welfare of Child Health both have published books describing the importance of preparing children for hospital and medical procedures, and methods and techniques for doing so (Rodin, 1989; Association for the Welfare of Child Health, 2005). Community health workers, in liaison with school teachers, can prepare primary and pre-school children for surgery by educating them about hospitalisation (Johnson, 1992). One technique is to use calico dolls on which children can draw their impression of what is happening to them. These are widely used in many countries (English & Bond, 1998), while some dolls are available which show the child the inner workings of the body and make explanations easier and more valuable. Some hospitals have play centres set up with hospital beds and equipment, so children can act out their own and anticipated experiences. It has been shown that the quality of a child's previous medical experiences influenced the child's anxiety levels for subsequent medical interventions. In an evaluation of preparation of children pre-day surgery admissions, children who had a previous negative experience were more anxious than children who had positive or neutral experiences (Dahlquist *et al.*, 1986).

History shows us that operating theatres and the surgery undertaken in them have progressed over time, but the basic principles of perioperative care remain the same. For many children it may be their first admission to a hospital, and their first experience of undergoing an anaesthetic or an operation. This can be a nerve-racking experience for both children and parents. Others may have had a previous traumatic experience in hospital, which could make them anxious. It is important for the admitting nurse on the ward, and the admitting OR nurse to alleviate such anxieties.

This section examines a number of aspects of admitting children to a ward and subsequently to theatre for surgery. The pre-operative admission provides an opportunity for any perceived complications for surgery to be considered. There are a number of procedures to follow depending on the type of admission, such as day of surgery admission (day surgery), pre-admission clinics and emergency admission. It is important to understand the difference between booked elective surgery and emergency admissions, and the difference between a theatre-classified emergency and an acute life-threatening emergency. However, it is beyond the scope of this book to give that sort of detail, and there are many excellent texts which cover just those topics (Paterson-Brown, 2005).

Procedures involved in an OR admission vary depending on the admission type but generally include a pre-operative check list which includes baseline observations, the child's weight, documentation of surgical and medical history, medications and allergies. The actual preparation for theatre includes fasting, body/site preparation and patient education. This chapter examines the OR nurse's role in theatre reception, and the protocol to be followed when admitting a patient into the operating suite.

Admission prior to surgery

Children and their families who arrive in the ward for pre-surgical admission will usually have received information by mail, telephone or from their local doctor regarding the time of their admission, and of the required fasting time. In children, fasting times are age dependent, and further explanation follows in this chapter. Most units use a standard checklist for all pre-operative admissions. Figure 3.1 shows an example of a standard pre-operative checklist.

Observation

Firstly, the child has to be fit for theatre, and so a set of baseline observations, including temperature, pulse, respiration and blood pressure are taken. While taking the observations, the OR nurse uses the opportunity to check on the child's skin integrity, particularly around the operating site. Rashes or sores can increase the risk of wound break down and infection following surgery and may result in the operation being cancelled (at the surgeon's discretion). Baseline observations are needed prior to the anaesthetist's review of the patient, and he or she is made aware of any untoward observations such as pyrexia, hypertension and cardiac arrhythmias, which may indicate that the patient is not fit for a general anaesthetic. As it can be unsafe to give an anaesthetic in the presence of fever or an upper respiratory tract infection, the operation may be cancelled until the child is well.

Weight

The child's weight is needed for drug calculations and administration, and anaesthetic agents and analgesics are determined on a dose for weight (milligram per kilogram) ratio. The anaesthetist will need to see the child's weight before administering an anaesthetic, so if possible weigh her or him and record it on the anaesthetic chart, the medication chart and the name band. In an emergency, or in the unusual occurrence that the child is bed bound and unable to stand on scales or sit in a weighing chair, the anaesthetist will estimate the weight.

Surgical history

Taking the surgical and medical history is a doctor's responsibility, but the OR nurse needs to be aware of anything that can affect the patient's well being. The surgical history is important to ascertain any previous complications with anaesthetics or post-operative complications, as the child may have a history of a reaction to one of the anaesthetic agents. The previous surgery may have included the insertion of a device or prosthesis of some kind, e.g., a head plate, or heart valve replacement, for which a prophylactic antibiotic may be administered. Some children are susceptible to bouts of vomiting and nausea following a general anaesthetic, and if the anaesthetist is aware of this, he or she may order anti-emetic drugs to alleviate the symptoms. It is the nurse's responsibility to make sure that this information is provided to the anaesthetist. Information about all potential problems is important in determining post-operative complications likely to arise with each individual child who is undergoing surgery.

Medical history

The child's medical history may determine risk factors and if possible should include a family health history. Whether or not an underlying condition is related to the problem

PREOPERATIVE NURSING RECORD

Med Rec No: ....
Surname:...
Forename: ....
Sex:.........................D.O.B ....

AFFIX LABEL HERE

Date:........./........./..........   Ward:_____

ALLERGIES: YES/NO If yes, give details	Fasted from:	
....	Food/Milk	Time: ....
	Clear Fluids	Time: ....
Preferred Name:	Temperature if < 36 > 38	Time: ....
Language spoken, other than English:	Last voided/nappy change	Time: ....

(Circle appropriate response to the following and comment where applicable)

CHECKLIST:	WARD	COMMENTS	PRE-OP BAY	THEATRE
Identification bands x 2	Yes/No		Yes/No	Yes/No
Patient medical records	Yes/No		Yes/No	Yes/No
Patient stickers > 15	Yes/No			
Operation consent form	Yes/No		Yes/No	Yes/No
Premedication given	Yes/No		Yes/No	
Topical anaesthetic cream applied	Yes/No			
Intravenous order/fluid balance sheet	Yes/NA		Yes/No	
Weight recorded	Yes/No		Yes/No	
X-rays/scans	Yes/No		Yes/No	Yes/No
Isolation precaution card	Yes/NA	Pre-op bay notified?	Yes/No	
Skin lesions/nappy rash	Yes/No	Lesion site:		
Correct clothing as per policy	Yes/No			
Dental -- loose teeth/plates	Yes/No			
Nails clean / polish removed	Yes/No			
Hair tied back	Yes/NA			
Prosthesis insitu	Yes/No	Type:		
Jewellery removed	Yes/No			
Comfort object labelled	Yes/NA			
Surgical site marked	Yes/No		Yes/No	Yes/No

Additional handover information (including disabilities):

Ward Nurse Signature: Print Name:

Pre-op Nurse Signature: Print Name:

Theatre Nurse Signature: Print Name:

Time of admission to Pre-operative Bay:

PREOPERATIVE NURSING RECORD

Fig. 3.1 Pre-operative checklist.

for which the surgery is planned, it still may significantly influence both surgical and anaesthetic treatment (American Academy of Pediatrics, 1996). Frequently encountered conditions in children include, e.g., asthma, diabetes and obstructive sleep apnoea. Asthmatic children will require premedication with their salbutamol inhalers and steroid sprays, and if the surgery is a long case, their anaesthetic will have to be specially adjusted to take account of their sensitive airways and possible allergies. Diabetic children are potentially at risk due to the fasting required before theatre and are often given an intravenous infusion to maintain a sufficient level of glucose in their blood. It is important to monitor their blood sugar level before, during and following theatre. Children with obstructive sleep apnoea will require intensive monitoring and probably a restriction on the use of narcotics. Any child with a history of bleeding disorders such as haemophilia or thalassaemia will require intensive observation for excessive bleeding or abnormal clotting.

Medications

An allergy to medication (or to anything) must be known before a child has an anaesthetic and surgery, and if so, they must be recorded on the medication sheet, the child's chart and clearly marked on the child's name band. Many hospitals mandate that if a child has an allergy, an extra armband, usually red, with the allergic agent clearly written on it, must be put on the child's arm. For many children with pre-existing morbidity, there is a high likelihood that they will be taking some form of medication. These medications may not be compatible with some of the anaesthetic or analgesic agents. All medications need to be recorded, including over-the-counter medications. If known, the child's compliance with taking medications should also be recorded (Martinelli, 2000).

Body/site preparation

Maintaining skin integrity is a means of reducing the risk of infection, and children should be checked for cuts and any break in skin integrity. Lesions such as impetigo must be reported to the surgeon, as these are caused either by streptococci or staphylococci (Mayo Clinic Staff, 2007), and such infection may result in cancellation of the surgery. A pre-operative shower using antimicrobial skin wash is an important means of reducing surgical site infection, though for many surgical procedures in children, which do not require incisions to the skin, this is not needed. There are many different skin preparation techniques and these are described in full in generic surgical nursing textbooks (Rothrock & McEwan, 2007).

Jewellery must be removed or covered with tape if unable to be removed, as any metal in contact with the patient's skin has the potential to cause burns from the diathermy current. Loose teeth and dental plates must be removed as they can dislodge during the anaesthetic intubation, and so children of the age to be losing their milk teeth must be asked about this.

Pre-admission clinic

Children and their parents sometime attend a pre-admission outpatients clinic, or their private doctor's rooms prior to surgery for the pre-admission examination. This provides an alternative to the costs of an overnight admission prior to theatre. Tests and blood cross matching may be required if the child is to undergo major surgery and are often done at the pre-admission visit. Baseline observations are recorded in the clinic as well as on admission to the ward. Pre- and post-operative education are given at the clinic, and often consent for theatre is signed. The child's detailed history will be recorded, including medications and allergies, surgical and medical history and any complications of previous surgery or anaesthetics. The pre-admission clinic provides a non-stressful environment in which questions regarding surgery can be clarified. On the day of surgery, there is often less time to alleviate anxieties than there may be in a clinic setting. In some children's hospitals, an integral part of the pre-admission clinic is a visit to the playroom, which holds miniature theatre equipment and medical equipment such as stethoscopes and IV cannulae, so the children can play and become familiar with them. The children have the opportunity, then, to ask questions about what is going to happen to them, and a specially trained nurse, play therapist or early childhood teacher will be able to give them explanations in ways the children can understand. Such techniques alleviate anxiety for both child and parent (Woon, 2004).

Emergency admission

In acute surgery, an emergency admission includes any procedure which requires treatment within 12 to 24 hours. An example could be a fractured limb, or abdominal pain with suspected appendicitis. In such cases, there is time for the ward staff to perform the standard pre-operative admission, observations, and surgical and family history. Emergency patients will often be admitted to the ward while waiting for theatre time to become available. The child will arrive directly from the accident and will be taken to the emergency department. Routine theatre cases delayed until the emergency case has been completed. In the case of a multiple trauma (such as a motor vehicle accident), the patient may need to undergo X-rays and CT scans prior to admission to theatre to ascertain the extent of the trauma, particularly in the case of head injury.

There are some extremes of acute emergency admission, (and the legal and ethical issues surrounding these will be mentioned in Chapter 13), e.g., a true emergency such as an acute airway obstruction where an emergency tracheostomy may need to be performed would bypass pre-admission checks and come directly into the OR. Scenario 3.1 describes an acute emergency admission to the OR. In these acute emergency admissions, allergies and medical history may be obtained from parents, friends or whoever can be found if time permits; if not, the anaesthetist and surgeon will be cautious and conservative about possible allergic agents, until information can be provided by the parents once they have been contacted.

All operating theatre suites will have dedicated rooms set up to receive any emergency at any time (or in smaller hospitals, at least one theatre). In most cases, OR staff will have time to set up a theatre in preparation for the procedures involved, and this includes organising the equipment and instruments required. On some occasions, there is little warning or preparation time so it is essential to leave all theatres set up to the extent that the bed and anaesthetic machine are in the correct place, that the theatre is properly stocked, and that the oxygen, suction, diathermy, lighting and anaesthetic machine are all functioning and ready for use.

Scenario 3.1 Acute emergency admission

> Sanjeev, aged 12, lived near the children's hospital. One morning on his way to school, he was knocked off his bike right in front of the hospital. A team from the Emergency Department ran out with a trolley and, after stabilising the boy, transported him into the resuscitation bay. He was unconscious, his vital signs were dropping fast and his visibly, rapidly expanding abdomen indicated profuse internal bleeding. A ruptured liver and spleen was the most likely cause, but there was no time to take an X-ray, so he was rushed to the OR where he was immediately anaesthetised and opened by the surgical team, as the anaesthetist poured in blood expanders through his IV. The blood was sucked out of his abdomen, the lacerations to his liver ligated and his spleen removed. Sanjeev was saved and made a full recovery. However, in the rush to access his bleeding internal organs, there was no time to find his parents or to have them sign a consent form. Under such circumstances, this was perfectly legal.

Day of surgery admission

Detailed explanation of day of surgery admission (variously called "day surgery", "day admission", "day procedure", etc.) can be found in generic perioperative texts (Rothrock & McEwan, 2007). With advances in surgical expertise and technology, length of hospital stay has been markedly reduced, and this is particularly true for children, where a consideration of the emotional effects of hospitalisation on children lead paediatric practitioners to believe that being in hospital for as short a time as possible is best for the child and family. However, there is little empirical evidence that, in the long term, day stay is best for children and families, and this is a ripe field for research. Because children (and adults) are discharged so early, we now have little information on even the most basic sequelae and complications, such as infection rates.

Procedures which once may have required a two to three day hospitalisation can now be performed laparoscopically and the patient discharged either the same day or after one night's stay. Procedures which allow children to be discharged on the same day of surgery significantly reduce the cost of health care and limit unnecessary bed occupancy. The type of procedures suitable for day surgery must have a minimal risk of post-operative haemorrhage, a minimal risk of post-operative airway compromise and controllable pain that can be managed with oral analgesics at home (Australia New Zealand College of Anaesthetists, 2006). To be fit for discharge on the day of surgery, the child needs to be able to tolerate food and fluids, to have voided post-operatively, have no bleeding and to be relatively free from pain and discomfort. The day surgery child must have a responsible adult to transport them home in a suitable vehicle, and a responsible person at home for at least the first night after discharge.

Procedures for a day surgery admission include the standard pre-operative checklist, including baseline observations, surgical and medical history, allergies, medications, fasting times and understanding of procedures. Each unit has standard times for morning and afternoon theatre lists, to ensure enough time for surgical and anaesthetic review prior to theatre. In some cases, the children have been surgically reviewed prior to admission and they and their parents may have already signed a consent form for surgery. The anaesthetist reviews the child on the day of surgery to ensure they are fit for an anaesthetic.

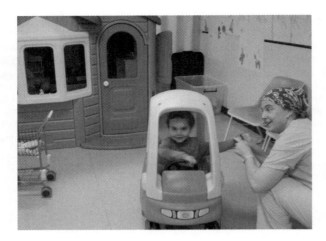

Fig. 3.2 A "child friendly" theatre suite.

Reception in the operating suite

Entering an OR can be a daunting experience for children about to undergo surgery and their parents. Theatre reception is the public face of theatre. It is important to introduce yourself and confirm the operative details with the patient using the preoperative checklist. Figure 3.2 shows a reception area in an operating theatre in a children's hospital which has been made as "child friendly" as possible, though still looks very foreign to anyone not used to such an environment.

Despite significant preparation, the child and her or his parents may be extremely anxious at this stage, some may claim they do not understand the surgical procedure or the anaesthetic they are about to undergo. In such cases, it is the theatre nurse's responsibility to ensure that the patient can speak with the surgeon or anaesthetist before going into the theatre. The perioperative nurse may be the last health care professional a child and parents encounter before the child undergoes surgery. Understanding the legal and ethical implications of informed consent enables perioperative nurses not only to act as patient advocate and facilitate solutions to dilemmas, but also to fulfil their legal responsibilities (Pryor, 1997).

On arrival in the theatre reception, a theatre nurse completes the child's preoperative checklist which has already been completed once by the nurse on the ward (see Figure 3.1). This checklist includes confirming with the child and parents that his or her identification band is correct in all details as to name (including correct spelling) and date of birth, both of which must correlate with the child's chart. Verification of any known allergies, and the child's and parents' understanding of the exact surgery the child is about to undergo is done here. This may include either written or verbal consent, the side of the body it is on and if the child and parents are well informed and understand the ramifications of the surgery as well as confirm when the child last ingested any food or fluids, and check if any premedication has been given (this may include the application of local anaesthetic cream to the hands for IV insertion). Relevant X-rays and pathology results must be available in the OR. Once these details are established and the correct patient is to undergo the correct procedure, the child can be accepted into theatre and transferred into the operating room.

Registration on entrance to the OR

In most countries, for children under 18 years of age, parental consent is required for surgery (although the concept of Gillick competence, which is accepted in many countries, means that a child who can reason and understand what is happening to him or her has the right to give their own consent (Miola, 2007)). Usually, a child requires a parent or legal guardian to be present when informed consent is explained and given. Parents are usually required to identify the child and are quizzed about the operation to ensure they understand the procedure their child is having, and to confirm the operative site.

Advocacy is an important part of the perioperative nurse's role and has particular relevance for paediatrics. There are certain safety factors that are important during admission to the OR:

Right procedure

When the child is checked in, the child (according to age) and parent are asked to state their understanding of the operation the child is having, and on what part of the body. Their explanation must agree with the documentation on the consent form. If discrepancy occurs, the doctors must ensure the child and parents are fully informed and the consent form re-signed. If a parent (or child) has questions or needs more information then this must be arranged as quickly as possible pre-operatively. Any relevant X-rays should be taken into the OR with the child.

Consent – the operation to be performed must have been fully explained to the parent and child (where appropriate) and signed for by both the parent and child, and the surgeon (according to local policy). Legalities of children signing their own consent form differ from country to country, but the autonomy of an older child can be enhanced by allowing her or him to sign the consent form in conjunction with a parent or guardian.

Right patient

In the near future, we may see children labelled by eye signature, DNA, fingerprint technology or some other form of identification technology not yet invented. However, the most common form of identification used in hospitals today is still wristbands or labels. While each health facility may use different methods, the child coming into the OR must have an identification band or label securely attached to his or her body. It must accurately state, as a minimum, the child's name, date of birth, any allergies and weight. It is the perioperative nurse's responsibility to check that this identification agrees fully with the child's other documentation such as hospital notes and consent form, and the child and parent must confirm the identity of the child with the nurse in the OR reception. In situations where a child is unaccompanied by a parent or guardian, the person accompanying the child assumes this responsibility, and the nurse must determine that legal consent has been obtained.

Fasting

For all pre-booked elective surgery, it is essential to fast prior to a general anaesthetic, and for emergency surgery, the child will not be allowed any food or drink during

the admission and assessment period, allowing for a passage of time prior to administration of an anaesthetic. If the patient has not fasted, there is a risk of vomiting
and aspirating food and fluids once she or he is paralysed. The general rule is to fast
from all fluids and foods for six hours before theatre, but children fast for periods
relevant to their age. Drinks or food must be removed from the child's bedside for
the fasting period and a fasting sign placed on the bed to alert others not to provide
anything, and children often wear a "fasting sticker" or vest. Within the fasting time,
the child may be ordered an oral premedication (usually analgesia or sedation) with
a minimal amount of water (20–30 mls). For acute, severe emergencies, where time
is of the essence (e.g., see Scenario 3.1), the anaesthetic will go ahead and a nasogastric tube will be passed once the child is unconscious and any stomach contents
aspirated.

Fasting in preparation for surgery is a contentious issue for children, particularly
for infants. If a child is hungry, he or she will become distressed, making it harder to
give an anaesthetic. Young children cannot rationalise why they are being deprived of
food and fluid, while babies can go into electrolyte imbalance if they are deprived
of fluid for prolonged periods.

On admission to the OR, the nurse must check with the child and/or parent when
the child actually fasted from and what she or he last ate and drank. While parents
and carers may have been informed of fasting times, sometimes the child will have
been given a drink or snack by mistake. This information must be communicated as
early as possible to the anaesthetist.

Other things to check on admission to the OR

Usually, the same pre-operative check list that is used for adults can be used for children, and checks for things such as "false teeth" can be changed to "loose teeth"
(Figure 3.1). Other things looked for prior to admission to the OR, and which must be
enquired about of the parent, or the child as appropriate, are current or recent infections, recent contact with infectious diseases such as chicken pox, presence of a rash
or break in skin integrity, any medications being taken, any known allergies, if medication has been ordered while in hospital (and this must be recorded on the medication sheet which must be in the child's chart). If an IV is *in situ* this must be noted
and checked for patency, and fluid orders and the fluid balance chart checked and the
child's vital signs taken and recorded. All charts, X-rays and pathology test results
must be taken into theatre with the child.

Anything that will affect the child in the PPACU must be communicated to the staff
there, and they must be made aware of where the parents can be reached during the
child's time in OR (it is a good idea to ensure that the parents' mobile phone numbers are written in the chart and confirmed with the parents during OR admission).
The parents need to be escorted from the OR and taken to the parents' waiting room,
where tea and coffee making facilities may be provided, or to the ward.

The safety of the child in the OR is paramount, and this covers all aspects of his or
her passage through the perioperative suite. There are generic safety issues, and those
in relation to particular aspects of the surgical experience.

Safety of children in the operating theatre

Children's physiology, metabolism, relative size and developmental stages are important considerations for anaesthesia, surgery and post-operative care. Anaesthetics which are suitable for adults may not be so for children or infants. Drugs, techniques and equipment for anaesthesia require a different approach to that used in adult anaesthetics. This is the same for both major and minor procedures.

Safety is a primary concern when caring for children and their families in the OR.

Safety during anaesthetic induction

Induction of anaesthetic can be commenced with or without the parent present, depending on local policy, the type of procedure and requirements of the individual anaesthetist. If a 'rapid sequence anaesthetic' is required, it may be considered inappropriate to have parents present. Consequently, this may leave the child in a frightening environment, so it is important for a nurse to stay with, talk to and comfort the child at all times. Parents need equal consideration, and their safety must also be considered. Many parents can feel anxious, distressed or even faint, and a nurse is required to stand with the parent while the child is being anaesthetised. Importantly, parents need a great deal of preparation about what their child is going to look like, how he or she will go limp very rapidly, and that this is a normal part of the anaesthetic induction.

It is important to reduce the amount of extraneous noise associated with setting up for procedures and preparing the theatre for the operation.

Specific safety issues for children during induction

- Keep bed rails and cot sides up at all time and ensure a nurse, parent or volunteer worker stays with the child to prevent falls from trolleys or theatre beds.
- Secure IV lines, arterial lines and epidural catheter lines safely and appropriately for the child's age and according to hospital policy.
- Check that any airway is appropriately secured.
- Connect monitoring devices, particularly oximeter, ECG and blood pressure as quickly as possible once the child is asleep. (For short procedures, ECG and blood pressure monitoring may not be required on children). A child with an obstructed airway from, e.g., a dislodged endotracheal tube will desaturate and become bradycardic within seconds.
- Neonates and smaller children in particular lose body heat quickly and attention to keeping them warm during induction is important. Body temperature can be controlled with the use of warm blankets and swaddling.
- If a child is known to be sensitive or allergic to latex, latex free equipment must be used according to local policy and practice.
- Children who are allergic to sticking plasters and tapes must have their eyes and lines taped with other material and devices.

Intraoperative safety issues

Within the OR other issues come into play:

- The temperature of the operating room needs to be adjusted so that the child stays warm (as required). Forced air body warmers, warmed skin preparation, warmed wash solutions and warm IV solutions should be used when appropriate. However, care must be taken not to overheat or burn the child while using these measures.
- Infants and some older children need temperature probes inserted, either rectally or through airway thermometer readings.
- Apply the diathermy plate carefully and correctly, ensuring the correct size for the weight of the child and positioning on a fleshy part of the body, e.g., thigh, abdomen or lower back.
- When applying the skin preparation, take care that fluid does not pool underneath or around the body.
- Remove anything metal: nappy pins, metal buttons and press-studs to prevent possible burns caused by diathermy.
- During the procedure, carefully and accurately measure blood and fluid losses, report them to the anaesthetist and document them on a fluid record sheet. Used swabs (pre-weighed while dry) should be weighed to ascertain blood loss, particularly with infants, and paediatric sucker catchment bottles with millilitre measurements should be used. The blood volume of a healthy 10 kg infant is approximately 800 mls (10 mls/kg) (Morgan & Mikhail, 1996), and a blood loss of 200 mls would equal a quarter of the child's total volume.
- Pay close attention to positioning of equipment and circulating/scrub staff at the operating table once the patient has been draped. Ensure they do not get in the way of the surgical team, that they do not lean on or touch the operating table and that they do not come into contact with the sterile area.
- Ensure that protective equipment such as a lead apron is placed over the child who requires X-ray intraoperatively, e.g., children having central lines inserted or fractures manipulated. Lead aprons are also required for any staff who have to stay close to the child when any radiographic procedure is being undertaken.
- Positioning the child on the operating table is important but it is generally the same as for adults (Rothrock & McEwan, 2007). However, there are some particular paediatric positions which require special safety considerations, e.g., the 'flying fetus' position used in craniofacial surgery, which involves lying the child prone, neck extended and face facing out. Too much extension can lead to venous congestion from blood pooling at the back of the neck. Once the child is anaesthetised, he or she is placed prone on a special beanbag which is moulded to shape and the air extracted. At this point, there must be no ridges or wrinkles that will cause pressure.
- Secure drains and indwelling catheters. Young children, when awake or when regaining consciousness will often try to remove or pull out tubes that frighten them or cause discomfort.

Post anaesthetic/post operative

Each hospital has its own process for moving patients out of the OR and into the PPACU (Figure 3.3). Children are moved from the OR to PPACU in various anaesthetic

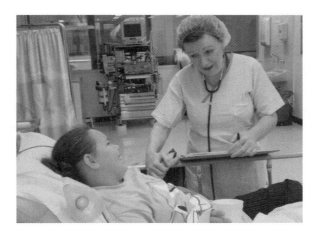

Fig. 3.3 A child in PPACU.

stages ranging from fully ventilated to extubated and rousable, or even wide awake. Special safety issues for children in this phase include the following.

- Place the child on a paediatric recovery trolley and ensure the side rails are up. Ensure the head is not hyper- extended. Children have short, narrow airways which easily obstruct as a result of extension or occlusion e.g. swelling, mucous and vomit, and are particularly susceptible to airway irritation causing laryngospasm.
- Oxygen, mask and T-piece and suction must be immediately available and oxygen saturation monitoring attached once the child arrives in PPACU. An obstructed airway or apnoea in a child can result in sudden respiratory arrest.
- A child must never be left alone on a bed or trolley in PPACU. Small children, because of their rapid metabolism, can wake rapidly, and find themselves in a totally unfamiliar room with unfamiliar people around them. They can be experiencing pain and be hungry, thirsty, confused and frightened. They can jump, fall or crawl off beds that do not have adequate safety rails and an adult (nurse or parent) with them at all times.
- IV access and IV lines must be secured as quickly as possible using arm boards and taping. Small children in particular often try and pull IV lines out. The same is true for drains such as indwelling catheters and wound drains. Secure taping with arm splints will ensure the IV lines cannot be dislodged, and constant watching by an adult is needed to ensure the newly-wakened child does not dislodge drains and other tubing.
- Distressed, confused children who are not fully awake can hurt themselves with self-harming behaviour such as scratching their faces or other body parts.
- Arm splints may be ordered and required for some children such as babies who have had palate or lip surgery. These also need to be applied as quickly as possible, ideally before the child has woken up.
- A child whose limb is splinted for safe IV access, or to prevent them harming operation sites, must have the circulation in their limb checked regularly.

- Ongoing monitoring of body temperature is important. Hypothermia will cause periodic breathing, apnoea and delays in rousing a post-operative child.

Standing orders

Standing orders are often used in PPACU, where nurses work autonomously and without immediate medical backup. Standing orders for medication management provide guidelines from which nurses can work. To be legally binding, these must be written in conjunction with the anaesthetist in charge of the PPACU, and are most often designed by a committee comprised of the head anaesthetist, nurse in charge of the PPACU and/or the nurse in charge of the OR. A sample of standing orders for the post-operative recovery of children who have had adeno-tonsillectomy for obstructive sleep apnoea are shown in Box 3.1.

Box 3.1   Sample of standing orders

Tonsils and Adenoids with Obstructive Sleep Apnoea (OSA)

In the post-operative phase a child with OSA who has had an ENT procedure is at risk due to post-op swelling and oedema. They should be closely monitored for signs of respiratory failure in addition to routine post-op observation.

Post-operative oxygen:
If Oxygen Saturation drops below 90%:

(1)   Attempt to rouse the child
(2)   Give oxygen
(3)   If the child is unrousable commence resuscitation as per resuscitation code procedure
(4)   Call the consultant or registrar concerned
(5)   Nurse the child individually until review by medical staff.

N.B. The child must not be left unattended with oxygen *in situ* while awaiting medical review

Post-op pain relief orders for children who cannot have narcotics.
It may be necessary for a child who usually cannot tolerate narcotics to be ordered narcotic pain relief and very close observation must then be undertaken for a minimum of 2 hours post-administration. The child should be on pulse oximetry, and visual observations should include rousability and respiratory rate.
   If a 'Not-For-Narcotic' child is in pain and requires stronger pain relief than ordered:

(1)   Call the ENT consultant or registrar concerned for a review of respiratory status and pain relief order.
(2)   Give pain relief as ordered if oxygen saturation drops below 90%.
(3)   Monitor oxygen saturations, respiratory rate and depth and rousability 1. 3.3.3.
   - 5 minutely for 15 mins
   - 15 minutely for 2 hours
(4)   If oxygen saturation drops below 90%:
   - Rouse the child
   - Give oxygen
   - If unrousable commence resuscitation as per resuscitation code procedure
   - Call ENT registrar or consultant concerned
   - Special the child until medical review

Conclusion

When children come into an OR, they have a range of requirements that are often quite different to those of adults in the same circumstances. Safety issues around their body size and metabolism, activity and emergence levels, and the presence of their parents mean that approaches that are used in the care of adults are inappropriate and insufficient for the care of children – in other words, the care of children in the perioperative area is a highly specialised field.

References

American Academy of Pediatrics. (1996). Evaluation and preparation of pediatric patients undergoing anesthesia. *Pediatrics,* 98: 502–508.

Association for the Welfare of Child Health (2005). *The psychosocial care of children and their families in hospital: AWCH national survey report.* Section 2: Preparation for admission. Available from http://www.awch.org.au/AWCH%20Psychosocial%20Survey%20Report%202005/PDF/2005%20AWCH%20NSR%20Section%202.pdf (accessed 11 January 2008).

Australia New Zealand College of Anaesthetists. (2006). *Review PS15 Recommendations for the perioperative care of patients selected for day care surgery.* Australian and New Zealand College of Anaesthetists. Melbourne, 2006. Available from http://www.anzca.edu.au/resources/professional-documents/professional-standards/ps15.html Accessed 12 January, 2008.

Dahlquist, L.M., Gil, K.M., Armstrong, D., DeLawyer, D.D., Greene, P. & Wuori, D. (1986). Preparing children for medical examinations: The importance of previous medical experience. *Health Psychology,* 5: 249–259.

Eckhardt, L.O. & Prugh, D.G. (1978). Preparing children psychologically for painful medical and surgical procedures. In: Gellert, E. (ed.). *Psychosocial aspects of pediatric care.* Grune & Stratton, New York.

English, C. & Bond, S. (1998). Evidence based nursing: easier said than done. *Paediatric Nursing,* 10(7–8): 10–11.

Johnson, A. (1992). Children and their families in hospital. In: Clements, A. (ed.). *Infant and family health in Australia,* 2nd ed. Churchill Livingstone, Melbourne.

Johnson, B.H. (1974). Before hospitalization: A preparation program for the child and his family. *Child Today,* November–December, 18–21.

Kristensson-Hallström, I. (2000). Parental participation in pediatric surgical care. *Association of Operating Room Nurses Journal,* 71: 1021–1029.

Martinelli, A.M. (2000). Administering drugs and solutions. In: Phippen, M.L., Wells, M.P. (eds). *Patient care during operative and invasive procedures.* WB Saunders, Philadelphia.

Mayo Clinic Staff. (2007). *Impetigo.* MayoClinic.com. Available from http://www.mayoclinic.com/health/impetigo/DS00464/DSECTION=3 (accessed 12 January 2007).

Miola, J. (2007). *Medical ethics and medical law : A symbiotic relationship.* Hart, Oxford.

Morgan, G.E., Mikhail, M.S. (1996). *Clinical anesthesiology,* 2nd ed. Appleton & Lange, Stamford.

Paterson-Brown, S. (2005). *Core topics in general and emergency surgery,* 3rd ed. Elsevier-Saunders, Philadelphia.

Pryor, F. (1997). Key concepts in informed consent for perioperative nurses. *Association of Operating Room Nurses Journal,* 65: 1105–1110.

Rodin, J. (1989). *Will this hurt?: Preparing children for hospital and medical procedures.* NAWCH, London.

Rothrock, J.C., McEwan, D. (eds). (2007). *Alexander's care of the patient in surgery.* M.O. Mosby/Elsevier, St. Louis.

Woon, R. (2004). Hospital play therapy: Helping children cope with hospitalisation through therapeutic play. *Singapore Nursing Journal,* 31: 16–19.

4 Nursing care and management of children's perioperative pain

Bernie Carter and Denise Jonas

Introduction

The experience of pain is potentially an overwhelming, all-encompassing experience for a child (Carter, 2002). One of the most fundamental of all perioperative nursing responsibilities is to ensure that every child receives optimal management of their pain throughout the whole of the perioperative period (Gold *et al.*, 2006). Effective management involves a cycle of prevention, assessment, intervention, evaluation and documentation. All of these elements need to occur within a supportive environment which promotes the child's ability to share any of their fears and concerns relating to their pain.

Pain management is often described as challenging and this in many senses is true. However, this does not mean that nurses should leave pain management solely to specialists such as members of a pain team (Carter, 2004). Management of pain requires active engagement in decision-making; it is 24 h a day, 7 days a week and needs to continue even when pain specialists are not available. Pain management is the responsibility of every nurse involved in providing perioperative care to children. Every nurse needs to maintain and enhance their skills and knowledge so that they can provide optimal care to every child. It is an essential component of ethical and compassionate nursing care (Cummings *et al.*, 1996). Pain should be seen as a clinical priority; it has both short-term and long-term consequences (Grunau *et al.*, 2006).

Perioperative care is changing. Many of these changes reflect the advances in surgical procedures (such as laparoscopic techniques), anaesthesia and the availability of sophisticated technology. Procedures which used to require hospitalisation for days or weeks are now routinely carried out as day cases. Ambulatory/day-case care is now common for minor surgeries and the modality is expanding rapidly (Hamers & Huijer Abu-Saad, 2002; Lonnqvist & Morton, 2006). More sophisticated drug delivery systems, multi-modal approaches, improved technology, new drugs and different regimes have all impacted on pain management practices. Key to these changes is the developments in patient-controlled analgesia (PCA), epidural analgesia and local anaesthetic infusions. Other changes reflect the greater social awareness of pain and the imperative for pain to be a treatment priority (Finley *et al.*, 2005). The shift towards early discharge from hospital along with the emphasis on partnership and collaboration with parents has seen more and more post-operative care being undertaken within community settings. Parents now take considerable responsibility for their children's continuing post-operative pain management.

Pain control policies must reflect these changes and ensure that pain management for children receiving day-case surgery includes parental advice and the provision of effective take-home analgesia (Department of Health, 2003). Whilst it is essential to ensure that policies are in place for supporting parental roles, hospitals and other settings should have evidence-based protocols, policies and nursing practice guidelines in place for all specialised pain management techniques but especially for those using local anaesthetics and opioids. These should be reviewed on a regular basis through a clinical governance system and evaluated by regular audit of practice. Standardised protocols and pain management algorithms have been shown to provide more effective overall pain relief (Falanga *et al.*, 2006). Policies and guidelines should provide information regarding whom to contact should problems arise (National Health Service Quality Improvement Scotland, 2004). Training programmes for nursing and medical staff should be in place with competency-based frameworks for pain management infusion devices. The volume of information available on the intranet can provide the remotest of units with up-to-date guidelines and literature on children's pain management (see Box 4.1). Pain societies and groups frequently share information and provide links for units developing safe paediatric pain management (Royal College of Nursing, 1999, 2002; Royal College of Paediatrics and Child Health, 2001; GOSH/ICH, 2006; Paediatrics & Child Health Division, 2006; The Royal Australasian College of Physicians, 2006).

Box 4.1   Useful websites

American Pain Society http://www.ampainsoc.org/
Australian Pain Society http://www.apsoc.org.au/
British Pain Society www.britishpainsociety.org
Pediatric Pain Source book http://painsourcebook.ca
The children's pain assessment project. http://www.ich.ucl.ac.uk/cpap/index.html

Effective perioperative pain management requires the nurse to have a good understanding of a range of issues including the physiology of pain, the potential psychosocial-emotional impact of pain on the child/family and the sequelae of unrelieved or poorly managed pain. Nurses also need a clear appreciation of their role and the role of other members of the multi-disciplinary team throughout the child's care. This is regardless of whether care is being delivered by health care professionals within a clinical setting or by parents and carers in the child's own home. Appropriate nursing care can mediate and relieve pain, and nurses need to utilise their clinical judgement and critical thinking skills, reflect on their practice and be active in solving pain management problems.

The nursing contribution to perioperative pain management is immense as nurses are involved in taking a comprehensive pain history from the child/family, assessing a child's pain, providing comfort and support to the child/family, educating and preparing the child/family about pain/pain management, using techniques such as distraction and imagery (where appropriate to the child's age and condition), administering medication and evaluating the effectiveness of interventions. Documenting all aspects of the child's pain management (assessment scores, behaviour, interventions, outcome of intervention, evaluation) (Holaday *et al.*, 1999; Finley *et al.*, 2005;

Salanterä, 2006) is crucial as improved documentation has been shown to result in improved pain management (Faries *et al.*, 1991; Treadwell *et al.*, 2002; Currell & Urquhart 2003).

A substantive amount of pain management research focuses on analgesia-oriented issues with much less considering the other issues related to the comprehensive management of post-operative pain. Many of these studies have focused on day surgery or surgery requiring short hospital stays such as adeno-tonsillectomy (Sutters & Miaskowski, 1999; Hamers & Huijer Abu-Saad, 2002; Huth *et al.*, 2004; Kain *et al.*, 2006). Relatively few studies have examined more diverse surgical populations although some evidence exists for general surgery (Gillies *et al.*, 1999; Perrott *et al.*, 2004) and cardiac surgery (Huth *et al.*, 2003). Some studies such as that undertaken by Perrott *et al.* (2004) have had a primary focus on the examination of the assessment tool being used. The evidence base for the perioperative pain management of some groups of children, such as those who are critically ill (Coffman *et al.*, 1997) and those who are cognitively impaired (Breau *et al.*, 2002a, 2003), is much less substantive.

Preparing and teaching children and parents about pain

Preparation is a crucial aspect of effective pain management and fundamental to good preparation is the education of the child and their parents. Effective communication needs to occur between the child (wherever feasible), their family and the professionals/ the multi-disciplinary team (Craig *et al.*, 1996). A child's pain experience can be heightened if they are anxious and/or distressed, and effective psychosocial preparation of children and their parents can mediate these factors. Supportive pre-operative education and information about post-operative pain can reduce pain scores when compared to children receiving routine pre-operative care (Demirel & Cam, 2006).

Although therapeutic play has been reported through case studies to have value within clinical practice there is no substantive and rigorous research base to underpin its use. The study by Li *et al.* (2006) aimed to address this deficit and whilst they demonstrated that therapeutic play as part of a psycho-educational programme resulted in lower child and parent state anxiety scores, no differences were noted in children's post-operative pain scores between the control and the experimental (therapeutic play) groups. Whilst focusing on reducing pre-operative anxiety rather than pain, the use of clown doctors was found to be effective for children and their parents (Vagnoli *et al.*, 2005) although medical personnel perceived that the clown doctors were interfering with the procedures within the setting.

Individually tailored, perioperative psychosocial interventions have been suggested for specific groups of children, such as those with a diagnosis of autism, whose needs are both different and heightened compared to other children requiring surgery. Seid *et al.* (1997) emphasise the particular importance of minimising disruption to the child's routines, reducing separation from familiar caretakers and the value of using distractors to reduce anxiety.

Not only do children from specific diagnostic groups need tailored preparation and management but other factors such as gender may also need consideration. Studies on pain generally indicate that girls exhibit greater behavioural distress than boys (Liddell & Murray, 1989), report higher levels of pain than boys (Chambers *et al.*, 1999) and have lower pain treatment thresholds than boys (Demyttenaere *et al.*, 2001;

Gauthier *et al.*, 1998). However, the evidence is conflicting; some studies show that pain intensity is not significantly linked to gender (Cummings *et al.*, 1996). A study by Sutters and Miaskowski (1999) (3–12 years; *n*=48 boys; *n*=39 girls) on gender differences in the post-operative period suggests that boys and girls respond differently to pain following surgery. In this study, boys exhibited more overt pain behaviours than girls in the paediatric post-operative anaesthetic care unit (PPACU) but girls reported higher pain scores when they were discharged from PPACU in the first hour in the day-surgery area. However, no gender differences were noted in the amount of or response to analgesics between boys and girls, although nurses in the PPACU administered analgesics sooner to boys than girls.

Parents and other carers need appropriate information about their children's pain (Simons *et al.*, 2001) and consideration of their own beliefs about their children's pain, how their children express pain, the use and effects of analgesia and other interventions and how to avoid feelings of helplessness (Woodgate & Kristjanson, 1995). This is an important consideration for parents of children who have undergone day-case surgery as studies have demonstrated that children can suffer clinically significant post-operative pain at home which may be mismanaged as a result of parents being uninformed or lacking in confidence (Hamers & Huijer Abu-Saad, 2002). Whilst parental education is often emphasised as being an important part of care prior to discharge home, Sutters *et al.*, (2004) note that parents who were coached in pain management by nurses did not have increased adherence to an around-the-clock dosing schedule for children post-tonsillectomy when compared with parents in the control group.

Some studies have noted that good preparation and information is particularly important for parents of children who are cognitively impaired; these parents may mistakenly believe that their children's perception of pain may also be impaired (Breau *et al.*, 2003). Parents need appropriate information, teaching and confidence in the use of pain assessment tools if they are to be effective in assessing (and managing) their children's pain (Polkki *et al.*, 2002b; Breau *et al.*, 2003; Voepel-Lewis *et al.*, 2005). Some of this preparation may occur within pre-admission clinics but not all children have the opportunity to attend such clinics/sessions, and a number of different factors such as timing, type of information provided and degree to which it is individually tailored influences effectiveness. Smith and Callery (2005) note that children would like more information about pain.

Whilst ambulatory care brings some benefits, it now means that the burden of post-operative pain management rests with the children's parents. Information is an essential component in ensuring that parents feel confident about their role in managing their children's pain and ongoing post-operative care (Bergstrom *et al.*, 2000; Sanders 2002a; Huth *et al.*, 2003). Work by Jonas (2003) found that parents benefited from being given both verbal and written information prior to discharge and also from a follow-up telephone call which gave parents the opportunity to discuss specific concerns and the value of an information leaflet.

Agency, education and training of health care professionals

Many studies demonstrate that pain is under/poorly-assessed and/or poorly documented resulting in children being under-medicated and/or poorly managed

(Cummings *et al.*, 1996; Gillies *et al.*, 1999; Holaday *et al.*, 1999; Jacob & Puntillo 1999; Kohler *et al.*, 2001; Sittl *et al.*, 2006). Many factors including education, context, expectations, personal attributes and leadership have been shown to be influential and these need to be considered when developing strategies to improve perioperative pain management. Enhancing pain management is a multi-factorial process, and a systemic approach that addresses many factors is likely to have a better chance of success than one which focuses just on one area. The social ecology approach of Jordan-Marsh *et al.* (2004) adopted an intensive, comprehensive set of interventions which had positive and sustained outcomes, which makes it a good model for consideration.

Studies demonstrate that nurses often score pain lower than parents (Ericsson *et al.*, 2006; Knutsson *et al.*, 2006). Hamers *et al.*, (1997) note that although nurse expertise did not influence assessments of the intensity of pain experienced by children, their expertise (based on length of nursing experience) did impact on their confidence levels and they were more inclined to administer analgesics.

Health care professionals need appropriate levels of education about pain (Simons & Roberson, 2002) as a nurse's perception of children's pain is highly related to overt pain behaviour (Byrne *et al.*, 2001). They also need adequate training/preparation in the use of pain assessment tools and proficiency in using them (Treadwell *et al.*, 2002), changes in working practices (Boyd & Stuart, 2005); organisational commitment (Treadwell *et al.*, 2002); quality improvement (Treadwell *et al.*, 2002), reflexivity and a willingness to change in relation to their attitudes, beliefs and attributes about children's pain (Polkki, 2002; Polkki *et al.*, 2003; Salanterä, 2006). Studies have demonstrated that health professionals' assessment of children's pain is subject to a range of individual, social and contextual influences (Craig *et al.*, 1996). There is evidence that professionals may attempt to distance themselves from a child's pain (Carter, 2002), and work by Byrne *et al.* (2001) identified behavioural and cognitive strategies which deny the reality or urgency of children's pain and distress that were used by professionals to defend themselves emotionally against children's post-operative pain; the result being compromised communication and poor pain management.

Whilst there is much evidence to support the generic need for improved education of health care professionals in relation to managing children's pain, some groups of children may be more at risk of their pain being poorly managed than others. For example, Breau *et al.*, (2006) found that some nurses believe that the pain experience of neurologically impaired infants is reduced relative to non-impaired infants (Breau *et al.*, 2006). Simons and Roberson (2002) demonstrated that even a short programme of pain education could increase nurses' knowledge and confidence and contribute to them feeling more assertive about managing children's pain. Van Hulle Vincent (2005) also notes that nurses with more knowledge and more positive attitudes towards pain reported greater ability in overcoming pain management barriers.

Assessing children's pain

Pain assessment is an essential contribution to ensuring that pain is both prevented and relieved (Howard, 2003; Finley *et al.*, 2005), and is enshrined in current pain management guidelines (Australian and New Zealand College of Anaesthetists, 2005;

American Academy of Pediatrics, Committee on Fetus and Newborn, Committee on Drugs, Section on Anesthesiology, Section on Surgery, Canadian Paediatric Society Fetus and Newborn Committee, 2000; Paediatrics & Child Health Division, 2006; Royal College of Paediatrics and Child Health, 2001; Howard *et al.*, 2008).

Many acute pain assessment tools exist. These tools vary in relation to child-related factors (e.g., child's language, ethnic origin, age, cognitive level), user-related factors (e.g. whether they have been designed for use by professionals or parents and their utility within a clinical or home/other setting) and structural factors (e.g, whether they are self-report or behavioural, use a rating scale or checklist, the dimensions they measure and the items they include) (Merkel *et al.*, 2002; Mathew & Mathew, 2003; von Baeyer, 2006; Stinson *et al.*, 2006; von Baeyer & Spagrud, 2007). Some acute pain tools have been developed for the assessment of post-operative pain; however, none has been identified as being specific to perioperative pain. These factors need to be taken into consideration when making choices about which acute pain assessment tool to use with an individual child/family during the perioperative period.

Core approaches to pain assessment

There are three fundamental approaches upon which pain assessment tools are based. Whilst all/most approaches purport to be measuring pain, each different approach may be measuring a different construct (Walco *et al.*, 2005; von Baeyer, 2006; von Baeyer & Spagrud, 2007). A number of tools draw on a combination of elements (e.g, heart rate and grimacing).

- **Physiological assessment:** measures the physiological arousal (e.g. heart rate, respiratory rate and changes in salivary cortisol levels) consequent to the pain rather than the actual pain.
- **Observational (behavioural) assessment:** measures the observable behavioural distress (e.g., grimacing, limb movements, crying) associated with the pain rather than actual pain.
- **Self-report by the child:** reflects the child's expressed experience of their pain rather than the pain itself.
- **Parent/carer-report:** reflects the perceived experience of pain as reported by someone who knows the child.

Only child-oriented, self-report tools attempt to gain an appreciation of the subjective experience of pain. Observational and child/parent/carer reports are surrogate ways of assessing pain (Australian and New Zealand College of Anaesthetists, 2005).

Children's self-report of pain is often seen as the gold standard and in most circumstances it is the preferred approach. However, it needs to be recognised that self-report is complex (Stinson *et al.*, 2006; von Baeyer, 2006), dependent on the child's age/cognition (Stanford *et al.*, 2006), subject to a range of social and other influences (de C Williams *et al.*, 2000) including biases (de C Williams *et al.*, 2000; Hodgins 2002). Whilst age can be used to guide the choice of tool to be used, other factors also need to be considered as these may impact (either in short or long term) on the child's ability to actively contribute self-reports or they may mask behaviour(s) and/or physiological response(s) (Table 4.1).

No individual observational (von Baeyer, 2006), self-report (Stinson *et al.*, 2006), or physiological measure is broadly recommended for pain assessment across all children or all contexts. Therefore, health care professionals need to make informed choices about which tool to use to assess each individual child's individual pain (see Tables 4.2 and 4.3). Composite measures using self-report and at least one other measure would be a more ideal approach (Stinson *et al.*, 2006).

Table 4.1 Overview of behavioural (observational) pain assessment tools suitable for use with postoperative pain

COMFORT	Has eight indicators (scored between 1 and 5)	alertness; calmness/agitation; respiratory response; physical movement; blood pressure; heart rate; muscle tone; facial tension
CRIES	Has five indicators (scored between 0 and 2)	crying; requirement for O_2 for $SaO_2 < 95\%$; increased vital signs (blood pressure and heart rate BP); facial expression; sleepless
PIPP	Has seven indicators (scored between 0 and 3)	gestational age; behavioural state before painful stimulus; change in heart rate during painful stimulus; change in oxygen saturation during painful stimulus; brow bulge during painful stimulus; eye squeeze during painful stimulus; nasolabial furrow during painful stimulus
NCCPC-PV	Has six indicator areas (scored between 0 and 3 and with option of not applicable)	vocal; social; facial; activity; body and limbs; physiological
NCCPC-R	Has seven indicator areas (scored between 0 and 3 and with the option of not applicable)	vocal; social; facial; activity; body and limbs; physiological; eating and sleeping
FLACC	Has five indicators (scored between 0 and 2)	face; legs; activity; cry; consolability
CAAS	Has four indicators (scored between 0 and 2)	pupillary size; heart rate; mean blood pressure; respiratory and motor response

Table 4.2 Overview of self-report pain assessment tools suitable for use with post-operative pain

The Pieces of Hurt Tool	Uses four poker chips that are described as being 'pieces of hurt' and which children use to help them describe the number of pieces of hurt they feel
The Faces Pain Scale – Revised	Uses six faces showing no pain to very much pain and scored 0-2-4-6-8-10
The Coloured Analogue Scale	Is a pocket sized tool with a long triangular shape that is coloured from light pink to dark red. The child moves a plastic marker along the length of the scale to locate the amount of pain they have. On the other side of the scale is a corresponding 0 to 10 numerical scale.

What tools to consider using with particular groups of children

Neonates: A number of assessment tools are being used within practice settings, although it is worth noting that Stevens and Gibbins (2002) note that these have not been rigorously tested for construct validity, feasibility and clinical utility. These tools which are most commonly used in practice include the **COMFORT** scale (Ambuel *et al.*, 1992; van Dijk *et al.*, 2000); **CRIES** (Krechel & Bildner, 1995) and **PIPP** (Premature Infant Pain Profile) (Stevens *et al.*, 1996; Ballantyne *et al.*, 1999; Jonsdóttir & Kristjánsdóttir, 2005; Pasero, 2002).

Cognitively impaired children: There are fewer tools available for children who are cognitively impaired, and it is generally accepted that pain assessment for children within this group is complex as their responses are often individualistic and need to be contextualised against the child's usual non-pain behaviour (Carter *et al.*, 2002; Breau *et al.*, 2003; Hunt *et al.*, 2004). Only one tool, the **NCCPC-PV** (Non-Communicating Children's Pain Checklist – Post-operative Version) (Breau *et al.*, 2002b), has been specifically developed to support the assessment of the post-operative pain experienced by children with cognitive impairment. However, other tools such as Hunts PPP (Paediatric Pain Profile) and the **NCCPC-R** (Non-Communicating Children's Pain Checklist) (Breau *et al.*, 2000, 2001, 2002b, 2003) which have been designed for assessment of generic pain may have value in the perioperative period. For cognitively impaired children who are being nursed within a critical care setting, the **COMFORT** scale (Ambuel *et al.*, 1992; van Dijk *et al.*, 2000) is a sound tool.

Children who cannot self-report but who are not cognitively impaired: This group of children requires the use of behavioural (observational) tools. The **FLACC** (Merkel *et al.*, 1997) is suitable for assessment of post-operative pain in the hospital setting. The **PPPM** (Parents Post-operative Pain Measure) (Chambers *et al.*, 1996, 2003; Finley *et al.*, 2003) is a useful tool for post-operative pain being managed by parents at home.

Preschool children who can self-report: This group of children can use the **Pieces of Hurt Tool** (Hester 1979, Hester *et al.*, 1990) and the **MSPCT** (The Multiple Size Poker Chip Tool) (St-Laurent-Gagnon *et al.*, 1999), although these have not been specifically designed for perioperative situations.

School-aged children who can self-report: This group has access to a range of acute pain assessment tools. Tools such as the **Wong and Baker FACES Pain Scale** (Wong & Baker, 1988) and the **Faces Pain Scale-Revised** (Hicks *et al.*, 2001) can be used with children older than about 5 years. **Visual analogue** and **numerical rating scales** and the **Coloured Analogue Scale** (McGrath *et al.*, 1996) can be used with children from about 8 years old.

Children undergoing surgery for specific conditions: A small subset of tools exists that have been developed for pain management of specific conditions such as cardiac surgery where the **CAAS** (Cardiac Analgesia Assessment Scale) has been developed (Suominen *et al.*, 2004). Generally such tools are not in widespread use and have limited evidence for reliability and validity.

Non-pharmacological interventions

Whilst pharmacological intervention is fundamental, non-pharmacological measures have the potential to make a substantive contribution to pain management.

Many studies show psychological techniques such as distraction, imagery and hypnosis, and comforting interventions such as holding, rocking and soothing can result in significant decreases in children's pain but most of these have focused on acute procedural pain (Lambert, 1999; Salanterä *et al.*, 1999; Liossi & Hatira, 2003). Whilst it is likely that these techniques will have similar effects in post-operative pain, they are not necessarily directly transferable as pain management involves recovery from anaesthetic; the pain experience lasts longer than procedural pain and is more often associated with pharmacological intervention. A few studies have focused on imagery and its role in managing post-operative pain (Lambert, 1996; Huth *et al.*, 2006). Another study of children who had undergone tonsillectomy and/or adenoidectomy showed that children in the experimental (imagery) group had reduced post-operative pain scores compared to the control group whilst they were in hospital but that this effect did not persist post-discharge (Huth *et al.* 2004). Interestingly the study showed no significant differences in combined opioid and non-opioid use between the control and imagery groups.

Other studies have examined the types of non-pharmacological approaches used by children and their parents and have found that distraction is a method that is commonly used (Polkki *et al.*, 2001, 2002a, 2003; Idvall *et al.*, 2005). Often distraction involves watching television, playing and reading (Idvall *et al.*, 2005) or talking with their parents (He *et al.*, 2006). A study by Hatem *et al.* (2006) demonstrated that music reduced pain scores, post-cardiac surgery, and had beneficial effects on heart rate and respiratory rate.

Overview of pharmacological intervention

Despite many advances in relation to pharmacological management of children's pain in general and perioperative pain in particular, pharmacodynamic knowledge of analgesic agents in children remains relatively neglected and a considerable amount of knowledge has been extrapolated from adult data (Anderson & Palmer, 2006). However, there is substantive evidence that children's pain should be managed using a multi-modal and multi-disciplinary approach whenever possible based on four analgesics: local anaesthetics, non-steroidal anti-inflammatory drugs (NSAIDs), Paracetamol and opioids (Lonnqvist & Morton, 2005), however most mild to moderate post-operative pain can be well managed without the use of opioids (See Table 4.3). The aim of effective pain management is to control pain rapidly and maintain steady serum concentrations to prevent breakthrough pain (Tom, 2005). This is best achieved with optimum loading doses, titration of medication depending on the child's response and subsequent round-the-clock administration. Preference of which analgesic to use will depend on the age of the child, type and severity of the pain, expected duration, any underlying disease and the availability of the pharmacological agent. Infants metabolise medication differently to older children and adults as they have immature liver and renal functions which delay the absorption and elimination of many analgesics (Berde *et al.*, 2005; Tom, 2005; Ward *et al.*, 2006); these issues need to be carefully considered but this should not preclude active pain management (Anand *et al.*, 2006). Significant pain in infants undergoing surgery without adequate analgesia can produce a pain memory which may result in an exaggerated response to pain later in childhood (Taddio *et al.*, 1997; Howard, 2003; Grunau *et al.*, 2006). The WHO analgesia ladder was originally devised for the management of cancer pain

(Zernikow *et al.*, 2006) but can easily be adapted to manage post-operative pain using a step-down approach (Cunliffe & Roberts, 2004; World Health Organization, 2006).

Routes of administration

Except in unusual or extreme circumstances, intramuscular pain relief should not be used in infants and children as it is painful and the absorption rate can be variable (Hagan *et al.*, 2001). The oral route is inexpensive and convenient. Whilst younger children tolerate rectal analgesia, the rectal route can result in embarrassment and distress and can be culturally and individually inappropriate; the nurse must gain informed consent from the child and parents before administration of rectal analgesia. Use of epidural and caudal routes is becoming more popular in response to increasing evidence of efficacy and safety (Sanders, 2002b; Patel, 2006). The intravenous route is used in children who have severe pain or those unable to tolerate oral analgesia. Intravenous cannulae should be inserted with adequate topical analgesia such as Ametop or EMLA (Lander *et al.*, 2006) as this can reduce the pain associated with venepuncture (Tak & van Bon, 2006) and other cutaneous procedures (O'Brien *et al.*, 2005). The subcutaneous route can also be used, an indwelling subcutaneous cannula can be considered as a suitable alternative to an intravenous cannula or intramuscular analgesia (Charlton, 1997; Lamacraft *et al.*, 1997; Vijayan, 1997).

All analgesic drugs should be calculated according to the child's weight to avoid over-dosage.

Pre-emptive analgesia

The use of pre-emptive analgesia (generally seen as analgesia given prior to surgery/intervention) is considered an important aspect of pain management (Newstead, 2005), although its efficacy has been challenged (Aida & Shimoji, 2000). Some of the recent debate about the efficacy of pre-emptive analgesia is said to relate to how the term pre-emptive is defined. However, it is generally agreed that *preventive* perioperative analgesia has a role in reducing the central and peripheral sensitisation which arises from noxious pre-operative, intra-operative and post-operative inputs (Katz & McCartney, 2002; Pogatzki-Zahn & Zahn, 2006). The aim of a pre-emptive approach is to administer the analgesic agent before the onset of painful stimulus. This prevents windup of pain receptors and results in a smoother post-operative course with reduced levels of pain (Berry, 1998). Many children now receive Paracetamol and Ibuprofen as pre-medication rather than sedative agents as used in the past. Hannallah (1997) suggests that there should be no need for sedative pre-medication if the child has received proper psychological preparation.

Paracetamol and NSAIDs

The main aim of NSAIDs and Paracetamol type drugs is to manage mild to moderate pain. When used in conjunction with local anaesthetic blocks they promote early ambulation with minimal sedation. They are also useful in preventing breakthrough pain when weaning children from opioid analgesics and providing beneficial synergistic effects when used with opioids (Morton & O'Brien, 1999).

Paracetamol (Acetaminophen) is a safe and effective mild analgesic with an anti-pyretic effect; it has few side-effects when used in healthy children. Care should be considered in children under 3 months of age and those with renal or liver impairment (Howell, 2000). Recent evidence has suggested that loading doses may be required followed by regular maintenance doses to ensure optimum serum plasma levels (Morton, 1999). Rectal absorption is also variable in children and may require higher loading doses than those administered orally (Tobias, 2000; Howell & Patel, 2003). Use of intravenous Paracetamol provides a useful route especially for children who are nil-by-mouth. It offers increased dosing accuracy and avoids absorption and bioavailability variability (Anderson & Palmer, 2006). Evidence suggests it has a significant morphine-sparing effect (Lonnqvist & Morton, 2005).

NSAIDs are increasingly used in children as they have an anti-inflammatory effect as well as anti-pyretic and analgesic effects. NSAIDs work by inhibiting the cyclo-oxygenase enzyme and thus inhibiting prostaglandin synthesis and decreasing pain intensity. Common NSAID agents include Ibuprofen, Diclofenac and Ketolorac. Aspirin (which is used commonly in adults) is contraindicated in children due to the risk of Reye's syndrome (McGovern *et al.*, 2001).

NSAIDs should be avoided in infants under 6 months of age, children with renal or hepatic impairment, coagulation disorders, gastrointestinal disorders such as history of gastritis or ulcer and dehydration or hypovolaemia (Kokki, 2003; Morris *et al.*, 2003; Moghal *et al.*, 2004). Despite these contraindications, a systematic review found no evidence of increased bleeding following tonsillectomy due to pre-operative and intra-operative use of NSAIDs (Cardwell *et al.*, 2005). Bronchospasm induced by NSAID use in children with asthma is rare (Short *et al.*, 2000; Body & Potier, 2004), but evidence suggests that NSAID use should be limited or avoided in children requiring systemic steroid treatment for asthma or those known to be sensitive to NSAIDs (Ray & Basu, 2000). There is no substantive evidence of delayed bone osteogenesis in children; however, long-term use of NSAIDs should be avoided when extensive bone healing is required (Verghese & Hannallah, 2005). Limited evidence is available for the use of COX2 inhibitors in children; so recommendations cannot be made.

Mild opioids

Codeine is a weak opioid which is metabolised in the liver where approximately 10% of the drug is converted into morphine. When codeine is used in combination with Paracetamol, it is more effective (Moore *et al.*, 1997). Recent evidence suggests that its use as an analgesic in infants and children is limited due to the variation in metabolism in the population (Williams *et al.*, 2001, 2002).

Tramadol is a weak synthetic opioid with a lower tolerance for sedation and respiratory depression. It can be used in older children for mild to moderate pain; however, there is the potential for increased incidence of nausea and vomiting (Khosravi *et al.*, 2006).

Stronger opioids

Morphine is the most widely used opioid for children's post-operative pain management. Oral and sublingual morphine is well tolerated by children and provides suitable analgesia for moderate to severe pain (Engelhardt & Crawford, 2001).

Table 4.3 Suggested analgesia for various types of surgery in children

Operation	Type of Pain	Intra-operative	Post-operative
Appendectomy	Moderate–severe	Opioid, LWI	Oral Opioid (IV PCA, NCA or continuous opioid infusion if severe), Paracetamol, NSAID when drinking
Circumcision	Mild	Caudal or dorsal penile block, fentanyl – In awake neonates, oral sucrose and local anaesthetic gel such as Emla (Taddio *et al.*, 1999)	Paracetamol, NSAID (see notes), consider local anaesthetic gel
Cleft lip and palate	Mild for lip, moderate for palate	Dexamethasone, infra-orbital block, LWI and adrenaline for lip, bilateral greater palatine nerve block for palate. Remifentanyl, titrate IV morphine in recovery. Some areas use Clonidine or Ketamine	Paracetamol, NSAID (see notes), oral opioid for breakthrough pain (Jonas *et al.*, 2003). Some hospitals use NCA
Craniotomy	Moderate–severe	Remifentanyl, titrate IV morphine	Paracetamol, morphine infusion or PCA or oral opioid, NSAID after 24 h (see notes)
Dental	Mild–moderate	LWI and epinephrine, Fentanyl	Paracetamol, NSAID
Femoral/lower leg procedures	Moderate–severe	Epidural or sciatic/femoral nerve block, opioid	Paracetamol, local anaesthetic sciatic/femoral nerve infusion, NSAID (avoid regular use in leg-lengthening procedures)
Grommets	Mild	Opioid	Paracetamol
Hip surgery	Moderate–severe	Caudal block or epidural opioid	Epidural or opioid infusion, Paracetamol, NSAID (see notes)
Hypospadias	Moderate	Caudal, opioid	Oral opioid, Paracetamol, NSAID (see notes)
Inguinal hernia	Mild–moderate	Caudal or ilioinguinal block, fentanyl	Paracetamol, NSAID (see notes)
Insertion new gastrostomy	Mild	LWI, fentanyl	Paracetamol, NSAID when taking fluids (see notes)
Lacerations	Mild	LWI, fentanyl, morphine if severe	Paracetamol, NSAID (see notes)
Laparoscopy	Mild	LWI, opioid	Paracetamol, NSAID (see notes)
Laparotomy	Moderate–severe	Epidural (unless septic), opioid	Epidural or opioid infusion/PCA, Paracetamol, NSAID when no longer nil-by-mouth

Procedure	Severity	Intraoperative technique	Postoperative analgesia
Mastoidectomy	Moderate	LWI or block, fentanyl	Paracetamol, NSAID (see notes)
Orchidopexy	Mild	Caudal block, fentanyl	Paracetamol, NSAID (see notes)
Pinnaplasty	Mild–moderate	LWI or block, opioid,	Paracetamol, NSAID (see notes)
Pyloromyotomy	Mild–moderate	Opioid, LWI	Paracetamol
Renal/ureteric surgery	Moderate–severe	Paravertebral block or LWI, opioid. Epidural for ureteric surgery reduces pain from spasm	Paravertebral infusion, Paracetamol, oral opioid. Or epidural and Paracetamol, consider NSAID if no renal contraindication. Oxybutamine for bladder spasm
Scopes	Mild	Fentanyl	Paracetamol, NSAID unless contraindicated due to poor renal function
Spinal fusion	Severe	Remifentanyl, morphine towards end of surgery, IV Paracetamol	Epidural, or Ketamine infusion, morphine infusion or PCA/NCA, Paracetamol, NSAID when weaning off morphine or for breakthrough pain
Ophthalmic surgery	Mild–moderate	Fentanyl, local anaesthetic eye drops, anti-emetic	Paracetamol, NSAID oral or as eye drops (see notes)
Testicular torsion	Moderate	Opioid, LWI	Paracetamol, NSAID, oral opioid for breakthrough pain
Thoracotomy	Severe	Epidural unless septic, consider interpleural block/infusion	Epidural or IV opioid infusion/interpleural infusion, Paracetamol, NSAID (see notes)
Toenail removal	Mild	Local Anaesthetic Ring block, fentanyl	Paracetamol, NSAID
Tonsillectomy	Moderate	Transmucosal fentanyl for premed (Howell *et al.*, 2002). Opioid, possible tonsillar block, dexamethasone. White and Nolan (2005) suggest avoiding opioids to decrease PONV	Paracetamol, NSAID, oral opioid for breakthrough pain
Trigger thumb	Mild–moderate	LWI or brachial plexus block, fentanyl (Fisher *et al.*, 2006)	Paracetamol, NSAID (see notes)
Umbilical hernia	Mild	Rectus sheath block, fentanyl	Paracetamol, NSAID (see notes)
VP shunt	Mild	LWI or block, fentanyl	Paracetamol, NSAID (see notes)

Notes:

1. All caudal blocks with or without additive.
2. LWI = Local Wound Infiltration.
3. NSAIDs – Ibuprofen may be used over 3 months of age and Diclofenac over 6 months of age.
4. Analgesia doses available from British National Formulary for Children (2006). Always take into account age and disease process of child when prescribing analgesia.
5. Analgesia may differ in individual organisations and according to individual anaesthetic practice.

Intravenous doses provide fast and effective pain relief within 10 min and should be titrated with repeated smaller doses to an acceptable pain level (Lundeberg & Lonnqvist, 2004). Side-effects of morphine include increased sedation, respiratory depression, nausea and vomiting, confusion or hallucinations, reduction in gastric motility leading to constipation, pruritus, urine retention and muscle spasm. Regular monitoring of intravenous opioids, prompt recognition and early intervention by nursing staff can significantly reduce these adverse effects.

Diamorphine in children tends to be restricted to palliative care but it has an effective place via the intranasal route in the management of acute trauma (Kendall *et al.*, 2001).

Pethidine is not commonly used in children because when it is given in multiple doses its metabolite – norpethidine – can accumulate and act as a CNS irritant, ultimately causing convulsions (Nagle & McQuay, 1990).

Fentanyl is used in infants and children. It provides a decreased histamine response and reduced haemodynamic changes compared to morphine but it is more potent. Therefore its use is limited to intensive care, high-dependency and theatre areas due to an increased risk of respiratory depression. Its short duration means that it should not be used as a sole analgesic, and additional local anaesthetic and NSAIDs should be considered.

Whilst opioids play a major role in the pain management of children, the dose must be adjusted to take into account age and underlying illness. Opioid boluses are useful for occasional doses but superior pain relief is obtained through continuous infusions or PCA.

Intravenous **Naloxone** is a pure opioid antagonist and has the ability to rapidly reverse the adverse effects of opioids. All settings where children are receiving opioids should have immediate access to this reversal agent.

Continuous morphine infusion (CMI) provides the child with a constant and steady level of pain relief. The infusion rate is titrated by the nurse according to the child's individual need and the prescription. This form of pain relief avoids the peaks and troughs associated with bolus doses of morphine. CMIs can also be used safely in ward areas when PCA/NCA is unavailable. Opioid infusions should only be managed by appropriately trained nursing staff. Guidelines, specific charts and protocols should be in place to support nursing staff. Information leaflets for both parent and child provide additional written reinforcement to verbal information. Regular observations (minimum hourly) of pain scores, respiratory rate, sedation scores, nausea and vomiting, heart rate and oxygen saturation are also recommended and should be formally documented on an appropriate chart. Increasing sedation score is a clear predictor of respiratory depression (National Health Service Quality Improvement Scotland, 2004). Infants under 6 months should have additional apnoea monitoring in place.

PCA or NCA (Nurse-controlled analgesia) can be used and the choice of patient- or nurse-control depends on the age and cognitive ability of the child.

Pain is always subjective and therefore difficult for others to control; PCA allows the child to have their own control over their pain relief. Using the PCA device means the child can provide a steady level of pain relief by delivering a dose of morphine when they feel pain, thus significantly reducing anxiety. A programmed lockout period prevents the child from receiving excess amounts of an opioid. Effective use of PCA is variable; cognitive ability rather than age is usually an indicator of ability to understand the concept of PCA. Children as young as 5 years can use PCA effectively with support, and individual assessment of each child is required. Parents should be advised about the dangers of activating the PCA device for the child and be actively discouraged from doing so.

NCA provides a higher background opioid infusion that, in addition, allows the nurse to activate the device according to strict criteria. Lockout periods are usually longer than with PCA.

With all PCA/NCA devices, dedicated infusion lines that incorporate anti-reflux and anti-siphon valves should be used. It is important to ensure side-effects are managed adequately so that good pain relief is not compromised by the child becoming distressed by the side-effects. Persistent nausea will discourage the child from activating PCA devices and thus result in uncontrolled pain. Anti-emetics such as Ondansetron should be administered because anti-emetics are not routinely added to opioid infusions in children's pain management. The use of anti-histamines to treat pruritus should only be administered with caution as this increases the risk of sedation.

Whilst a background infusion on PCA may improve sleep patterns, the risk of respiratory depression and sedation is significantly increased (Doyle *et al.*, 1993). Additional, regular Paracetamol should be given to children receiving opioid infusions as the combined effect is synergistic resulting in a significant opioid-sparing effect (Lonnqvist & Morton, 2005). Discontinuation of PCA/NCA should occur only after the individual assessment of the child and the instigation of oral analgesia. CMI should be gradually reduced to prevent breakthrough pain or withdrawal rather than stopped abruptly.

Local anaesthetics

Infiltration of local anaesthetic agents can provide pain relief for several hours (Ray & Basu, 2000). Local anaesthetic blocks have become the main analgesic requirement for children and should be considered in all surgical cases unless there is a specific contraindication. A large survey of more than 24,000 paediatric regional anaesthetic blocks found an overall incidence of complications of 0.9 in 1000 blocks, with no complications of the technique (Giaufre *et al.*, 1996). Peripheral nerve blocks such as penile block, inguinal block and sciatic/femoral nerve block have been demonstrated to be as effective as single-shot caudal block and produce long-lasting analgesia. Caudal epidural block is widely used in children to provide analgesia following surgery below the level of the umbilicus; a single injection provides long-lasting postoperative analgesia (Ray & Basu, 2000). Hollis *et al.* (1999) found little beneficial evidence for the use of tonsillar blocks during tonsillectomy in reducing post-operative pain.

Caudal additives

The use of various additives to caudal blocks can increase the duration of the local anaesthetic block up to twofold, this not only decreases the need for anaesthetic agents but also for supplementary analgesics in the recovery period. Opioid additives tend to be reserved for major surgery as side-effects have been noted up to 24h post-surgery (Ansermino *et al.*, 2003). Clonidine, an alpha-2-receptor agonist, has been associated with increased incidence of sedation, dry mouth, whilst preservative-free Ketamine, a NMDA antagonist, has been noted for adverse behavioural side-effects (Semple *et al.*, 1996; Ansermino *et al.*, 2003). Ketamine infusion is increasingly being used as an additional analgesic in children with severe pain. When used along-side opioid infusions, its action reduces opioid requirements, thus reducing risk of sedation and respiratory depression (Royal Children's Hospital Melbourne, 2006). However, both Clonidine and Ketamine have been noted to delay discharge after day surgery; if the criteria are for the child to walk and pass urine before discharge, parents should be informed by nursing staff of the possibility of transient numbness before discharge (Charlton, 1997). Interestingly, the study by Bergendahl *et al.* (2004) showed that the calming and sedating effects of Clonidine in the first 24 h post-operatively were viewed positively by parents of children who had undergone adeno-tonsillectomy.

Regardless of the type of analgesia prescribed, parents need comprehensive written and verbal information relating to pain management before discharge (Jonas & Worsley-Cox, 2000; Action for Sick Children, 2006). This information should include the possible adverse effects of local anaesthetic blocks as complications following diminished sensation have been noted (Cooper *et al.*, 2000).

Epidural analgesia

An epidural is the administration of local anaesthetic solution into the epidural space (with or without an adjuvant such as Clonidine or Fentanyl) via an epidural catheter. This specialist technique enables analgesics to infuse close to the spinal nerves where they exert a powerful analgesic effect. Evidence suggests epidurals provide a superior form of pain relief when compared to intravenous opioids (Werawatganon & Charuluxanun, 2005; Wu *et al.*, 2005). Contraindications include systemic sepsis, coagulation disorder, local anaesthetic allergy and raised intracranial pressure. Education and training of nursing staff with support of guidelines and protocols means that these techniques do not need to be restricted to high-dependency settings (Lovett, 1997; Pasero, 2003).

Epidural catheters are normally inserted when the child is anaesthetised in theatre by a trained anaesthetist. Lower doses of local anaesthetic and additional opioid provide effective analgesia and minimises complications such as sedation and complications as a result of reduced bowel motility. This technique has been found to be suitable for cognitively impaired children in reducing the incidence of post-operative muscle spasm (Nolan *et al.*, 2000). Good quality analgesia is more likely with continuous epidural infusion rather than with intermittent bolus doses. However, if bolus doses are used, observation and monitoring should be the same as for continuous infusion.

Any local anaesthetic infusion should be infused through a dedicated pump with colour-coded infusion lines to avoid the inadvertent intravenous administration. Hourly observations of sedation scores, respiratory rates, heart rate, pain scores, oxygen saturation, blood pressure and assessment of level of block are mandatory. In addition, the nurse should be alert for the possible development of motor block, pressure sores from diminished sensation, pruritus (if opioid is used) and urinary retention. The site of insertion of the epidural catheter and securing of bacterial filter must be observed regularly for any leakage or disconnection. Guidelines must be in place to support the nurse should any of these complications arise. The Royal College of Anaesthetists (2004) recommends that there is access to an on-site anaesthetist for nursing staff to contact should problems arise.

Major complications from epidural infusions are uncommon in children but do happen. Epidural abscess are a rare but a potentially catastrophic complication (Patel & McComsey, 2001). Any redness around the site, back pain, motor block or purulent discharge should be treated seriously. MR scan may be necessary to exclude the presence of an epidural abscess. Dural puncture is managed in the majority of children with analgesics, bed rest and hydration. However, a small proportion of children may require an epidural blood patch; this involves injecting a small amount of the child's own blood into the epidural space to seal the dural puncture and prevent further leakage of spinal fluid (Ylönen & Kokki, 2002). Local anaesthetic toxicity may result in muscle twitching, irritability, excessive sedation, hypotension, convulsions or cardiac arrhythmias. The early signs of toxicity are difficult to detect in younger children. The prolonged half-life of local anaesthetic drugs renders infants more susceptible to the side-effects of local anaesthetic toxicity. To minimise the risk of toxicity, epidural catheters are sited as close as possible to the dermatome level that needs to be blocked and the duration limited to 36–48 h in infants (Morton, 1999). Ropivacaine and Levobupivacaine are newer agents that have less systemic toxicity than bupivacaine (European Society of Regional Anaesthesia and Pain Therapy [ESRA] 2006).

Other local anaesthetic infusions

The recent developments in local anaesthetic techniques have seen a rise in the use of paravetebral, intrapleural, sciatic/femoral nerve and brachial plexus infusions (Vas, 2005). However, insertion is usually best achieved when the child is asleep during general anaesthesia; disposable infusion devices for this purpose are available. These infusions can be managed safely in ward areas by following guidelines and protocols. Regular monitoring is mandatory with particular attention to local anaesthetic toxicity.

Intrathecal analgesia is commonplace in neonatal surgery in place of general anaesthesia and intrathecal diamorphine can provide pain relief for up to 24 h. However, during this time the child should be carefully monitored for the adverse effects of the opioid and so it is not a suitable analgesia for day-case surgery (Morton, 1999).

Discharge home

Increased use of Paracetamol, NSAIDs and local anaesthetics have significantly reduced the incidence of pain, sedation and post-operative nausea and vomiting in children following surgery. Children's day surgery has continued to flourish as it is considered beneficial to organisations, children and their families. However, the success of day surgery depends upon the parent managing the child's care at home. Discharge protocols must include the provision of adequate analgesia. Telephone follow-up should be considered for all children after discharge from hospital (Jonas, 2003) as this can identify adverse events and provide additional parental support. Pain management in children will improve as education of health professionals expands, with the increase in ambulatory surgery this education needs to be directed towards parents and carers to avoid unnecessary suffering.

Conclusion

Effective management of a child's pain is a crucial contribution to the overall success of perioperative management. Nurses and other health professionals have a responsibility to maintain and enhance their skills and knowledge about pain and to share this, as appropriate, with the children and their families. New techniques and new technologies go some way to ensuring that children's perioperative pain management is improving and that children are not suffering unnecessary pain. However, the heart of good pain management is a nurse who listens to and believes the child, uses their clinical skills and judgement, engages empathically with the child and their family and who sees that effective pain management is a clinical priority.

References

Action for Sick Children. (2006). *Helping children deal with pain*. Available from http://www.actionforsickchildren.org/parentspain. html (accessed 29 November 2006).

Aida, S., Shimoji, K. (2000). Pre-emptive analgesia: Recent findings. *Pain Reviews*, 7: 105–117.

Ambuel, B., Hamlett, K.W., Marx, C.M., Blumer, J.L. (1992). Assessing distress in pediatric intensive-care environments – the Comfort Scale. *Journal of Pediatric Psychology*, 17: 95–109.

American Academy of Pediatrics, Committee on Fetus and Newborn, Committee on Drugs, Section on Anesthesiology, Section on Surgery, Canadian Paediatric Society Fetus and Newborn Committee. (2000). Prevention and management of pain and stress in the neonate. *Pediatrics*, 105: 454–461.

Anand, K.J., Aranda, J.V., Berde, C.B., Buckman, S., Capparelli, E.V., Carlo, W., Hummel, P., Johnston, C.C., Lantos, J., Tutag-Lehr, V., Lynn, A.M., Maxwell, L.G., Oberlander, T.F., Raju, T.N., Soriano, S.G., Taddio, A., Walco, G.A. (2006). Summary proceedings from the neonatal pain-control group. *Pediatrics*, 117: S9–S22.

Anderson, B.J. Palmer, G.M. (2006). Recent developments in the pharmacological management of pain in children. *Current Opinion in Anaesthesiology*, 19: 285–292.

Ansermino, M., Basu, R., Vandebeek, C. Montgomery, C. (2003). Nonopioid additives to local anaesthetics for caudal blockade in children: A systematic review. *Paediatric Anaesthesia*, 13: 561–573.

Australian and New Zealand College of Anaesthetists. (2005). *Acute pain management: Scientific evidence*, 2nd ed. Australian and New Zealand College of Anaesthetists and Faculty of Pain Medicine, Melbourne.

von Baeyer, C.L. (2006). Children's self-report of pain intensity: Scale selection, limitations and interpretation. *Pain Research Management*, 11: 157–162.

von Baeyer, C.L., Spagrud, L.J. (2007). Systematic review of observational (behavioral) measures of pain for children and adolescents aged 3 to 18 years. *Pain*, 127: 140–150.

Ballantyne, M., Stevens, B., McAllister, M., Dionne, K., Jack, A. (1999). Validation of the premature infant pain profile in the clinical setting. *Clinical Journal of Pain*, 15: 297–303.

Berde, C.B., Jaksic, T., Lynn, A.M., Maxwell, L.G., Soriano, S.G. Tibboel, D. (2005). Anesthesia and analgesia during and after surgery in neonates. *Clinical Therapeutics*, 27: 900–921.

Bergendahl, H.T.G., Lonnqvist, P.A., Eksborg, S., Ruthstro, M.E., Nordenberg, L., Zetterqvist, H., Oddby, E. (2004). Clonidine versus midazolam as premedication in children undergoing adeno-tonsillectomy: A prospective, randomized, controlled clinical trial. *Acta Anaesthesiologica Scandinavica*, 48: 1292–1300.

Bergstrom,Y., Carlson, T. Jonsson, A. (2000). Nursing care for ambulatory day surgery: The concept and organization of nursing care. *Ambulatory Surgery*, 8: 3–5.

Berry, F.A. (1998). Preemptive analgesia for postop pain. *Paediatric Anaesthesia*, 8: 187–188.

Body, R., Potier, K. (2004). Non-steroidal anti-inflammatory drugs and exacerbations of asthma in children. *Emergency Medicine Journal*, 21: 713–714.

Boyd, R.J., Stuart, P. (2005). The efficacy of structured assessment and analgesia provision in the paediatric emergency department. *Emergency Medicine Journal*, 22: 30–32.

Breau, L.M., McGrath, P.J., Camfield, C., Rosmus, C. Finley, G.A. (2000). Preliminary validation of an observational pain checklist for persons with cognitive impairments and inability to communicate verbally. *Developmental Medicine and Child Neurology*, 42: 609–616.

Breau, L.M., Camfield, C., McGrath, P.J., Rosmus, C., Finley, G.A. (2001). Measuring pain accurately in children with cognitive impairments: Refinement of a caregiver scale. *Journal of Pediatrics*, 138: 721–727.

Breau, L.M., Finley, G.A., McGrath, P.J., Camfield, C.S. (2002a). Validation of the non-communicating children's pain checklist-postoperative version. *Anesthesiology*, 96: 528–535.

Breau, L.M., McGrath, P.J., Camfield, C.S. Finley, G.A. (2002b). Psychometric properties of the non-communicating children's pain checklist – revised. *Pain*, 99: 349–357.

Breau, L.M.P., MacLaren, J.B., McGrath, P.J.P., Camfield, C.S.M.F. Finley, G.A.M. (2003). Caregivers' beliefs regarding pain in children with cognitive impairment: Relation between pain sensation and reaction increases with severity of impairment. *Clinical Journal of Pain*, 19: 335–344.

Breau, L.M., McGrath, P.J., Stevens, B., Beyene, J., Camfield, C., Finley, G.A., Franck, L., Gibbins, S., Howlett, A., McKeever, P., O'Brien, K., Ohlsson, A. (2006). Judgments of pain in the neonatal intensive care setting: A survey of direct care staffs' perceptions of pain in infants at risk for neurological impairment. *Clinical Journal of Pain*, 22: 122–129.

British National Formulary for Children. (2006). The British Medical Association and The Royal Pharmaceutical Society of Great Britain. BMJ Publishing Group, London.

Byrne, A., Morton, J., Salmon, P. (2001). Defending against patients' pain: A qualitative analysis of nurses' responses to children's postoperative pain. *Journal of Psychosomatic Research*, 50: 69–76.

Cardwell, M., Siviter, G., Smith, A. (2005). Non-steroidal anti-inflammatory drugs and perioperative bleeding in paediatric tonsillectomy. *Cochrane Database of Systematic Reviews*, Issue 2. Art. No.: CD003591. DOI: 10.1002/14651858.CD003591.pub2.

Carter, B. (2002). Chronic pain in childhood and the medical encounter: Professional ventriloquism and hidden voices. *Qualitative Health Research*, 12: 28–41.

Carter, B. (2004). *Management of fever and pain in babies and children*. RCN Forum Accredited Education Unit, Royal College of Nursing, London.

Carter, B., McArthur, E., Cunliffe, M. (2002). Dealing with uncertainty: Parental assessment of pain in their children with profound special needs. *Journal of Advanced Nursing*, 38: 449–457.

Chambers, C.T., Reid, G.J., McGrath, P.J., Finley, G.A. (1996). Development and preliminary validation of a postoperative pain measure for parents. *Pain*, 68: 307–313.

Chambers, C.T., Giesbrecht, K., Craig, K.D., Bennett, S.M., Huntsman, E. (1999). A comparison of faces scales for the measurement of pediatric pain: children's and parents' ratings. *Pain*, 83: 25–35.

Chambers, C.T., Finley, G.A., McGrath, P.J., Walsh, T.M. (2003). The parents' postoperative pain measure: Replication and extension to 2-6-year-old children. *Pain*, 105: 437–443.

Charlton, E. (1997). The management of postoperative pain. *Update in Anaesthesia*, 2–17.

Coffman, S., Alvarez, Y., Pyngolil, M., Petit, R., Hall, C., Smyth, M. (1997). Nursing assessment and management of pain in critically ill children. *Heart and Lung*, 26: 221–228.

Cooper, R., Nishina, K., Mikawa, K. (2000). Clonidine in paediatric anaesthesia [1] (multiple letters). *Paediatric Anaesthesia*, 10: 223–224.

Craig, K.D., Lilley, C.M., Gilbert, C.A. (1996). Social barriers to optimal pain management in infants and children. *Clinical Journal of Pain*, 12: 232–242.

Cummings, E.A., Reid, G.J., Finley, G.A., McGrath, P.J., Ritchie, JA. (1996). Prevalence and source of pain in pediatric inpatients. *Pain*, 68: 25–31.

Cunliffe, M., Roberts, S.A. (2004). Pain management in children. *Current Anaesthesia and Critical Care*, 15: 272–283.

Currell, R., Urquhart, C. (2003). Nursing record systems: Effects on nursing practice and health care outcomes. *Cochrane Database of Systematic Reviews* 2003, Issue 3. Art. No.: CD002099. DOI: 10.1002/14651858.CD002099.

Demirel, D., Cam, O. (2006). Effect of preoperative education given by nurses on post-operative pain in children. *Cocuk Cerrahisi Dergisi*, 20: 98–104.

Demyttenaere, S., Finley, G.A., Johnston, C.F., McGrath, P.J. (2001). Pain treatment thresh-olds in children after major surgery. *Clinical Journal of Pain*, 17: 173–177.

Department of Health. (2003). *Getting the right start: National Service Framework for Children*. Standard for Hospital Services, London.

van Dijk, M., de Boer, J.B., Koot, H.M., Tibboel, D., Passchier, J., Duivenvoorden, H.J. (2000). The reliability and validity of the COMFORT scale as a postoperative pain instrument in 0 to 3-year-old infants. *Pain*, 84: 367–377.

Doyle, E., Robinson, D., Morton, N.S. (1993). Comparison of patient-controlled analgesia with and without a background infusion after lower abdominal surgery in children. *British Journal of Anaesthesia*, 71: 670–673.

Engelhardt, T., Crawford, M. (2001). Sublingual morphine may be a suitable alternative for pain control in children in the postoperative period. *Paediatric Anaesthesia*, 11: 81–83.

Ericsson, E., Wadsby, M., Hultcrantz, E. (2006). Pre-surgical child behavior ratings and pain management after two different techniques of tonsil surgery. *International Journal of Pediatric Otorhinolaryngology*, 70: 1749–1758.

European Society of Regional Anaesthesia and Pain Therapy (ESRA). (2006). *Postoperative pain management guidelines*. Available from http://www.esraeu rope.org/gu idelines. html (accessed 29 November 2006).

Falanga, I.J., Lafrenaye, S., Mayer, S.K., Trault, J.P. (2006). Management of acute pain in children: Safety and efficacy of a nurse-controlled algorithm for pain relief. *Acute Pain*, 8: 45–54.

Faries, J.E., Mills, D.S., Goldsmith, K.W., Phillips, K.D., Orr, J. (1991). Systematic pain records and their impact on pain control – a pilot study. *Cancer Nursing*, 14: 306–313.

Finley, G.A., Chambers, C.T., McGrath, P.J., Walsh, T.M. (2003). Construct validity of the Parents' Postoperative Pain Measure. *Clinical Journal of Pain*, 19: 329–334.

Finley, G.A., Franck, L., Grunau, R., von Baeyer, C.L. (2005). Why children's pain matters. *Pain: Clinical Updates*, XIII: 1–6.

Fisher, P., Wilson, S.E., Brown, M., Ditunno, T. (2006). Continuous infraclavicular brachial plexus block in a child. *Paediatric Anaesthesia*, 16: 884–886.

Gauthier, J.C., Finley, G.A., McGrath, P.J. (1998). Children's self-report of postoperative pain intensity and treatment threshold: Determining the adequacy of medication. *Clinical Journal of Pain*, 14: 116–120.

Giaufre, E., Dalens, B., Gombert, A. (1996). Epidemiology and morbidity of regional anesthesia in children: A one-year prospective survey of the French-Language Society of Pediatric Anesthesiologists. *Anesthesia and Analgesia*, 83: 904–912.

Gillies, M.L., Smith, L.N., Parry-Jones, W.L. (1999). Postoperative pain assessment and man-agement in adolescents. *Pain*, 79: 207–215.

Gold, J.I., Townsend, J., Jury, D.L., Kant, A.J., Gallardo, C.C., Joseph, M.H. (2006). Current trends in pediatric pain management: From preoperative to the postoperative bedside and beyond. *Seminars in Anesthesia, Perioperative Medicine and Pain*, 25: 159–171.

GOSH/ICH. (2006). *The children's pain assessment project*. Available from http://www.ich.ucl.ac.uk/cpap/index.html (accessed 29 November 2006).

Grunau, R.E., Holsti, L., Peters, J.W.B. (2006). Long-term consequences of pain in human neonates. *Seminars in Fetal and Neonatal Medicine*, 11: 268–275.

Hagan, J.F., Coleman, W.L., Foy, J.M., Goldson, E., Howard, B.J., Navarro, A., Tanner, J.L., Tolmas, H.C., Walco, G.A., Broome, M.E., Schechter, N.L., Shapiro, B.S., Strafford, M., Zeltzer, L.K. (2001). The assessment and management of acute pain in infants, children, and adolescents. *Pediatrics*, 108: 793–797.

Hamers, J.P.H., van den Hout, M.A., Halfens, R.J.G., Abu-Saad, H.H., Heijltjes, A.E.G. (1997). Differences in pain assessment and decisions regarding the administration of analgesics between novices, intermediates and experts in pediatric nursing. *International Journal of Nursing Studies*, 34: 325–334.

Hamers, J.P.H., Huijer Abu-Saad, H.H. (2002). Children's pain at home following (adeno)tonsillectomy. *European Journal of Pain*, 6: 213–219.

Hannallah, R.S. (1997). Paediatric quality assurance. *Ambulatory Surgery*, 5: 109–112.

Hatem, T.P., Lira, P.I.C., Mattos, S.S. (2006). The therapeutic effects of music in children following cardiac surgery. *Journal of Pediatrics*, 82: 186–192.

He, H.G., Polkki, T., Pietila, A.M., Vehvilainen-Julkunen, K. (2006). Chinese parent's use of nonpharmacological methods in children's postoperative pain relief. *Scandinavian Journal of Caring Sciences*, 20: 2–9.

Hester, N.K.O. (1979). Preoperational child's reaction to immunization. *Nursing Research*, 28: 250–255.

Hester, N.O., Foster, R., Kristensen, K. (1990). Measurement of pain in children – generalizability and validity of the Pain Ladder and the Poker Chip Tool. *Advances in Pain Research and Therapy*, 15: 79–84.

Hicks, C.L., von Baeyer, C.L., Spafford, P.A., van Korlaar, I., Goodenough, B. (2001). The Faces Pain Scale – Revised: Toward a common metric in pediatric pain measurement. *Pain*, 93: 173–183.

Hodgins, M.J. (2002). Interpreting the meaning of pain severity scores. *Pain Research & Management*, 7: 192–198.

Holaday, B., Salanterä, S., Lauri, S., Salmi, T.T., Aantaa, R. (1999). Nursing activities and outcomes of care in the assessment, management, and documentation of children's pain. *Journal of Pediatric Nursing*, 14: 408–415.

Hollis, L.J., Burton, M.J., Millar, J.M. (1999). Perioperative local anaesthesia for reducing pain following tonsillectomy. *Cochrane Database of Systematic Reviews*, Issue 4. Art. No.: CD001874. DOI: 10.1002/14651858.CD001874.

Howard, R.F. (2003). Current status of pain management in children. *JAMA – Journal of the American Medical Association*, 290: 2464–2469.

Howard, R., Carter, B., Curry, J., Morton, N., Rivett, K., Rose, M., Tyrell, J., Walker, S., Williams, G. (2008). Good practice in postoperative and procedural pain management. *Paediatric Anaesthesia*, 18: 1–81.

Howell, T.K. (2000). Paracetamol-induced fulminant hepatic failure in a child after 5 days of therapeutic doses. *Paediatric Anaesthesia*, 10: 344–345.

Howell, T.K., Patel, D. (2003). Plasma paracetamol concentrations after different doses of rectal paracetamol in older children: A comparison of 1 g versus 40 mg kg^{-1}. *Anaesthesia*, 58: 69–73.

Howell, T.K., Smith, S., Rushman, S.C., Walker, R.W.M., Radivan, F. (2002). A comparison of oral transmucosal fentanyl and oral midazolam for premedication in children. *Anaesthesia*, 57: 798–805.

Hunt, A., Goldman, A., Seers, K., Crichton, N., Mastroyannopoulou, K., Moffat, V., Oulton, K., Brady, M. (2004). Clinical validation of the paediatric pain profile. *Developmental Medicine & Child Neurology*, 46: 9–18.

Huth, M.M., Broome, M.E., Mussatto, K.A., Morgan, S.W. (2003). A study of the effectiveness of a pain management education booklet for parents of children having cardiac surgery. *Pain Management Nursing*, 4: 31–39.

Huth, M.M., Broome, M.E., Good, M. (2004). Imagery reduces children's post-operative pain. *Pain*, 110: 439–448.

Huth, M.M., Van Kuiken, D.M., Broome, M.E. (2006). Playing in the park: What school-age children tell us about imagery. *Journal of Pediatric Nursing*, 21: 115–125.

Idvall, E., Holm, C., Runeson, I. (2005). Pain experiences and non-pharmacological strategies for pain management after tonsillectomy: A qualitative interview study of children and parents. *Journal of Child Health Care*, 9: 196–207.

Jacob, E., Puntillo, K.A. (1999). Pain in hospitalized children: Pediatric nurses' beliefs and practices. *Journal of Pediatric Nursing*, 14: 379–391.

Jonas, D., Worsley-Cox, K. (2000). Information giving can be painless. *Journal of Child Health Care*, 4: 55–58.

Jonas, D., Perkins, R., Bland, J. (2003). Audit of pain management following cleft lip and palate surgery. Abstracts of the annual scientific meeting of the Association of Paediatric Anaesthetists of Great Britain and Ireland, 15–16 March 2002, Dublin. *Pediatric Anesthesia*, 13: 856.

Jonas, D.A. (2003). Parent's management of their child's pain in the home following day surgery. *Journal of Child Health Care*, 7: 150–162.

Jonsdóttir, R.B., Kristjánsdóttir, G. (2005). The sensitivity of the premature infant pain profile – PIPP to measure pain in hospitalized neonates. *Journal of Evaluation in Clinical Practice*, 11: 598–605.

Jordan-Marsh, M., Hubbard, J., Watson, R., von Hall, R., Miller, P., Mohan, O. (2004). The social ecology of changing pain management: Do I have to cry? *Journal of Pediatric Nursing*, 19: 193–203.

Kain, Z.N., Mayes, L.C., Caldwell-Andrews, A.A., Karas, D.E., McClain, B.C. (2006). Preoperative anxiety, postoperative pain, and behavioral recovery in young children undergoing surgery. *Pediatrics*, 118: 651–658.

Katz, J., McCartney, C.J.L. (2002). Current status of pre-emptive analgesia. *Current Opinion in Anaesthesiology*, 15: 435–441.

Kendall, J.M., Reeves, B.C., Latter, V.S. (2001). Multicentre randomised controlled trial of nasal diamorphine for analgesia in children and teenagers with clinical fractures. *British Medical Journal*, 322: 261–265.

Khosravi, M.B., Khezri, S., Azemati, S. (2006). Tramadol for pain relief in children undergoing herniotomy: A comparison with ilioinguinal and iliohypogastric blocks. *Paediatric Anaesthesia*, 16: 54–58.

Knutsson, J., Tibbelin, A., Von Unge, M. (2006). Postoperative pain after paediatric adenoidectomy and differences between the pain scores made by the recovery room staff, the parent and the child. *Acta Oto-Laryngologica*, 126: 1079–1083.

Kohler, H., Schulz, S., Wiebalck, A. (2001). Pain management in children: Assessment and documentation in burn units. *European Journal of Pediatric Surgery*, 11: 40–43.

Kokki, H. (2003). Nonsteroidal anti-inflammatory drugs for postoperative pain: A focus on children. *Pediatric Drugs*, 5: 103–123.

Krechel, S.W., Bildner, J. (1995). Cries – a new neonatal postoperative pain measurement score – initial testing of validity and reliability. *Paediatric Anaesthesia*, 5: 53–61.

Lamacraft, G., Cooper, M.G., Cavalletto, B.P. (1997). Subcutaneous cannulae for morphine boluses in children: Assessment of a technique. *Journal of Pain and Symptom Management*. 13: 43–49.

Lambert, S.A. (1996). The effects of hypnosis/guided imagery on the postoperative course of children. *Journal of Developmental and Behavioral Pediatrics*, 17: 307–310.

Lambert, S.A. (1999). Distraction, imagery, and hypnosis. Techniques for management of children's pain. *Journal of Child and Family Nursing*, 2: 5–15.

Lander, J.A., Weltman, B.J., So, S.S. (2006). EMLA and Amethocaine for reduction of children's pain associated with needle insertion. *Cochrane Database of Systematic Reviews*, Issue 3. Art. No.: CD004236. DOI: 10.1002/14651858.CD004236.pub2.

Li, H.C.W., Lopez, V., Lee, T.L.I. (2006). Psychoeducational preparation of children for surgery: The importance of parental involvement. *Patient Education and Counseling*, 65: 34–41.

Liddell, A., Murray, P. (1989). Age and sex-differences in children's reports of dental anxiety and self-efficacy relating to dental visits. *Canadian Journal of Behavioural Science–Revue Canadienne des Sciences du Comportement*, 21: 270–279.

Liossi, C., Hatira, P. (2003). Clinical hypnosis in the alleviation of procedure-related pain in pediatric oncology patients. *International Journal of Clinical and Experimental Hypnosis*, 51: 4–28.

Lonnqvist, P.A., Morton, N.S. (2005). Postoperative analgesia in infants and children. *Acta Anaesthesiologica Italica/Anaesthesia and Intensive Care in Italy*, 56: 440–458.

Lonnqvist, P.A., Morton, N.S. (2006). Paediatric day-case anaesthesia and pain control. *Current Opinion in Anaesthesiology*, 19: 617–621.

Lovett, P. (1997). Planning and implementing an epidural analgesia teaching programme for orthopaedic nurses. *Journal of Orthopaedic Nursing*, 1: 127–130.

Lundeberg, S., Lonnqvist, P.A. (2004). Update on systemic postoperative analgesia in children. *Paediatric Anaesthesia*, 14: 394–397.

Mathew, P.J., Mathew, J.L. (2003). Assessment and management of pain in infants. *Postgraduate Medical Journal*, 79: 438–443.

McGovern, M.C., Glasgow, J.F.T., Stewart, M.C. (2001). Lesson of the week: Reye's syndrome and aspirin: Lest we forget. *British Medical Journal*, 322: 1591–1592.

McGrath, P., Seifert, C.E., Speechley, K.N., Booth, J.C., Stitt, L., Gibson, M.C. (1996). A new analogue scale for assessing children's pain: An initial validation study. *Pain*, 64: 435–443.

Merkel, S.I., Voepel-Lewis, T., Shayevitz, J.R., Malviya, S. (1997). The FLACC: A behavioral scale for scoring postoperative pain in young children. *Pediatric Nursing*, 23: 293–297.

Merkel, S.M., Voepel-Lewis, T.M.R., Malviya, S.M. (2002). Pain assessment in infants and young children: The FLACC Scale: A behavioral tool to measure pain in young children. *American Journal of Nursing*, 102: 55–58.

Moghal, N.E., Hegde, S., Eastham, K.M. (2004). Ibuprofen and acute renal failure in a toddler. *Archives of Disease in Childhood*, 89: 276–277.

Moore, A., Collins, S., Carroll, D., McQuay, H. (1997). Paracetamol with and without codeine in acute pain: A quantitative systematic review. *Pain*, 70: 193–201.

Morris, J.L., Rosen, D.A., Rosen, K.R. (2003). Nonsteroidal anti-inflammatory agents in neonates. *Pediatric Drugs*, 5: 385–405.

Morton, N.S. (1999). Prevention and control of pain in children. *British Journal of Anaesthesia*, 83: 118–129.

Morton, N.S., O'Brien, K. (1999). Analgesic efficacy of Paracetamol and Diclofenac in children receiving PCA morphine. *British Journal of Anaesthesia*, 82: 715–717.

Nagle, C.J., McQuay, H.J. (1990). Opiate receptors: Their role in effect and side-effect. *Current Anaesthesia and Critical Care*, 1: 247–252.

National Health Service Quality Improvement Scotland. (2004). *Postoperative Pain Management. Best Practice Statement*. Available from http://www.nhshealthquality.org/nhsqis/files/Post_Pain_COMPLETE.pdf (accessed 25 January, 2008).

Newstead, B. (2005). Premedication drugs useful for children. *Update in Anaesthesia*, 6–7.

Nolan, J., Chalkiadis, G.A., Low, J., Olesch, C.A., Brown, T.C.K. (2000). Anaesthesia and pain management in cerebral palsy. *Anaesthesia*, 55: 32–41.

O'Brien, L., Taddio, A., Lyszkiewicz, D.A., Koren, G. (2005). A critical review of the topical local anesthetic amethocaine (Ametop?) for pediatric pain. *Pediatric Drugs*, 7: 41–54.

Paediatrics and Child Health Division TRACoP. (2006). Management of procedure-related pain in children and adolescents: Paediatrics & Child Health Division, The Royal Australasian College of Physicians. *Journal of Paediatrics & Child Health*, 42: S2–S29.

Pasero, C. (2002). Pain assessment in infants and young children: Premature infant pain profile – The PIPP is a tool for assessing pain in premature and term neonates. *American Journal of Nursing*, 102: 105–106.

Pasero, C. (2003). Epidural analgesia for postoperative pain, part 2: Multimodal recovery programs improve patient outcomes. *American Journal of Nursing*, 103: 43–45.

Patel, D. (2006). Epidural analgesia for children. *Continuing Education in Anaesthesia, Critical Care and Pain*, 6: 63–66.

Patel, S.S., McComsey, G. (2001). Medical management of spinal epidural abscesses in children: A case report and review of the literature. *International Pediatrics*, 16: 176–181.

Perrott, D.A., Goodenough, B., Champion, G.D. (2004). Children's ratings of the intensity and unpleasantness of post-operative pain using facial expression scales. *European Journal of Pain*, 8: 119–127.

Pogatzki-Zahn, E.M., Zahn, P.K. (2006). From preemptive to preventive analgesia. *Current Opinion in Anaesthesiology*, 19: 551–555.

Polkki, T. (2002). Nurses' perceptions of parental guidance in pediatric surgical pain relief. *International Journal of Nursing Studies*, 39: 319–327.

Polkki, T., Vehvilainen-Julkunen, K., Pietila, A.M. (2001). Nonpharmacological methods in relieving children's postoperative pain: A survey on hospital nurses in Finland. *Journal of Advanced Nursing*, 34: 483–492.

Polkki, T., Vehvilainen-Julkunen, K., Pietila, A.M. (2002a). Parents' roles in using nonpharmacological methods in their child's postoperative pain alleviation. *Journal of Clinical Nursing*, 11: 526–536.

Polkki, T., Pietila, A.-M., Vehvilainen-Julkunen, K., Laukkala, H., Ryhanen, P. (2002b). Parental views on participation in their child's pain relief measures and recommendations to health care providers. *Journal of Pediatric Nursing*, 17: 270–278.

Polkki, T., Laukkala, H., Vehvilainen-Julkunen, K., Pietila, A.M. (2003). Factors influencing nurses' use of nonpharmacological pain alleviation methods in paediatric patients. *Scandinavian Journal of Caring Sciences*, 17: 373–383.

Ray, M., Basu, S.M. (2000). Postoperative analgesia in paediatric day case surgery. *Update in Anaesthesia*, 34–37.

Royal Children's Hospital Melbourne. (2006). *Anaesthesia and pain management – Ketamine Infusion*. Available from http://www.rch.org.au/anaes/pain/index.cfm?doc_id=848 (accessed 12 May 2009).

Royal College of Anaesthetists. (2004). *Good practice in the management of continuous epidural analgesia in the hospital setting.* Available from http://www.rcoa.ac.uk/docs/Epid-Analg .pdf (accessed 25 January 2008).

Royal College of Nursing (1999). *The recognition and assessment of acute pain in children. Technical report.* Available from http://www.rcn.org.uk/development/practice/clinical-guidelines/pain (accessed 25 January 2008).

Royal College of Nursing (2002). *Clinical practice guidelines. The recognition and assessment of acute pain in children: Audit protocol.* Available from http://www.rcn.org.uk/__data/ assets/pdf_file/0005/109823/001597.pdf (accessed 25 January 2008).

Royal College of Paediatrics and Child Health. (2001). *Guidelines for good practice: Recognition and assessment of acute pain in children.* Royal College of Paediatrics and Child Health, London.

Salanterä, S. (2006). Finnish nurses' attitudes to pain in children. *Journal of Advanced Nursing,* 29: 727–736.

Salanterä, S., Lauri, S., Salmi, T.T., Helenius, H. (1999). Nurses' knowledge about pharmacological and nonpharmacological pain management in children. *Journal of Pain and Symptom Management,* 18: 289–299.

Sanders, C. (2002a). A review of current practice for boys undergoing hypospadias repair: From pre-operative work up to removal of dressing post-surgery. *Journal of Child Health Care,* 6: 60–69.

Sanders, J.C. (2002b). Paediatric regional anaesthesia, a survey of practice in the United Kingdom. *British Journal of Anaesthesia,* 89: 707–710.

Seid, M., Sherman, M., Seid, A.B. (1997). Perioperative psychosocial interventions for autistic children undergoing ENT surgery. *International Journal of Pediatric Otorhinolaryngology,* 40: 107–113.

Semple, D., Findlow, D., Aldridge, L.M., Doyle, E. (1996). The optimal dose of ketamine for caudal epidural blockade in children. *Anaesthesia,* 51: 1170–1172.

Short, J.A., Barr, C.A., Palmer, C.D., Goddard, J.M., Stack, C.G., Primhak, R.A. (2000). Use diclofenac in children with asthma. *Anaesthesia,* 55: 334–337.

Simons, J., Roberson, E. (2002). Poor communication and knowledge deficits: Obstacles to effective management of children's postoperative pain. *Journal of Advanced Nursing,* 40: 78–86.

Simons, J., Franck, L., Roberson, E. (2001). Parent involvement in children's pain care: Views of parents and nurses. *Journal of Advanced Nursing,* 36: 591–599.

Sittl, R., Likar, R., Grieinger, N. (2006). Management of postoperative pain in children. *Monatsschrift fur Kinderheilkunde,* 154: 755–763.

Smith, L., Callery, P. (2005). Children's accounts of their preoperative information needs. *Journal of Clinical Nursing,* 14: 230–238.

Stanford, E.A., Chambers, C.T., Craig, K.D. (2006). The role of developmental factors in predicting young children's use of a self-report scale for pain. *Pain,* 120: 16–23.

Stevens, B., Gibbins, S. (2002). Clinical utility and clinical significance in the assessment and management of pain in vulnerable infants. *Clinics in Perinatology,* 29: 459–468.

Stevens, B., Johnston, C., Petryshen, P., Taddio, A. (1996). Premature infant pain profile: Development and initial validation. *Clinical Journal of Pain,* 12: 13–22.

Stinson, J.N., Kavanagh, T., Yamada, J., Gill, N., Stevens, B. (2006). Systematic review of the psychometric properties, interpretability and feasibility of self-report pain intensity measures for use in clinical trials in children and adolescents. *Pain,* 125:143–157.

St-Laurent-Gagnon, T., Bernard-Bonnin, A.C., Villeneuve, E. (1999). Pain evaluation in preschool children and by their parents. *Acta Paediatrica,* 88: 422–427.

Suominen, P., Caffin, C., Linton, S., McKinley, D., Ragg, P., Davie, G., Eyres, R. (2004). The Cardiac Analgesic Assessment Scale (CAAS): A pain assessment tool for intubated and ventilated children after cardiac surgery. *Pediatric Anesthesia*, 14,: 336–343.

Sutters, K., Miaskowski, C. (1999). Gender differences in children's pain experience following tonsillectomy with or without adenoidectomy and/or myringotomy. *Acute Pain*, 2: 79–88.

Sutters, K.A., Miaskowski, C., Holdridge-Zeuner, D., Waite, S., Paul, S.M., Savedra, M.C., Lanier, B. (2004). A randomized clinical trial of the effectiveness of a scheduled oral analgesic dosing regimen for the management of postoperative pain in children following tonsillectomy. *Pain*, 110: 49–55.

Taddio, A., Katz, J., Ilersich, A.L., Koren, G. (1997). Effect of neonatal circumcision on pain response during subsequent routine vaccination. *Lancet*, 349: 599–603.

Taddio, A., Ohlsson, K., Ohlsson, A. (1999). Lidocaine-prilocaine cream for analgesia during circumcision in newborn boys. *Cochrane Database of Systematic Reviews*, Issue 3. Art. No.: CD000496. DOI: 10.1002/14651858.CD000496.

Tak, J.H., van Bon, W.H.J. (2006). Pain- and distress-reducing interventions for venepuncture in children. *Child: Care, Health and Development*, 32: 257–268.

The Royal Australasian College of Physicians P&CHD. (2006). Management of procedure-related pain in neonates. *Journal of Paediatrics & Child Health*, 42: S31–S32.

Tobias, J.D. (2000). Weak analgesics and nonsteroidal anti-inflammatory agents in the management of children with acute pain. *Pediatric Clinics of North America*, 47: 527–543.

Tom, C.M. (2005). *Management of acute pain in hospitalized children*. Available from http://www.uspharmacist.com/index.asp?show=article&page=8_1557.htm (accessed 25 January 2008).

Treadwell, M.J., Franck, L.S., Vichinsky, E. (2002). Using quality improvement strategies to enhance pediatric pain assessment. *International Journal for Quality in Health Care*, 14: 39–47.

Vagnoli, L., Caprilli, S., Robiglio, A., Messeri, A. (2005). Clown doctors as a treatment for preoperative anxiety in children: A randomized, prospective study. *Pediatrics*, 116.

Van Hulle Vincent, C.P.R. (2005). Nurses' knowledge, attitudes, and practices: Regarding children's pain. *MCN, American Journal of Maternal Child Nursing*, 30: 177–183.

Vas, L. (2005). Continuous sciatic block for leg and foot surgery in 160 children. *Paediatric Anaesthesia*, 15: 971–978.

Verghese, S.T., Hannallah, R.S. (2005). Postoperative pain management in children. *Anesthesiology Clinics of North America*, 23: 163–184.

Vijayan, R. (1997). Subcutaneous morphine a simple technique for postoperative analgesia. *Acute Pain*, 1: 21–26.

Voepel-Lewis, T., Malviya, S., Tait, A.R. (2005). Validity of parent ratings as proxy measures of pain in children with cognitive impairment. *Pain Management Nursing*, 6: 168–174.

Walco, G.A., Conte, P.M., Labay, L.E., Engel, R., Zeltzer, L.K. (2005). Procedural distress in children with cancer – Self-report, behavioral observations, and physiological parameters. *Clinical Journal of Pain*, 21: 484–490.

Ward, R.M., Benitz, W.E., Benjamin, J., Blackmon, L., Giacoia, G.P., Hudak, M., Lasky, T., Rodriguez, W., Selen, A. (2006). Criteria supporting the study of drugs in the newborn. *Clinical Therapeutics*, 28: 1385–1398.

Werawatganon, T., Charuluxanun, S. (2005). Patient controlled intravenous opioid analgesia versus continuous epidural analgesia for pain after intra-abdominal surgery. *Cochrane Database of Systematic Reviews*, Issue 1. Art. No.: CD004088. DOI: 10.1002/14651858. CD004088.pub2.

White, M.C., Nolan, J.A. (2005). An evaluation of pain and postoperative nausea and vomiting following the introduction of guidelines for tonsillectomy. *Pediatric Anesthesia*, 15: 683–688.

de C Williams, A., Davies, H.T., Chadury, Y. (2000). Simple pain rating scales hide complex idiosyncratic meanings. *Pain*, 85: 457–463.

Williams, D.G., Hatch, D.J., Howard, R.F. (2001). Codeine phosphate in paediatric medicine. *British Journal of Anaesthesia*, 86, 413–421.

Williams, D.G., Patel, A., Howard, R.F. (2002). Pharmacogenetics of codeine metabolism in an urban population of children and its implications for analgesic reliability. *British Journal of Anaesthesia*, 89, 839–845.

Wong, D., Baker, C. (1988). Pain in children: Comparison of assessment scales. *Pediatric Nursing*, 14, 9–17.

Woodgate, R., Kristjanson, L.J. (1995). Young children's behavioral responses to acute pain – Strategies for getting better. *Journal of Advanced Nursing*, 22, 243–249.

World Health Organization. (2006). *WHO's pain ladder*. Available from http://www.who .int/cancer/pal liative/pai nladder/en/ (accessed 29 November 2006).

Wu, C.L., Cohen, S.R., Richman, J.M., Rowlingson, A.J., Courpas, G.E., Cheung, K., Lin, E.E., Liu, S.S. (2005). Efficacy of postoperative patient-controlled and continuous infusion epidural analgesia versus intravenous patient-controlled analgesia with opioids: A meta-analysis. *Anesthesiology*, 103, 1079–1110.

Ylönen, P., Kokki, H. (2002). Management of postdural puncture headache with epidural blood patch in children. *Paediatric Anaesthesia*, 12, 526–529.

Zernikow, B., Smale, H., Michel, E., Hasan, C., Jorch, N., Andler, W. (2006). Paediatric cancer pain management using the WHO analgesic ladder – results of a prospective analysis from 2265 treatment days during a quality improvement study. *European Journal of Pain*, 10, 587–595.

5   Surgical procedures on children

Linda Shields and Ann Tanner

Introduction

Surgical procedures performed on the neonate, infant, child and adolescent are generally significantly different from those procedures performed on the adult. A child can be defined thus:

- *Premature infant*: born after a gestation period of less than 37 weeks.
- *Neonate*: born from 38 weeks gestation till 28 days (1 month) old.
- *Baby*: from 1-month-old to 12 months of age.
- *Infant*: a child in the first period of life.
- *Child*: a young person between infancy and adolescence.
- *Adolescent*: the period of life from puberty to maturity terminating legally at the age of majority.

Common surgical procedures performed on children

The same type of instruments are used for surgery on children as on adults; however, paediatric instruments are often smaller and more delicate with less pronounced curves and lighter in weight. The smaller the child, the smaller the instrument the surgeon is likely to use. Laparoscopic surgery is becoming popular in the paediatric setting (Esposito, 1998), and size of instruments is an important consideration for ease of use and evaluation shows it to be a cost-efficient alternative to regular procedures (Luks *et al.*, 1999).

Paediatric surgery, like adult surgery, is divided into areas of specialty. These specialities include the following: general, ear, nose and throat (ENT), neurosurgery, urology, orthopaedics, ophthalmology and plastic and craniofacial surgery. Paediatric general surgery includes chest and abdominal problems in neonates, infants, children and adolescents. Some common surgical procedures performed on children are explained in further detail.

Abdominal paediatric surgery

Appendicectomy

Appendicitis is a common, important and sometimes fatal disease in childhood (Ein *et al.*, 2000). Consequently, an appendicectomy (or appendectomy in North American parlance) is a relatively common paediatric procedure. The appendix can be removed either by an incisional, open operation or, more recently, by laparoscopy. In both procedures, the appendix is located, tied off from its stump and excised, and each surgeon has a specific method of doing this. The abdominal cavity is then washed out and closed.

Perioperative nursing implications
- The child will receive a general anaesthetic.
- The child will lie supine on the operating table.
- The child will require a patient return electrode/diathermy plate.
- A basic laparotomy set of instruments will be used.
- The peritoneal cavity may require washing out with normal saline prior to the abdomen being closed.

Atresia

'Atresia' means 'the absence of a normal body opening, duct or canal...' (Anderson *et al.*, 1994, p. 144). Intestinal atresias occur most frequently in the ileum, but can also occur in the duodenum, jejunum or colon. Intestinal atresia can be found by ultrasound during pregnancy, or on the first or second day of life, when the abdomen becomes distended – the infant fails to pass stools and, finally, begins to vomit – all being signs of gut obstruction. Radiological examination will detect the deformity. Other common atresias are oesophageal and tracheal. A tracheal atresia will often involve the oesophagus, forming a tracheo-oesphageal fistula (TOF), where there is a common passage joining the trachea and oesophagus (Filston & Shorter, 2000). Oesophageal atresia (OA) and TOF are related conditions found in the neonate, usually detected soon after birth by the inability to pass a nasogastric catheter into the oesophagus (Wilson *et al.*, 2008). These conditions are of unknown aetiology, but occur in early fetal life (Figure 5.1).

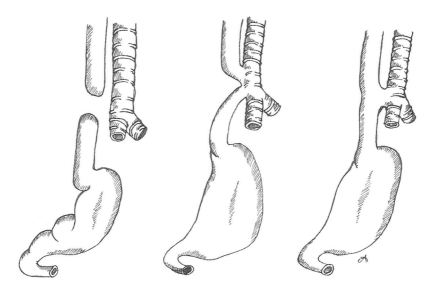

Fig. 5.1 Structures of TOF.

As OA is lethal, operative repair is done as soon as possible after detection. A thoracotomy incision is performed and the defects repaired with anastomosis of the oesophageal ends. If a TOF exists, repair will include ligature of the tracheal branch (Wilson *et al.*, 2008). Repair of OA or TOF may require repeated operations over a period of years.

Perioperative nursing implications
- The child will receive a general anaesthetic.
- The child will lie supine on the operating table.
- The child will require a patient return electrode/diathermy plate.
- A basic laparotomy set of instruments will be used requiring extra retractors for the chest, ligating clips dilators, vessel loops and an infant chest drain.
- Warming mattress will be required, the temperature of the room set high and fluids warmed.

Gastroschisis and omphalocele

Gastroschisis and omphalocele are similar conditions found at birth, the aetiology of which is poorly understood (Figures 5.2 and 5.3). Gastroschisis is the herniation

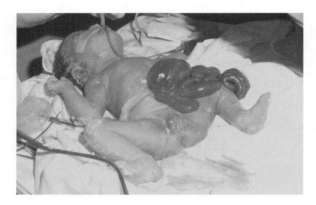

Fig. 5.2 Gastroschisis, with abdominal organs protruding lateral to umbilicus. Note visible stomach, bowel and fallopian tubes. *Source*: Photograph courtesy of Mater Health Services.

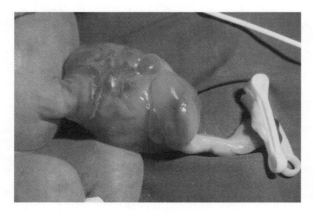

Fig. 5.3 Omphalocele, with abdominal organs protruding through the umbilicus. *Source*: Photograph courtesy of Mater Health Services.

of abdominal contents through the abdominal wall lateral to a normal umbilical cord, whereas an omphalocele is a congenital malformation in which the intestines protrude from the abdominal wall and are covered by a sac from which the umbilical cord begins (Gaines *et al.*, 2000).

These defects are often detected by ultrasound before birth, and it is unusual for a child born with gastroschisis to have other serious birth defects; however, undescended testis is common in these children. Omphalocele, on the other hand, is often associated with chromosome abnormalities which include syndromes such as Beckwith–Wiedemann and Down's syndromes (Gaines *et al.*, 2000). Rupture of the omphalocele constitutes an emergency requiring immediate surgery.

Operative treatment depends on the severity of the condition, the size of the omphalocele and the health of the infant. A simple closure is rarely possible as the organs have to be pushed back into the abdomen. Often, a series of operations over a long period of years is necessary. To prevent increased pressure in the abdomen, a pouch, or 'silo' of Silastic™ sheeting is often used to contain the gut and over a period of time, as gravity allows the organs to fall back into the infant's growing abdominal cavity, the pouch is shortened until it can be removed and the abdominal wall closed (Islam, 2008). In the case of omphaloceles with large openings, surgery may be contraindicated, and these lesions are allowed to epithelialise over a long period (Figures 5.4 and 5.5).

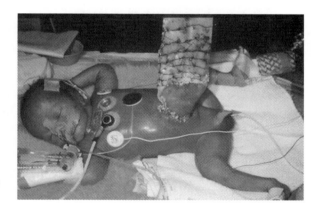

Fig. 5.4 Surgical reduction of omphalocele. 'Silo' containing infant's abdominal contents for treatment of omphalocele. *Source*: Photograph courtesy of Mater Health Services.

Perioperative nursing implications
- The child will receive a general anaesthetic.
- The child will lie supine on the operating table.
- The child will require a patient return electrode/diathermy plate.
- A basic laparotomy set of instruments will be used.
- Sterile Silastic™ sheets must be available.

Imperforate anus

Imperforate anus is the absence of a normal anal opening. Clinically, it is divided into three main categories – low anomalies, intermediate anomalies and high anomalies.

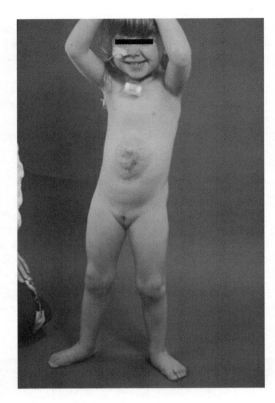

Fig. 5.5 Closed omphalocele. This 3-year-old was born with a large omphalocele which was allowed to epithelialise and eventually grow and cover the abdominal organs. *Source*: Photograph courtesy of Mater Health Services.

Low anomalies occur where most of the rectum has developed normally and sphincters are present, but the anus itself is non-existent. Intermediate anomalies consist of those where the rectum ends at or below the level of the puborectalis muscle without passing into an anal passage. High anomalies occur when the rectum ends above the *puborectalis* muscle, and the internal and external sphincters are absent. Genito-urinary fistulae usually occur with high anomalies (Wilson *et al.*, 2008). Diagnosis is usually made shortly after birth when routine physical examination reveals no anal opening, or when a neonate fails to pass meconium stool in the first 24–48 hours after birth. Imperforate anus occurs in about 1 in 5000 births and its cause is unknown (Hutson *et al.*, 1999).

Surgical treatment of infants with imperforate anus depends upon the severity of the condition and can range from a simple perineal anoplasty to make a passage in the perineum for the anus, to complicated procedures for the reconstruction of bowel, vagina and urethral walls. Colostomy is often part of the operative procedures for high anomalies (Figure 5.6).

Perioperative nursing implications
- The child will receive a general anaesthetic.
- The child will be lying supine on the operating table with legs taped up into a lithotomy position in order to operate on the perineum.

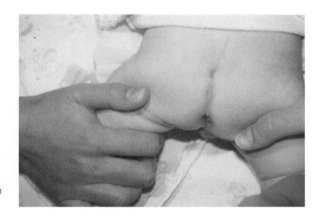

Fig. 5.6 Imperforate anus. *Source*:
Photograph courtesy of Mater Health
Services.

- The child will require a patient return electrode/diathermy plate.
- A basic laparotomy set of instruments will be used with the addition of anal retractors, dilators and lubricant gel and a nerve and muscle stimulator.
- The child may require an indwelling catheter to be inserted during the procedure.

Hernia

A hernia is the protrusion of an organ through an abnormal opening in the muscle wall of a body cavity (Anderson *et al.*, 1994). Two types of hernia found in children are umbilical and inguinal. Umbilical hernias are of small clinical consequence and often resolve spontaneously. Usually, they are repaired for cosmetic reasons. Operative repair is often done in day surgery or as an outpatient procedure, often with a caudal anaesthetic block (Maldonado *et al.*, 1999). Inguinal hernia is common in children, but has more serious consequences than umbilical hernia. A loop of intestine enters the inguinal canal and can become obstructed, and strangulation of the hernia can occur (Wilson *et al.*, 2008).

Inguinal hernias account for about 80% of all hernias and are the most common surgical procedures done in infancy. These hernias appear more frequently in boys than in girls. Repair consists of repairing the protrusion in the hernial sac and anchoring it in the inguinal canal (Garcia, 2000). Inguinal hernia can be associated with hydrocele (Figure 5.7).

Perioperative nursing implications
- The child will receive a general anaesthetic.
- The child will be lying supine on the operating table.
- The child will require a patient return electrode/diathermy plate.
- A basic minor set of instruments will be used.

Intussusception

Intussusception is the telescoping of one segment of bowel into the lumen of another (Anderson *et al.*, 1994) and is one of the most common causes of gut obstruction in

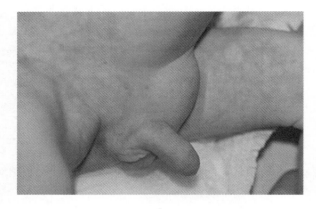

Fig. 5.7 Child with bilateral inguinal hernias. *Source*: Photograph courtesy of Mater Health Services.

infancy (Wilson *et al.*, 2008). About 80% of intussusceptions are in the ileocolic region of the bowel (Fallat, 2000). It can occur at any age but is most frequently seen in children between 5 and 10 months old, and 70% of them are male. As the bowel telescopes, it becomes compressed, resulting in oedema of the bowel wall, compromised circulation and, if left untreated, strangulation of the gut (Figure 5.8).

Treatment begins with insertion of a nasogastric tube to deflate the stomach, and insertion of an IV line and fluid administration. It is sometimes possible to correct

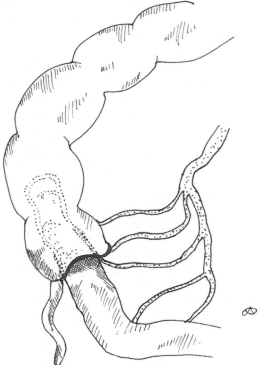

Fig. 5.8 Intussusception.

the invagination of the loops of bowel using barium or air under radiological control. If this is unsuccessful – or the intussusception recurs – surgery will be required to access the affected bowel, massage it back into normal alignment and, if the bowel has been damaged, removal of the affected areas may be necessary (Fallat, 2000). An appendicectomy is usually done at the same time because the site of the scar is often the same as that for an appendicectomy. In later life, if the person presents with abdominal pain and an 'appendix' scar, treatment for appendicitis may be delayed (Fallat, 2000).

Perioperative nursing implications
- The child will receive a general anaesthetic.
- The child will be placed supine on the operating table.
- The child will require a patient return electrode/diathermy plate.
- A basic minor set of instruments will be used with the addition of some retractors.

Necrotising enterocolitis

The incidence of necrotising enterocolitis (NEC) has increased with technological advances which support the lives of infants born prematurely as over 90% of children with NEC are premature newborns (Abdullah, 2008). The cause of NEC is unknown, and suggestions include immaturity of bowel wall function and motility (Gregory, 2008), hypoxia and infection, and there has been a suggested link between NEC and infant formula feeding (Wilson *et al.*, 2008) while breast milk is thought to provide some protection against NEC (Nair *et al.*, 2008). However, all these are speculative and more research is needed to clarify all the issues (Tyson & Kennedy, 2005).

The infant presents with abdominal distension and bloody stools soon after enteral feeding has begun. Diagnosis is based on the clinical picture and radiological review. Treatment can be either medical, which involves nasogastric suction and antibiotics; or surgical, (required in up to 50% of cases) to repair perforation or severe necrosis of the gut (Caty & Azizkhan, 1990).

Perioperative nursing implications
- The child will receive a general anaesthetic.
- The child will be lying supine on the operating table.
- The child will require a patient return electrode/diathermy plate.
- A major laparotomy set of instruments will be used with the addition of bowel clamps such as Debakey clamps.

Pyloric stenosis

Pyloric stenosis is a commonly seen paediatric condition and is caused by thickening of the gastric outlet musculature, although the aetiology of this is unknown (Wilson *et al.*, 2008). It occurs in up to three infants per thousand, and is more common in males than females (Dillon & Cilley, 2000). Its characteristic presentation of projectile vomiting in a previously well infant and visible peristalsis on the abdominal wall makes clinical diagnosis simple, though varying degrees of these symptoms can cloud the issue and X-ray or ultrasound can be used to confirm the findings (Dillon & Cilley, 2000). Surgery to open the thickened pylorus (pyloromyotomy or Ramstedt's operation) involves splitting the muscle fibres (Moushey *et al.*, 2000) to ensure free passage of food into the duodenum (Figure 5.9).

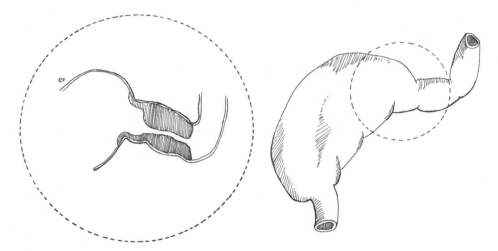

Fig. 5.9   Pyloric stenosis. Diagram shows thickened muscle in the pylorus.

Perioperative nursing implications

- The child will receive a general anaesthetic.
- The child will be lying supine on the operating table.
- The child will require a patient return electrode/diathermy plate.
- A basic minor set of instruments will be used with the addition of a hernia director that some surgeons prefer to split the pylorus.

Genito-urinary paediatric surgery

Circumcision

Circumcision is one of the oldest operations and provokes much controversy (Dickson *et al.*, 2008). Sometimes it is done because a specific problem with the foreskin (prepuce) exists, other times it is done for family, cultural or religious reasons. Although routine circumcision was once advocated for all newborn males, current feeling is that it is not necessary, as understanding and performance of hygiene has improved in modern times. As with all surgery, it carries some risks to the child and complications, such as penile adhesions (Ponsky *et al.*, 2000) and inconspicuous penis (Williams *et al.*, 2000) occur (Figures 5.10, 5.11 and 5.12).

Clinical indicators for circumcision include narrowing at the tip of the penis (phimosis, Figure 5.13), infections (posthitis, balanitis) (Raynor, 2000) or paraphimosis, where the prepuce cannot be returned to its normal position after being retracted down the glans (Raynor, 2000).

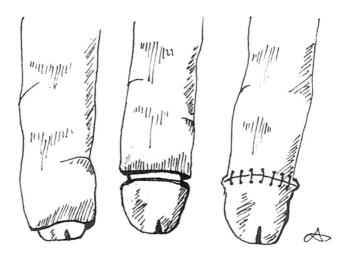

Fig 5.10 Diagram shows procedure for circumcision.

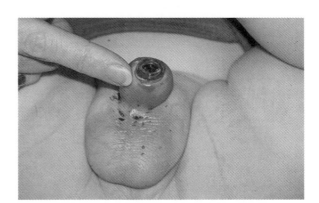

Fig. 5.11 Bleeding following circumcision. *Source*: Photograph courtesy of Mater Health Services.

The procedure, if done on older boys, involves a general anaesthetic and the foreskin is lifted, excised and rejoined to the shaft skin. Neonatal circumcision, on which debate rages, is usually done with local anaesthetic, often with devices which include a bell arrangement around which the foreskin is cut away. Complications of neonatal circumcision include bleeding and infection, though the incidence of these is low (Raynor, 2000).

Perioperative nursing implications
- The child will receive a general anaesthetic and sometimes with a caudal block.
- The child will be lying supine on the operating table.
- The child will require a patient return electrode/diathermy plate.
- A basic minor set of instruments will be used.

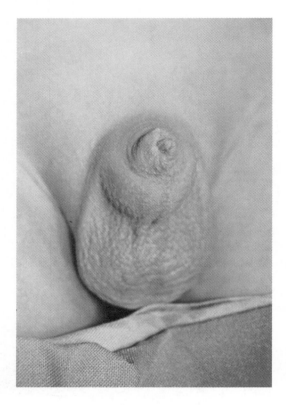

Fig. 5.12 'Inconspicuous' penis. *Source*: Photograph courtesy of Mater Health Services.

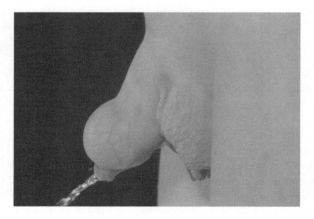

Fig. 5.13 Phimosis. *Source*: Photograph courtesy of Mater Health Services.

Hydrocele

A hydrocele (Figure 5.14) is a collection of fluid around the testicle, which occurs in infants when the canal between the peritoneal cavity and the scrotum fails to close during fetal development (Anderson *et al.*, 1994). The condition often resolves spontaneously, but sometimes requires surgical intervention. Hydroceles are often related

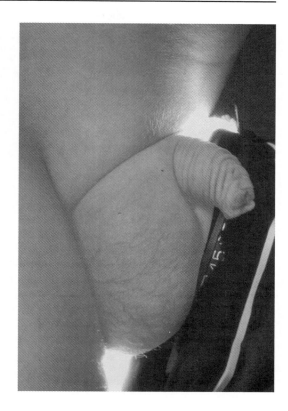

Fig. 5.14 Hydrocele. *Source*: Photograph courtesy of Mater Health Services.

to inguinal hernias and the surgical procedure for their repair is similar, with drainage of the fluid in the sac (Moushey *et al.*, 2000).

Perioperative nursing implications
- The child will receive a general anaesthetic and sometimes with a caudal block.
- The child will lie supine on the operating table.
- The child will require a patient return electrode/diathermy plate.
- A basic minor set of instruments will be used.

Undescended testicles (Orchidopexy)

If the testis does not descend into the scrotum during fetal development, the infant may be born with an undescended testis (Figure 5.15). Some descend spontaneously in the first year of life. However, surgery may be necessary to ensure that complications, such as torsion of the testis and malignancy (Wallen & Shortliffe, 2000), does not occur later in life. The operation is known as 'orchidopexy'. The procedure involves finding the testis in the groin or the abdomen (made easier by laparoscope), pulling it down into the scrotal sac and anchoring it there (Esposito *et al.*, 2008).

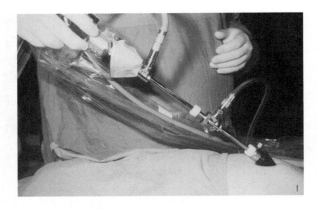

Fig. 5.15 Minimally invasive surgery for undescended testis. Laparoscopic testicular localisation. *Source*: Photograph courtesy of Mater Health Services.

Perioperative nursing implications
- The child will receive a general anaesthetic and sometimes with a caudal block.
- The child will be lying supine on the operating table.
- The child will require a patient return electrode/diathermy plate.
- A basic minor set of instruments will be used.

Hypospadias repair

Some boys are born with their urinary meatus situated somewhere along the shaft of their penis, rather than at its tip. The incidence is about 1 in every 125 live male births (Duckett, 1989), and the incidence is said to be increasing in many countries (Silver, 2000; Nassar *et al.*, 2007), with many suggestions as to why this is so, including exposure to maternal (Nelson *et al.*, 2007; Akre *et al.*, 2008) and environmental factors (Abdullah *et al.*, 2007).

Repair depends on the position of the lesion and its size. Repair may take one operation, or many, and is usually done in the first year of life. The techniques used are many and varied, including the use of laser and tissue solder (Borer & Retik, 1999; Kirsch *et al.*, 2001), but their aim is always to place the urethral meatus in the tip of the penis to correct curvature, create a conical glans and to ensure cosmetic acceptability (Ellsworth *et al.*, 1999).

Perioperative nursing implications
- The child will receive a general anaesthetic and sometimes with a caudal block.
- The child will be lying supine on the operating table.
- The child will require a patient return electrode/diathermy plate.
- A basic minor set of instruments will be used.
- Dressings as per the surgeon's preference must be available as some can be very elaborate and time consuming.
- Have a urinary catheter available in the room.

Paediatric urology

Urology encompasses diseases and malformation of the adrenal glands, kidneys, ureter, bladder, female and male genitalia including for the male, the penis, urethra, prostate gland and scrotum. Some of the more common procedures in paediatric urology are outlined below.

Cystoscopy and urethroscopy

Cystoscopy and urethroscopy involve inserting a scope into the bladder and urethra respectively. In children, these procedures are usually performed under a general anaesthetic. The child's legs will be placed in stirrups, so that the urethra is easily accessed. The perianal area is prepared, and a window sheet is used as a drape, along with small drapes, to cover the child's legs. The scope has a telescope, light source and irrigation line attached. The telescope may or may not be connected to a television monitor. In children, the urethral valves may need dissecting. The surgeon may use a paediatric resectoscope, and may perform diathermy to overcome the urethral obstruction (Hendren, 2000). The child needs a diathermy plate for this procedure. Because the diathermy is performed in a liquid field, the irrigation solution used must be non-conductive to prevent burns. Usually glycine 1.5% solution is used. For all other cystoscopies and urethroscopies not involving diathermy, normal saline is used for irrigation.

Ureteropelvic junction obstruction

An ureteropelvic junction obstruction (UPJ) obstruction occurs when there is insufficient drainage of urine from the renal pelvis into the upper ureter. This can result in distension of the renal pelvis, raised intra pelvic pressure and kidney damage from the stasis of urine in the collecting ducts (Coplen & Snyder, 2000). UPJ obstruction results from a narrowing of the ureteropelvic junction which may form a partial or complete obstruction. The surgical treatment is by means of a pyeloplasty in which the renal pelvis is reduced, the ureter divided below the obstruction, then re-anastomosed to the renal pelvis above the site of the obstruction.

Ureteric reimplantation

Ureteric reimplants are indicated when the ureters are significantly dilated (often termed 'megaureter') (Coplen & Snyder, 2000). The ureter can be refluxing, obstructed, non-refluxing or non-obstructed. The reflux can be congenital or as a result of the urethral valves or a neurogenic bladder. The obstruction may be primary (adynamic segment) or secondary to a urethral obstruction, mass or tumour. Ureteric reimplants can be unilateral or bilateral. For the procedure, a longitudinal segment of the ureter is excised and closed over a 10French or 12French catheter, the ureter is then tunnelled submucosally into the bladder. There is an 85%–95% success rate for a non-refluxing, non-obstructive reimplantation.

Some general paediatric surgical procedures

Diaphragmatic hernia

Diaphragmatic hernia occurs due to failed closure of the diaphragm in embryonic development (Arensman & Bambini, 2000). Gut and other organs find their way through the defect and sit in the chest, displacing the heart and lungs (Hartnett, 2008). Prenatal diagnosis allows preparation for treatment after birth. This usually includes ventilation, as respiration can be seriously compromised, and ventilation must be maintained until the abnormality is surgically corrected and the child's chest grows to allow room for correct placement of the organs. Once the baby's condition is stable, surgery can go ahead. Surgery may need to be done in stages depending on the severity and extent of the abnormality and its effect on the heart and lungs; however, its aim is to anchor the abdominal organs in the abdominal cavity and provide room for normal growth and function of the thoracic organs (Figure 5.16).

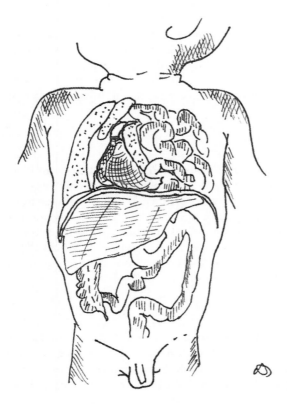

Fig. 5.16 Diaphragmatic hernia.

Perioperative nursing implications
- The child will receive a general anaesthetic.
- The child will be laid supine on the operating table.
- The child will require a patient return electrode/diathermy plate.
- A basic major laparotomy set of instruments will be used.
- Use of patient warming equipment for preventing hypothermia is of utmost importance because of the length of surgical time.
- A chest drain and water seal drain will be required.
- Silastic™ sheeting or mesh may be required.

Insertion of central venous line

A 'central line' is an intravenous catheter placed into a large, central vein such as the superior vena cava. A central line is needed to give the medical team access to a large vein that can be used to give fluids, including total parenteral nutrition, measure the amount of fluid in the body or give medication that might irritate smaller veins. Older children are sedated for the central line insertion; younger children are usually given a general anaesthetic. Central lines are usually inserted in the OR, though in some situations, insertion can be done at the bedside or in the treatment room.

Perioperative nursing implications
- The child will receive a general anaesthetic or, if old enough and cooperative, a local anaesthetic can be used.
- The child will be lying supine on the operating table with a sandbag under the shoulder if the line is to be placed in the clavicular area.
- The child will require a patient return electrode/diathermy plate.
- A basic minor set of instruments will be used with a tunnelling device.
- Have ampoules of heparin available.

ENT surgery

ENT surgery constitutes a major part of paediatric surgery, as it treats some of the most common surgical illnesses such as otitis media, sinusitis, tonsillitis and adenoiditis and upper airway obstruction. Most children for ENT surgery are admitted as day stay patients as the operations are small, simple and quickly performed. They include adenoid and tonsillectomy, myringotomy and insertion of grommets. A few are outlined here.

Tonsillectomy and adenoidectomy

There is some controversy over the need for tonsillectomy and adenoidectomy (Burton *et al.*, 1999) and there is some suggestion that the operations are performed unnecessarily in some instances (Paediatrics & Child Health Division of The Royal Australasian College of Physicians and The Australian Society of Otolaryngology Head and Neck Surgery, 2008). In children, adenotonsillectomy or adenoidectomy are performed to treat recurrent tonsillitis, obstruction of the nasopharynx and obstructive sleep apnoea (Garetz, 2008). Adenoidectomy can be performed by itself and is usually done to relieve pressure from inflamed adenoids on the middle ear (Davis & Chaliar, 2000). Research has indicated that it is safe to perform adenoidectomy as outpatient or day case surgery (Segerdahl *et al.*, 2008), but complications, in particular post-operative haemorrhage, prevent children having tonsillectomy from going home the same day (Asiri *et al.*, 2006) though some contest this (Bennett *et al.*, 2005).

Traditionally, there have been two methods for tonsillectomy – using a tonsil snare (guillotine) which loops over the tonsil and cuts it off at its base (Homer *et al.*, 2000), and sometimes by sharp or blunt dissection (Korkmaz *et al.*, 2008). However, innovative methods are tried often with the main aims to decrease bleeding and post-operative pain. New methods include tonsillotomy using a carbon dioxide laser (Magdy *et al.*, 2008), an ultrasonic scalpel (Parsons *et al.*, 2006) and cryoanalgesia (Robinson & Purdie, 2000; Figure 5.17).

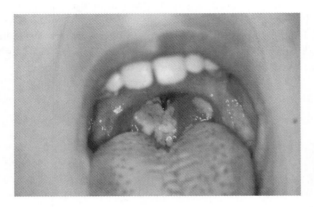

Fig. 5.17 Tonsillitis. Infected tonsils covered with pus. *Source*: Photograph courtesy of Mater Health Services.

Perioperative nursing implications
- The child will receive a general anaesthetic.
- The child will be lying supine on the operating table.
- The child will require a patient return electrode/diathermy plate.
- A tonsillectomy set of instruments will be used that will include tonsil snares, adenatomes and a mouth gag and blade.

Myringotomy and insertion of tympanostomy tubes (grommets)

Otitis media, where fluid builds up behind the ear drum, is very common and can take two forms in children – acute and chronic. A short and open eustachian tube predisposes young children to otitis media. Acute otitis media is a painful condition treated variously with nasal decongestant drops and antibiotics. Repeated, chronic episodes of otitis media often require surgical intervention.

Chronic suppurative otitis media and its variant, chronic serous otitis media, is a disease found most commonly in indigenous races of the world – Australian Aborigines (Dugdale *et al.*, 1978; Havas, 1984; Shields, 1990), Maori children (Tonkin, 1970), Canadian Inuit (Reed *et al.*, 1967) and American Indians (Johnson, 1967), to mention a few. It is a disease of particular importance for these children as their hearing is impaired and this negatively affects their school performance. It is treated by myringotomy, which affords proper hearing conduction by releasing fluid from behind the drum, and provides less scarring than if the drum were allowed to rupture spontaneously.

Myringotomy is a very common paediatric procedure in which a small incision is made into the tympanic membrane to release fluid and relieve pressure due to otitis media (Stow, 2007). Sometimes myringotomy is done by itself, at other times, it is supplemented by the insertion of tubes (grommets) which equalise pressure on both sides of the ear drum, allowing free passage of sound waves to the inner ear. The grommets fall out as the ear grows, and in about 1% of patients, a small hole is left which may require repair by tympanoplasty later. Insertion of grommets takes about 10 minutes, so an operation list with a preponderance of these operations is usually very busy.

Perioperative nursing implications
- The child will receive a general anaesthetic without intubation.
- The child will be lying supine on the operating table.
- A basic ear set of instruments will be used.
- The child's head will be placed in a head ring.

Paediatric eye surgery

Visual impairments are common in childhood, and the rate of children wearing glasses can be up to 3.5%, but only 0.5/1000 of those children will be legally blind (Wilson *et al.*, 2008). Good vision is vitally important for learning and development, and refractive errors are the most common types of paediatric visual disorders. These often require surgical correction. Only a small number of paediatric ophthalmic surgery procedures are outlined here.

Nasolacrimal duct obstruction

Six percent of infants have obstruction of their nasolacrimal duct, and 90% of these will clear spontaneously (Wright & Speigel, 1999). In babies under 6 months of age, massage of the duct may clear it, and parents can be taught to do this once a day. If this fails, probing is required. A fine dilator is passed down the duct under general anaesthetic and the duct irrigated. In rare cases, probing has to be repeated.

Perioperative nursing implications
- The child will receive a general anaesthetic without intubation.
- The child will be lying supine on the operating table.
- A set of lacrimal probes will be used to probe the tear duct.
- The child's head will be placed in a head ring.

Squint repair

Strabismus is a visual defect in which the extraocular muscles are unable to coordinate and direct the eyes in the same direction (Smith, 2007). It affects up to 4% of children in some countries (Abrahamsson *et al.*, 1999). Occlusive therapy to strengthen the eye muscles may be tried, but often surgery is required (Wilson *et al.*, 2008). The operative procedure to correct strabismus will depend on the muscles affected and which way the eye turns. Some muscles are shortened by resection, whereas others can be severed from their original attachment and replaced on a different position of the sclera to pull the eye in the required position (recession) (Abrahamsson *et al.*, 1999; Smith, 2007).

Perioperative nursing implications
- The child will receive a general anaesthetic.
- The child will be lying supine on the operating table.

- A basic eye set of instruments will be used including squint repair instrumentation such as princess clamps to hold eye muscles and eyelid retractors.
- The child's head will be placed in a head ring.
- Bipolar diathermy will be used, therefore no patient electrode/diathermy plate will be needed.
- Very small sutures will be used, so special care with the fine needles must be taken.

Paediatric neurosurgery

Paediatric neurosurgery has changed dramatically since the use of car seat belts has become widely accepted and the incidence of severe head injury has reduced, and with the successful treatment of conditions such as hydrocephalus.

Hydrocephalus

Hydrocephalus, 'water on the brain' occurs when there is an increase of cerebrospinal fluid (CSF) in the brain and spinal cord because of obstruction, excessive production of CSF or under-absorption (Figure 5.18). It was once a relatively common condition in infancy, and very visible because of the deformity of the head which kept growing

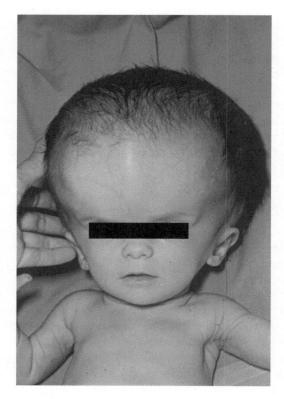

Fig. 5.18 Infant with untreated hydrocephalus. *Source*: Photograph courtesy of Mater Health Services.

as fluid built up, eventually killing the child. With screening procedures in child health such as routine head circumference measurement, hydrocephalus is found and treated with insertion of a shunt to carry the excess fluid into a vein or the abdominal cavity. Hydrocephalus is still seen in developing countries where screening may not be available in remote villages (Shields, 1999). Hydrocephalus is often associated with myelomeningocele (Wilson *et al.*, 2008).

Surgical treatment involves the removal of the cause of the obstruction (e.g. a tumour) or by insertion of a shunt mechanism which allows excess CSF to flow away (Wilson *et al.*, 2008). Most shunts consist of a catheter which is placed in the ventricles, a flush pump, a one-way valve and a distal catheter which is placed in the peritoneum or a cardiac atrium (Smith, 2007). Shunts must be changed as the child grows (Figure 5.19).

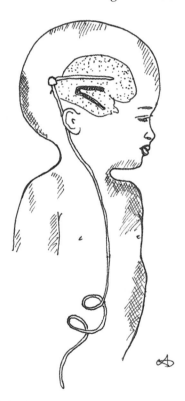

Fig. 5.19 Ventriculo-peritoneal shunt.

A different technique – third ventriculostomy – has been developed for use in children with hydrocephalus caused by obstruction. Endoscopically, the surgeon punctures a hole between the subarachnoid space and the third ventricle creating a drainage pathway for CSF (Decq *et al.*, 2000).

Craniotomy

Craniotomies are performed for a variety of reasons ranging from traumatic and closed head injuries to brain tumours, aneurysms and craniofacial surgery.

A craniotomy involves the removal of a section of the skull, also known as a flap. Depending on the site of the craniotomy, the child may be positioned prone or supine. In the case of a brain tumour, the operation may take many hours to complete, therefore, correct and safe patient positioning is required. This includes centring the patient on the bed, padding bony prominences, supporting limbs and using positioning devices where needed (Cordier & Sion, 2000).

Many surgical procedures involving the brain have an increased risk of morbidity or mortality. For the perioperative nurse scrubbing or scouting for the craniotomy, it is important to be prepared and commence setting up for the case as early as possible. In the larger booked cases, the anaesthetic preparation is much more involved. The patient will have a number of intravenous access lines and often will require an arterial line (Kerner, 2000). The airway is secured with occlusive and waterproof tapes. The eyes are protected with lubricant and covered by gauze and occlusive waterproof dressings. The patient may require a urinary catheter to monitor the output, and may have a rectally inserted temperature probe. For the emergency admissions such as subdural and extradural haematomas, the child may arrive via CAT scan already intubated. This means that for the OR nurse, there is less set up time, so speed and organisation are essential.

For the craniotomy, a neurosurgical headrest is often used, commonly the Mayfield head rest (Kerner, 2000), which consists of a head clamp in which three sterile pins are placed to pierce the scalp. The clamp is fixed to the head of the bed and immobilises the skull for surgery. The surgeon shaves the area of the head and marks the incision line with a permanent marker. The scrub nurse can then commence the skin preparation. A large semi-circular incision is made into the scalp, plastic skin clips (Leroy clips) are applied to the skin edges to maintain haemostasis as the skin over the skull is highly vascularised. A periosteal elevator is used to separate muscle from bone on the skull. The bone flap is removed using a powered drilling burr to make the initial hole in the skull, followed by a cutting drill bit, which cuts the bone in the same fashion as a jig saw. (The removed piece of bone is plated or wired back onto the skull following the surgery). The exposed dura can then be picked up with a dural hook and an incision made into it with a clean blade followed by dissection with scissors. The dura is retracted with stay sutures, leaving the brain exposed for surgery.

Emergency craniotomies can be performed in the case of subdural and extradural haematomas. These can occur following a substantial blow to the skull where venous or arterial vessels are disrupted and bleed (Gruber *et al.*, 2000). In the case of extradural haematomas, the bleed occurs between the skull and the dural space. These are more commonly arterial bleeds and, due to the rapidity of the bleed, are acute and life threatening, especially in children, if not surgically evacuated and the haemostasis controlled. The subdural bleeds are venous bleeds which occur between the brain and the dura. The surgical removal and control of subdural haematomas is the primary treatment of the brain injury, the ensuing intra cranial hypertension from the trauma often indicates if and how well the patient will recover. The injury caused to the brain tends to be more severe for subdural haematomas than extradural haematomas, and their recovery is related to their clinical presentation on arrival, including level of consciousness and pupillary reactions. The lower the neurological status on admission, the poorer the expected outcome to the surgery.

Perioperative nursing implications

There are a number of important issues to consider for the paediatric perioperative nurse. Organisation and preparation of the required equipment is essential. In the case of booked admissions, the child and their family may be extremely anxious prior to surgery. Older children with greater understanding of the procedure may have received a premedication prior to their admission to theatre to assist in the relief of anxiety. On admission to theatre, the perioperative nurse can help allay anxiety by introducing themselves to the child and their family, and establishing rapport with the parents. It is important that the OR staff have a contact number for the parents or have instructed them as to where they can wait whilst their child undergoes surgery, so that they are easily contacted should the surgeon need to speak to them during or after the procedure.

Spina bifida

Spina bifida (Figure 5.20) is a congenital defect in which the neural tube has failed to close and is not fully encased in the protective sheath of the meninges and spine. The failure of the neural tube closure occurs early in the development of the embryo (Wilson *et al.*, 2008), and this has been related to a deficiency of folate in early pregnancy (Molloy *et al.*, 1991; Morris & Wald, 1999). In a normal spine, the spinal cord is located in the spinal canal. It is an extension of the brain stem, commences in the first cervical vertebra (C1) and finishes at the second lumbar vertebra (L2). The lumbar spine encapsulates a vertical bundle of spinal nerves known as the *cauda equine*

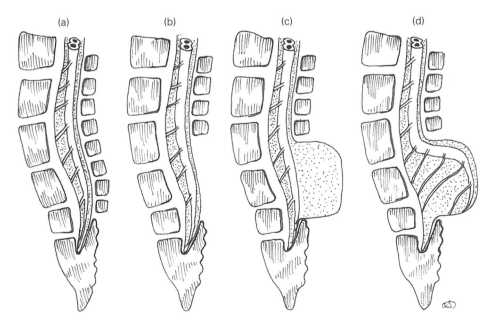

(a) (b) (c) (d)

Fig. 5.20 Spina bifida: (a) normal spine, (b) spina bifida occulta, (c) spina bifida with meningocele, (d) spina bifida with myelomeningocele.

(Kerner, 2000). Spina bifida usually occurs in the lumbar or lumbar sacral region of the spine. The aetiology has been linked to an abnormal increase in CSF pressure during the first trimester of pregnancy causing a split in the previously enclosed neural tube. Hydrocephalus is commonly associated with spina bifida (Wilson *et al.*, 2008).

There are varying degrees of severity of spina bifida. The mildest form is spina bifida occulta where there is a gap in the vertebra usually at the second lumbar vertebra, with no herniation of meninges or spinal cord and limited loss of sensation or function. Meningoceles (Figure 5.21) occur when the meninges have herniated out the gap in the vertebra without involving the spinal cord. The herniated meninges form a cyst-like sac filled with CSF (Wilson *et al.*, 2008). Children born with meningoceles can have varying degrees of sensory and motor impairment. Some may be able to walk but have impairment or paralysis to the bladder and anal sphincter.

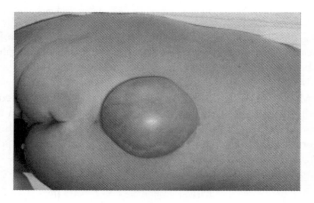

Fig. 5.21 Meningocele. *Source*: Photograph courtesy of Mater Health Services.

The most severe form of spina bifida is the myelomeningocele (sometimes called meningomyelocele). The meninges herniate out through the bony defect taking with them a portion of the spinal cord and nerves (Figure 5.22). These children can have full paralysis and complete sensory deficit below the region of the herniation (Wilson *et al.*, 2008).

Surgical treatment of both the meningocele and the myelomeningocele involves initial closure of the herniated meninges and spinal cord. Surgical closure reduces the risk of infection. The procedure often requires a multi-disciplinary approach involving a combination of neuro- and plastic surgeons. Children suffering from spina bifida often require multiple operations over many years. These range from ventriculo-peritoneal shunts for congenital hydrocephalus to the creation of stomas for the bladder and bowel, so that the child may self-catheterise via the abdomen, and may perform bowel washouts to prevent continuing incontinence. Some may need to undergo surgery for the placement of spinal rods or fusions to reduce curvature of the spine.

Perioperative nursing implications

It is important for the perioperative nurse to note that spina bifida children have a high incidence of latex allergies (Petsonk, 2000). This is possibly as a result of their high exposure to latex products with their daily intermittent urinary catheterisations, and their frequent hospital admissions and subsequent exposure to the latex in the

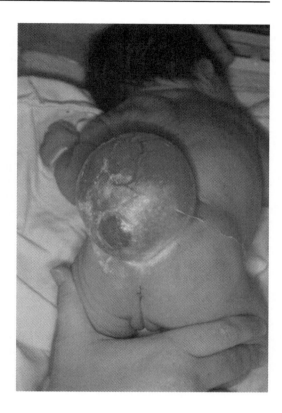

Fig. 5.22 Myelomeningocele. *Source*:
Photograph courtesy of Mater Health
Services.

gloves worn by staff. It is important for the perioperative nurse to be aware of latex allergies as at worst, they can result in anaphylaxis.

Paediatric orthopaedics

Children require orthopaedic surgery for the correction of congenital deformities, washout of infections of the bone or joints, for the removal of bone tumours and for the repair of injured or fractured limbs, joints, tendons or nerves as a result of trauma.

Perioperative nursing implications

For the perioperative nurse, there are a number of common factors involved. Orthopaedics generally involves a limb as spinal and neck surgery is considered a subspecialty of orthopaedics. The limb is fully prepared and draped with extra water-proof mackintosh drapes and extra small and medium drapes to ensure blood or fluids do not penetrate the drapes and risk contaminating the wound. In many instances (except in trauma cases), a tourniquet is applied to the limb to block the arterial blood supply so that the procedure can be carried out in a bloodless field (Murphy & Hahn, 2000). The tourniquet may remain on for up to 2 hours. It is important that the tourniquet cuff does not pinch the skin or the skin preparation fluid does not run under the cuff as both can cause significant burns to the child.

Orthopaedic surgery often requires the use of a number of powered instruments. For those not familiar with power tools, their use requires very much a 'hands on' education session. There is a whole range of nitrous cylinder-powered drills, taps, screws, burrs and saws to master for the perioperative nurse scrubbing for an orthopaedic case. An important point to remember is to always have the safety switch on when loading and unloading bone cutting instruments.

Infection of the bone or joint

When a child presents with acute commencement of pain, swelling or tenderness of any joint or limb, with an associated unwillingness to weight bear, the suspected prognosis is of osteomyelitis or septic arthritis (Williams & Cole, 1991). The surgical treatment for such infections involves opening the infected section of the limb or joint and washing out the infected area. The child is routinely given antibiotic coverage during the procedure, and a specimen of pus is taken to determine the most effective course of antibiotics and the nature of the infection.

Congenital deformities

There is a huge number of differing congenital abnormalities which may benefit from surgical orthopaedic intervention. Talipes, or 'club feet' (Figures 5.23 and 5.24) can be repaired by tendon release and transfers and a succession of plaster casts changed every 1–2 weeks to improve positioning (Williams & Cole, 1991).

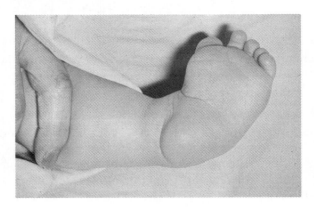

Fig. 5.23 Infant with 'club feet' – talipes. *Source*: Photograph courtesy of Mater Health Services.

Children with cerebral palsy often require tendon release surgery and splinting to assist in gait and stance. Children born with shortened, stunted limbs, fused joints, extra or missing digits, missing bones, fragile bones (osteogenesis imperfecta), bowed legs, deformed feet and hands and many more are all potential candidates for corrective orthopaedic surgery (Williams & Cole, 1991).

Bone tumours

Malignant bone tumours are more common in children than in adults, and the annual incidence is approximately 5.6 per million in children under 15 years (Arndt, 2000).

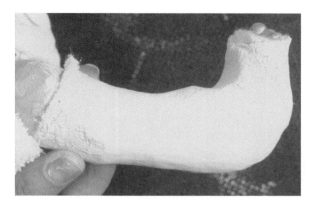

Fig. 5.24 Treated talipes in plaster cast following remedial surgery. *Source*: Photograph courtesy of Mater Health Services.

The age group most at risk are the 15–19 year olds. This is thought to be related to the increased rate of bone tissue growth during that age. The two major types of bone tumours that make up 85% of cases are Ewing's sarcoma and osteogenic sarcoma (Wilson *et al.*, 2008). Some of the clinical signs of a bone tumour are localised pain at the affected site, limping and generally limited activity. Occasionally, the child may present with a pathological fracture as the first indication of a tumour. Bone tumours are primarily suspected whenever there is a fracture following a trivial fall (Williams & Cole, 1991). Surgery is the primary method of treatment for a bone tumour. With increased technology, the limb can often be saved following excision of the affected bone (e.g. the femur) by means of a femoral prosthesis. Prior to such advances in prosthetic surgery, the limb would have been amputated.

Fractures in children

Due to children's natural curiosity and play behaviour, they are much more physically active than adults, and have a greater risk of falls and limb fractures (Figure 5.25). The cause of such fractures include falls from playground equipment, trampolines, bicycles, roller blades, skate boards, scooters, trees and more. Fractures in children differ from adults in that the growing child is at risk of growth plate injuries which can stunt the growth of the affected limb. One-third of fractures suffered by children involve the growth plate (Williams & Cole, 1991).

A commonly found fracture in children is a metaphyseal fracture to the distal radius, ulna or tibia. There are three types: (1) buckle fracture, where the compressed metaphyseal bone elevates the cortical surface of the bone, giving a buckled appearance; (2) greenstick fracture, an incomplete break where one side of the cortex is compressed and remains intact while the other side breaks, causing the bone to angulate and (3) a complete fracture, which can be displaced or undisplaced, and in severe trauma may be compound, in which the fracture protrudes from the skin (Williams & Cole, 1991). Treatment of fractures in children ranges from a closed reduction under a general anaesthetic, where the surgeon manipulates the fracture and provides traction on the limb until the bone is realigned. In more severe fractures, the child may require an open reduction and internal fixation of the fracture. The fixation can be in the form of wires, plates and screws.

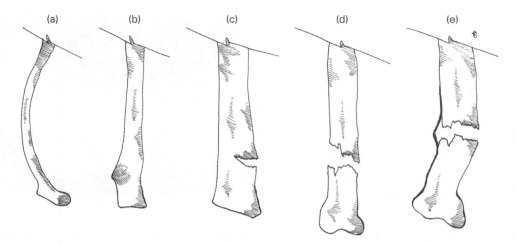

(a)   (b)   (c)   (d)   (e)

Fig. 5.25   Common fractures in children: (a) bend in bone (usually ulna and fibula), (b) buckle fracture, (c) greenstick fracture, (d) complete fracture, (e) periosteal hinge.

Congenital hip dysplasia

Congenital hip dysplasia is more commonly known as developmental dysplasia of the hip, as it is now recognised that at birth, the hips are rarely dislocated, but are easily 'dislocatable' (Thompson & Scoles, 2000). This is diagnosed soon after birth by routine examination of the hips, and is often treated conservatively with traction and splints (Wilson *et al.*, 2008). In older infants and more severe cases, surgical treatment to reposition the joint may be needed (Thompson & Scoles, 2000).

Paediatric plastic surgery

Paediatric plastic surgery involves the surgical reconstruction and repair of congenital abnormalities, injury (e.g. facial fractures), disfigurement and scarring. Plastic surgery is the process of restoring normal appearance and of achieving normal function where possible (Golden & Low, 2000). Some of the more common plastics procedures performed on children are outlined below.

Craniofacial surgery

Craniofacial surgery involves a team of plastic surgeons and neuro surgeons. The plastic surgery team is responsible for the remodelling of facial and cranial bones and structures; the neurosurgeon performs the craniotomy (see previous section describing craniotomy). The child may require craniofacial surgery because of premature fusion of the cranial sutures of the skull which need to be released and remoulded (Phillips, 2007). There may be an encephalocele (Kerner, 2000), a sack-like extrusion as a result of some form of facial cleft, usually from the midline of the nose, which can contain CSF and brain tissue, or may be independent of the brain. If there is neurological involvement, it can take many hours to surgically excise, and to realign the facial cleft.

Cleft lip and palate repair

Cleft lip and palate (Figure 5.26) are congenital abnormalities which can occur in 1:750 to 1:2500 live births, and are more common in males (Stow, 2007). They are facial malformations that occur during the development of the embryo, and while no one cause is known, inheritance (Bender, 2000), ethnicity and maternal drug exposure are thought to play a part. A cleft lip is the failure of the maxillary and median processes to fuse, while a cleft palate is a failure of fusion of the midline of the palate resulting in a fissure in the palate. Cleft lips can occur unilaterally or bilaterally, and can occur in conjunction with a cleft palate. Usually the more severe bilateral cleft lips occur with a cleft palate.

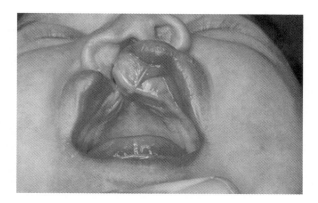

Fig. 5.26 Cleft lip and palate.
Source: Photograph courtesy of Mater Health Services.

The surgical treatment involves the repair of the cleft lip at about 3 months of age, when it is believed the infant has sufficient weight gain and lung function to withstand a general anaesthetic. The cleft palate is often repaired in two stages, initially with the hard palate repair followed by the soft palate repair, although other techniques are commonly used (Sadove *et al.*, 2004; Kobus, 2007). The severity of the cleft determines the amount of surgery required. The primary palate repair is usually performed at 6 months of age, with the secondary repair at 9 or 10 months of age. Many surgeons like to repair the palate before the child develops faulty speech patterns (Wilson *et al.*, 2008).

Setback otoplasty

A setback otoplasty is commonly referred to as correction of protruding ears, and is most often done for cosmetic reasons, as these children often become victims of mockery and abuse by their peers. Otoplasty often involves an incision to the back of the ear and the ear is resected down to the cartilage layer, the cartilage is scored with a blade or a specially designed raked forceps so that it can be reshaped and moulded closer to the head (Petersson & Friedman, 2008). The incision is closed and a head bundle dressing applied which remains intact until follow up review, usually 10 days after surgery, though some surgeons require the bandages to remain on for much shorter periods (Ramkumar *et al.*, 2006). The moulding created by the head bundle helps the ears to sit closer to the head as the wound heals. Some post-operative considerations include the fact that the child has a complete head bundle dressing occluding the ears, and can be slightly deaf, may suffer nausea and anti emetics are often ordered.

Hand and foot deformities

There are many deformities of the hands and feet which require plastic surgery intervention. In basic terms, syndactyly (Figure 5.27) occurs when digits are joined together by a web of skin, can be complete or incomplete, depending on the number of digits involved and can be complex or simple, depending on the level of bony union between the involved digits (Stow, 2007). Polydactyly (Figures 5.28 and 5.29) is the duplication of some digits, and can be simple or complex depending on bony involvement. In surgery for syndactyly, the digits are separated by a series of z-plasties, a series of zigzag incisions to divide the joined digits. These are resutured and each digit wrapped in a supportive dressing. The dressing forms an integral part of the repair

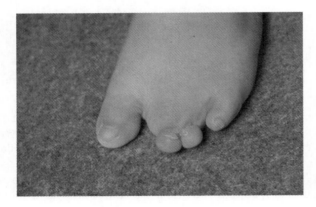

Fig. 5.27 Syndactyly of the foot. *Source*: Photograph courtesy of Mater Health Services.

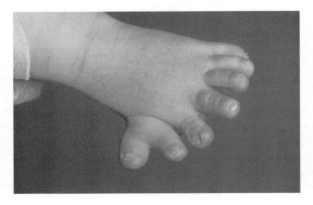

Fig. 5.28 Polydactyly of the foot. *Source*: Photograph courtesy of Mater Health Services.

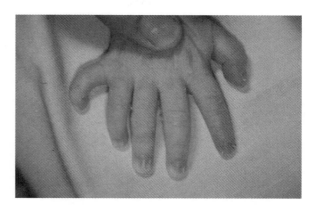

Fig. 5.29 Polydactyly of the hand.
Source: Photograph courtesy of
Mater Health Services.

as it helps to shape and mould the digit as the wound heals, and acts in a splinting capacity. Surgery for polydactyly can be a simple removal of extra digits or very complex reconstruction of the whole hand. This type of plastic surgery is very complicated and takes several hours to complete, especially if both hands/feet are affected (Hart *et al.*, 2005).

Disfiguring lesions

There are many types of skin lesions which can require plastic surgical intervention. Some of the most common are outlined below.

Dermoid cysts are congenital cysts, they are usually rounded, soft and often fixed to deep tissues or bone. In children, they are commonly found under the lateral part of the eyebrow, the scalp, the tip of the nose and the orbit (Laberge *et al.*, 2000). Naevus is a term applied to 'any skin lesion appearing at or after birth' (Jaksic *et al.*, 2000, p. 955) and covers a wide range of conditions, from the trivial to melanoma which may have the potential to become malignant (metastatic melanoma). They can be non-melanocytic in which case, there is very little risk of malignancy, and little need for excision unless the naevus is disfiguring. The naevus can range in size, pigmentation, colour and appear with or without hair, occasionally having a velvet texture (Jaksic *et al.*, 2000). Treatment for the melanocytic naevus usually involves surgical excision, with the specimen sent to pathology. This is particularly the case if there is a family history of malignant melanoma.

Haemangiomas (Stringel, 2000) are the most common tumours in infants and the term covers a wide complex of conditions from simple 'birth marks' to involvement of complex arterial systems and various organs (Figure 5.30). They are vascular in nature; some resolve spontaneously, some reposed to treatments such as compression, radiation, steroids and sclerotherapy. Some haemangiomas can be fatal, especially if they occlude vital organs. Surgical intervention is governed by the position, size and organ involvement and can include excision by conventional methods and laser.

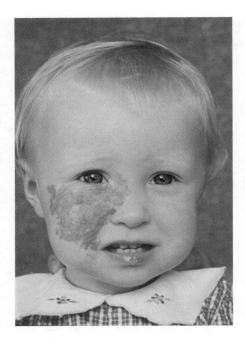

Fig. 5.30 Child with facial haemangioma. *Source*: Photograph courtesy of Mater Health Services.

Acknowledgement

This chapter is adapted from Herron, A., Shields, L., Tanner, A. (2003). Surgical procedures on children. In: Shields, L., Werder. H. (eds.). *Perioperative Nursing*. Greenwich Medical Media, London, pp. 193–214.

References

Abdullah, F. (2008). Necrotizing enterocolitis: Finding infants at highest risk. *Journal of Perinatology*, 28: 655–656.

Abdullah, N.A., Pearce, M.S., Parker, L., Wilkinson, J.R., McNally, R.J. (2007). Evidence of an environmental contribution to the aetiology of cryptorchidism and hypospadias? *European Journal of Epidemiology*, 22(9): 615–620.

Abrahamsson, M., Magnusson, G., Sjostrand, J. (1999). Inheritance of strabismus and the gain of using heredity to determine populations at risk of developing strabismus. *Acta Ophthalmolica Scandinavica*, 77: 653–657.

Akre, O., Boyd, H.A., Wilbrand, K., Westergaard, T., Hialgrim, H., Nordenskjöld, A., Ekbom, A., Melbye, M. (2008). Maternal and gestational risk factors for hypospadias. *Environmental Health Perspectives*, 116(8): 1071–1076.

Anderson, K.N., Anderson, L.E., Glanze, W.D. (eds.). (1994). *Mosby's medical, nursing and allied health dictionary*, 4th ed. Mosby, St. Louis.

Arensman, R.M., Bambini, D.A. (2000). Congenital diaphragmatic hernia and eventration. In: Ashcraft, K.W., Murphy, J.P., Sharp, R.J., Sigalet, D.L., Snyder, C.L. (eds.). *Pediatric surgery*, 3rd ed. WB Saunders Company, Philadelphia.

Arndt, C.A.S. (2000). Neoplasms of bone. In: Behrman, R.E., Kliegman, R.M., Jenson, H.B. (eds.). *Nelson textbook of pediatrics*, 16th ed. WB Saunders, Philadelphia.

Asiri, S.M., Abu-Bakr, Y.A., Al-Enazi, F. (2006). Paediatric ENT day surgery: Is it a safe practice? *Ambulatory Surgery*, 12(4): 147–149.

Bender, P.L. (2000). Genetics of cleft lip and palate. *Journal of Pediatric Nursing*, 15: 242–249.

Bennett, A.M.D., Clark, A.B., Bath, A.P., Montgomery, P.Q. (2005). Meta-analysis of the timing of haemorrhage after tonsillectomy: An important factor in determining the safety of performing tonsillectomy as a day case procedure. *Clinical Otolaryngology*, 30: 418–423.

Borer, J.G., Retik, A.B. (1999). Current trends in hypospadias repair. *Urology Clinics of North America*, 26: 15–37, vii.

Burton, M.J., Towler, B., Glasziou, P. (1999). Tonsillectomy versus non-surgical treatment for chronic/recurrent acute tonsillitis. *Cochrane Database of Systematic Reviews* Issue 3. Art. No.: CD001802. DOI: 10.1002/14651858.CD001802.

Caty, M.G., Azizkhan, R.G. (2000). Necrotizing enterocolitis. In: Ashcraft, K.W., Murphy, J.P., Sharp, R.J., Sigalet, D.L., Snyder, C.L. (eds.). *Pediatric surgery*, 3rd ed. WB Saunders Company, Philadelphia.

Coplen, D.E., Snyder, H.M. (2000). Ureteral obstruction and malformations. In: Ashcraft, K.W., Murphy, J.P., Sharp, R.J., Sigalet, D.L., Snyder, C.L. (eds.). *Pediatric surgery*, 3rd ed. WB Saunders Company, Philadelphia.

Cordier, P.L., Sion, B. (2000). Positioning the patient. In: Phippen, M.L., Wells, M.P. (eds.). *Patient care during operative and invasive procedures*. WB Saunders, Philadelphia.

Davis, C.L., Chaliar, A. (2000). Otolaryngological surgery. In: Phippen, M.L., Wells, M.P. (eds.). *Patient care during operative and invasive procedures*. WB Saunders Company, Philadelphia.

Decq, P., Le Geurinel, C., Palfi, S., Djindjian, M., Keravel, Y., Nguyen, J.P. (2000). A new device for endoscopic third ventriculostomy. *Journal of Neurosurgery*, 93: 509–512.

Dickson, N.P., van Roode, T., Herbison P., Paul, C. (2008). Circumcision and risk of sexually transmitted infections in a birth cohort. *Journal of Pediatrics*, 152(3): 383–387.

Dillon, P.W., Cilley, R.E. (2000). Lesions of the stomach. In: Ashcraft, K.W., Murphy, J.P., Sharp, R.J., Sigalet, D.L., Snyder, C.L. (eds.). *Pediatric surgery*, 3rd ed. WB Saunders Company, Philadelphia.

Duckett, J.W. (1989). Hypospadias. *Pediatric Reviews*, 11: 37–42.

Dugdale, A.E., Canty, A., Lewis, A.N., Lovell, S. (1978). The natural history of chronic middle ear disease in Australian Aboriginals: A cross-sectional study. *Medical Journal of Australia Supplement*, March 28: 6–8.

Ein, S.H. (2000). Appendicitis. In: Ashcraft, K.W., Murphy, J.P., Sharp, R.J., Sigalet, D.L., Snyder, C.L. (eds.). *Pediatric surgery*, 3rd ed. WB Saunders Company, Philadelphia.

Ellsworth, P., Cendron, M., Ritland, D., McCullough, M. (1999). Hypospadias repair in the 1990s. *AORN Journal*, 69: 148–150, 152–153, 155–156.

Esposito, C. (1998). One-trocar appendectomy in pediatric surgery. *Surgery and Endoscopy*, 12: 177–178.

Esposito, C., Caldamore, A.A., Settimi, A., El-Ghoneimi, A. (2008). Management of boys with nonpalpable undescended testis. *Nature Clinical Practice Urology*, 5(5): 252–260.

Fallat, M.E. (2000). Intussusception. In: Ashcraft, K.W., Murphy, J.P., Sharp, R.J., Sigalet, D.L., Snyder, C.L. (eds.). *Pediatric surgery*, 3rd ed. WB Saunders Company, Philadelphia.

Filston, H.C., Shorter, N.A. (2000). Esophageal atresia and tracheoesophageal malformations. In: Ashcraft, K.W., Murphy, J.P., Sharp, R.J., Sigalet, D.L., Snyder, C.L. (eds.). *Pediatric surgery*, 3rd ed. WB Saunders Company, Philadelphia.

Gaines, B.A., Holcomb, G.W., Neblett, W.W. (2000). Gastroschisis and omphalocele. In: Ashcraft, K.W., Murphy, J.P., Sharp, R.J., Sigalet, D.L., Snyder, C.L. (eds.). *Pediatric surgery*, 3rd ed. WB Saunders Company, Philadelphia.

Garcia, V.F. (2000). Umbilical and other abdominal wall hernias. In: Ashcraft, K.W., Murphy, J.P., Sharp, R.J., Sigalet, D.L., Snyder, C.L. (eds.). *Pediatric surgery*, 3rd ed. WB Saunders Company, Philadelphia.

Garetz, S.L. (2008). Behaviour, cognition and quality of life after adenotonsillectomy for pediatric sleep-disordered breathing: Summary of the literature. *Otolaryngology Head and Neck Surgery*, 138: S19–S26.

Golden, A., Low, D.W. (2000). Plastic surgery. In: Phippen, M.L., Wells, M.P. (eds.). *Patient care during operative and invasive procedures*. WB Saunders, Philadelphia.

Gregory, K.E. (2008). Clinical predictors of necrotizing enterocolitis in premature infants. *Nursing Research*, 57(4): 260–270.

Gruber, D.P., Brockmeyer, D.L., Walker, M.L. (2000). Head injuries in children. In: Ashcraft, K.W., Murphy, J.P., Sharp, R.J., Sigalet, D.L., Snyder, C.L. (eds.). *Pediatric surgery*, 3rd ed. WB Saunders Company, Philadelphia.

Hart, E.S., Grottkau, B.E., Rebello, G.N., Albright, M.B. (2005). The newborn foot: Diagnosis and management of common conditions. *Orthopaedic Nursing*, 24(5): 313–321.

Hartnett, K.S. (2008). Beyond the basics. Congenital diaphragmatic hernia: Advanced physiology and care concepts. *Advances in Neonatal Care*, 8(2): 107–115.

Havas, T. (1984). A longitudinal study of otitis media in the Aboriginal population of Groote Eylandt. *Journal of Otolaryngological Society of Australasia*, 5: 365–369.

Hendren, W.H. (2000). Urethral valves. In: Ashcraft, K.W., Murphy, J.P., Sharp, R.J., Sigalet, D.L., Snyder, C.L. (eds.). *Pediatric surgery*, 3rd ed. WB Saunders Company, Philadelphia.

Homer, J.J., Williams, B.T., Semple, P., Swanepoel, A., Knight, L.C. (2000). Tonsillectomy by guillotine is less painful than by dissection. *International Journal of Pediatric Otorhinolaryngology*, 52: 25–29.

Hutson, J.M., Woodward, A.A., Beasley, S.W. (1999). *Jones' clinical paediatric surgery: Diagnosis and management*, 5th ed. Blackwell Science Asia, Melbourne.

Islam, S. (2008). Clinical care outcomes in abdominal wall defects. *Current Opinion in Pediatrics*, 20(3): 305–310.

Jaksic, T., Nigro, J.F., Hicks, M.J. (2000). Nevus and melanoma. In: Ashcraft, K.W., Murphy, J.P., Sharp, R.J., Sigalet, D.L., Snyder, C.L. (eds.). *Pediatric surgery*, 3rd ed. WB Saunders Company, Philadelphia.

Johnson, R.L. (1967). Chronic otitis media in school age Navajo Indians. *The Laryngoscope*, 78: 1990–1995.

Kerner, M. (2000). Neurosurgery. In: Phippen, M.L., Wells, M.P. (eds.). *Patient care during operative and invasive procedures*. WB Saunders, Philadelphia.

Kirsch, A., Cooper, C.S., Gatti, J., Scherz, H.A.L.C., Canning, D.A., Zderic, S.A., Snyder, H.M., Hensle, T.W. (2001). Laser tissue soldering for hypospadias repair: Results of a controlled prospective clinical trial. Commentary. *The Journal of Urology*, 165(2): 574–577.

Kobus, K.F. (2007). Cleft palate repair with the use of osmotic expanders: A preliminary report. *Journal of Plastic, Reconstructive & Aesthetic Surgery*, 60(4): 414–421.

Korkmaz, O., Bektas, D., Cobanoglu, B., Caylan, R. (2008). Partial tonsillectomy with scalpel in children with obstructive tonsillar hypertrophy. *International Journal of Pediatric Otorhinolaryngology*, 72(7): 1007–1012.

Laberge, J.M., Nguyen, L.T., Shaw, K.S. (2000). Teratomas, dermoids and other soft tissue tumours. In: Ashcraft, K.W., Murphy, J.P., Sharp, R.J., Sigalet, D.L., Snyder, C.L. (eds.). *Pediatric surgery*, 3rd ed. WB Saunders Company, Philadelphia.

Luks, F.I., Logan, J., Breuer, C.K., Kurkchubasche, A.G., Wesselhoeft, C.W., Tracy, T.F. (1999). Cost-effectiveness of laparoscopy in children. *Archives of Pediatric and Adolescent Medicine*, 153: 965–968.

Magdy, E.A., Elwany, S., el-Daly, A.S., Abdel-Hadi, M., Morshedy, M.A. (2008). Coblation tonsillectomy: A prospective, double-blind, randomised, clinical and histopathological comparison with dissection–ligation, monopolar electrocautery and laser tonsillectomies. *The Journal of Laryngology and Otology*, 122(3): 282–290.

Molloy, A.M., Mills, J.L., Kirke, P.N., Weir, D.G., Scott, J.M. (1999). Folate status and neural tube defects. *Biofactors*, 10: 291–294.

Morris, J.K., Wald, N.J. (1999). Quantifying the decline in the birth prevalence of neural tube defects in England and Wales. *Journal of Medical Screening*, 6: 182–185.

Moushey, R., Hawley, C., Diomede, B. (2000). Care of the pediatric patient. In: Phippen, M.L., Wells, M.P. (eds.). *Patient care during operative and invasive procedures*. WB Saunders Company, Philadelphia.

Murphy, M., Hahn, G.V. (2000). Orthopedic surgery. In: Phippen, M.L., Wells, M.P. (eds.). *Patient care during operative and invasive procedures*. WB Saunders, Philadelphia.

Nair, R.R., Warner, B.B., Warner, B.W. (2008) Role of epidermal growth factor and other growth factors in the prevention of necrotizing enterocolitis. *Seminars in Perinatology*, 32(2): 107–113.

Nassar, N., Bower, C., Barker, A. (2007). Increasing prevalence of hypospadias in Western Australia, 1980–2000. *Archives of Disease in Childhood*, 92(7): 580–584.

Nelson, P., Nieuwenhuijsen, M., Jensen, T.K., Mouriquand, P., Wilcox, D., Elliott, P. (2007). Prevalence of hypospadias in the same geographic region as ascertained by three different registries. *Birth Defects Research. Part A, Clinical And Molecular Teratology*, 79(10): 685–687.

Paediatrics & Child Health Division of The Royal Australasian College of Physicians and The Australian Society of Otolaryngology Head and Neck Surgery (2008). *Indications to tonsillectomy and adenotonsillectomy in children*. Sydney.

Parsons, S.P., Cordes, S.R., Comer, B. (2006). Comparison of post-tonsillectomy pain using the *ultrasonic scalpel*, coblator, and electrocautery. *Otolaryngology – Head and Neck Surgery*, 134(1): 106–113.

Petersson, R.S., Friedman, O. (2008). Current trends in otoplasty. *Current Opinion in Otolaryngology & Head and Neck Surgery*, 16(4): 352–358.

Petsonk, E.L. (2000). Couriers of asthma: Antigenic proteins in natural rubber latex. *Occupational Medicine*, 15: 421–430.

Phillips, N. (2007). *Berry & Kohn's operating room technique*. Mosby Elsevier: St Louis.

Ponsky, L.E, Ross, J.H., Knipper, N., Kay, R. (2000). Penile adhesions after neonatal circumcision. *Journal of Urology*, 164: 495–496.

Ramkumar, S., Narayanan, V., Laing, J.H. (2006). Twenty-four hours or 10 days? A prospective randomised controlled trial in children comparing head bandages following pinnaplasty. *Journal of Plastic, Reconstructive & Aesthetic Surgery*, 59(9): 969–974.

Raynor, S.C. (2000). Circumcision. In: Ashcraft, K.W., Murphy, J.P., Sharp, R.J., Sigalet, D.L., Snyder, C.L. (eds.). *Pediatric surgery*, 3rd ed. WB Saunders Company, Philadelphia.

Reed, W., Struve, S., Maynard, J.E. (1967). Otitis media and hearing deficiency among Eskimo children: A cohort study. *American Journal of Public Health*, 57: 1657–1662.

Robinson, S.R., Purdie, G.L. (2000). Reducing post-tonsillectomy pain with cryoanalgesia: A randomized controlled trial. *Laryngoscope*, 110: 1128–1131.

Sadove, A.M., van Aalst, J.A., Culp, J.A. (2004). Cleft palate repair: Art and issues. *Clinics in Plastic Surgery*, 31(2): 231–241.

Segerdahl, M., Warrén-Stromberg, M., Rawal, N., Bratwall, M., Jakobsson, J. (2008). Children in day surgery: Clinical practice and routines. The results from a nation-wide survey. *Acta Anaesthesiologica Scandinavica*, 52(6): 821–828.

Shields, L. (1990). *The influence of the family on young children's growth and disease at Cherbourg Aboriginal Community, Australia.* Masters Thesis, University of Queensland, Brisbane.

Shields, L. (1999). *A comparative study of the care of hospitalized children in developed and developing countries.* Ph. D. Thesis, University of Queensland, 1999. Available from URL http://adt.library.uq.edu.au/public/adt-QU2001.0013/index.html (accessed 10 October 2008).

Silver, R.I. (2000). What is the etiology of hypospadias? A review of recent research. *Delaware Medical Journal*, 72: 343–347.

Smith. S.C. (2007). Ophthalmic surgery. In: Rothrock, J.C. (ed.). *Alexander's care of the patient in surgery*, 13th ed. Mosby Elsevier, St Louis.

Stow, J. (2007). Pediatric surgery. In: Rothrock, J.C. (ed.). *Alexander's care of the patient in surgery* 13th ed. Mosby Elsevier, St Louis.

Stringel, G. (2000). Hemangiomas and lymphangiomas. In: Ashcraft, K.W., Murphy, J.P., Sharp, R.J., Sigalet, D.L., Snyder, C.L. (eds.). *Pediatric surgery*, 3rd ed. WB Saunders Company, Philadelphia.

Thompson, G.H., Scoles, P.V. (2000). Bone and joint disorders. In: Behrman, R.E., Kliegman, R.M., Jenson, H.B. (eds.). *Nelson textbook of pediatrics*, 16th ed. WB Saunders, Philadelphia.

Tonkin, S. (1970). Maori infant health: 2. Study of morbidity and medico-social aspects. *New Zealand Medical Journal*, 72: 229–273.

Tyson, J.E., Kennedy, K.A. (2005). Trophic feedings for parenterally fed infants. *Cochrane Database of Systematic Reviews*, CD000504(3): DOI: 10.1002/14651858.CD000504.pub2.

Wallen, E.M., Shortliffe, L.M.D. (2000). Undescended testis and testicular tumors. In: Ashcraft, K.W., Murphy, J.P., Sharp, R.J., Sigalet, D.L., Snyder, C.L. (eds.). *Pediatric surgery*, 3rd ed. WB Saunders Company, Philadelphia.

Williams, C.P., Richardson, B.G., Bukowski, T.P. (2000). Importance of identifying the inconspicuous penis: Prevention of circumcision complications. *Urology*, 56: 140–143.

Williams, P.F., Cole, W.G. (1991). *Orthopaedic management in childhood.* Chapman and Hall, London.

Wilson, D., Hochenberry, M.J., Wong, D.L. (2008). *Wong's clinical manual of pediatric nursing*, 7th ed. Mosby Elsevier, St Louis.

Wright, K.W., Spiegel, P.H. (1999). *Pediatric ophthalmology and strabismus.* Mosby Elsevier, St Louis.

6 Day surgery for children

Ann Tanner

Day procedure centres

A significant area of change in paediatric surgery has been the increase in the number of cases performed as day procedures. Over the past 20 years, the percentage of elective admission day case surgery has more than doubled, with the trend continuing to rise (Jarrett, 2001). Also known as ambulatory surgery, the increase can be attributed to a multitude of medical and technological advancements. New anaesthetic drugs have a rapid onset coupled with a short duration of effect, a good control of analgesia, a rapid recovery and less incidence of post-operative pain and nausea (Aantaa & Manner, 1999). Advances in surgical techniques in which minimally invasive and laparoscopic surgery have replaced the previously 'open' procedures that involved a larger wound site and all associated extra risks of bleeding, infection and pain. There has been an improvement in facilities with the growth of specialised day procedure centres, staffed with nurses and clinicians familiar with day surgery protocol and procedures and adept in fast admissions, preparation for theatre and post-operative recovery and discharge.

Prerequisites for day surgery

Day case surgery should not be associated with excessive blood loss or fluid shifts, and any post-operative pain must be manageable at home (Prabhu & Chung, 2001). Neonates, low birth weight and very low birth weight babies have a higher risk of anaesthetic complications and post-operative complications, e.g. oxygen requirements pre- or post-operatively. As such they are not classified as suitable for day case surgery.

There are many benefits for the child and their families in undergoing day surgery as opposed to an overnight stay, with minimal disruption in routine for the child and their family. Day case admissions have been seen to reduce the psychological trauma of a hospital admission (Glasper & Haggarty, 2006). It is important to be aware of the child's anxiety particularly prior to surgery. The anxiety itself can initiate a stress response, which can delay wound healing and suppress the immune system (Koinig, 2002). In this chapter, we will be looking at the typical activities of a day procedure centre. This includes pre-admission phone calls and clinics, admissions, preparation for the OR, ward stage recovery, child and parental education and preparation for discharge. For an indication of the wide scope of surgical and medical admissions encountered in day procedure centres, see Table 6.1.

Table 6.1   Examples of day case surgical and medical procedures

DAY PROCEDURE SURGICAL PROCEDURES (Gwinn *et al.*, 2004)

1. General Surgical Procedures
Insertion of PEG: a safe technique for establishing enteral feeding (Avitsland *et al.*, 2006).
Circumcision: cultural or medical: excision of foreskin from the penis.
Cystoscopy: Insertion of rigid cystoscope into bladder via urethra.
Hernia repair: inguinal: a segment of the intestine along with fluid, protrudes through the muscle of the abdominal wall.
Hydrocele repair: similar to hernia with collection of fluid from abdominal cavity around the testicle, no small bowel involvement (Anderson *et al.*, 1994).
Hypospadias repair: malformation of the urethral meatus in which it is situated along the shaft of the penis, repair to reposition at the tip of the penis (Ellsworth *et al.*, 1999).
Orchidopexy: laparoscopic retrieval of undescended testes from the groin which is then pulled down into the scrotal sac (Maldonado and Nygren, 1999).
Removal/insertion of central venous lines and ports: a central venous catheter inserted into the superior vena cava or a port or central venous implantable access device (Heron *et al.*, 2002).
Removal of skin lesions: dermoid cysts, naevus: dermoid cysts are soft and rounded and often fixed to deep tissue or bone (Laberge *et al.*, 2000), Naevus can be any skin lesion appearing at or after birth (Jaksic *et al.*, 2000).
Removal of thyroglossal cysts: thyroglossal duct cysts (TDCs) a soft lump in the centre of the throat an embryological remnant of the thyroglossal tract (Sprinzl *et al.*, 2000).
Willets procedure: ingrown toenail excision.

2. Ear, nose and throat surgery (ENT)
Adenoidectomy (curettage of adenoidal tissue in post-nasal space).
Bronchoscopy (rigid bronchoscope examination of upper airways, removal of foreign body).
Cautery inferior turbinates (CIT) of nose.
Cautery of Littles Area (treatment of chronic nose bleeds).
Examination under anaesthetic (EUA) ears.
Examination under anaesthetic (EUA) nose.
Grommets (insertion or removal of a ventilation tube to the eardrum).
Laser microlaryngoscopy (laser microsurgery to lesions which may cause airway obstruction).
Reduction of fractured nose.
Removal of foreign body (nose, throat, ear).

3. Ophthalmology
Excision of chalazion: cyst like growth located near the eye lashes caused by a blockage of one of the meibomian glands (these produce the fluid that lubricates the eye) (Medline Encyclopaedia, 2006).
Insertion of Crawford tubes (creates tear duct).
Dacrocystogram: injecting dye via the tear ducts and X-ray to determine blockages (Gwinn *et al.*, 2004).
Electroretinogram (tests visual preceptors of the eyes).
Examination under anaesthetic (EUA) eyes.
Probe and syringe of tear ducts (unblocks nasolacrimal ducts).
Ptosis repair (drooping upper eyelid).
Squint repair (malalignment of the eyes on the object of gaze).

4. Orthopaedic
Removal of K-wires, pins and plates.
Change of plaster.
Removal of hip spica.
Re-manipulation of existing fracture.

5. Plastic surgery
Set back otoplasty: correction of prominent ears usually cosmetic as children can become a victim of ridicule by their peers (Palmer, 1988).
Removal of extra digit: polydactyly or release of webbed fingers/toes: syndactyly (Tanner, 2002).
Repair of laceration.

Table 6.1 (*Continued*)

Revision of scars: excision of existing scar and re-suturing.
Debriding and grafting burns scars.
Steroid injections to keloid scars.

6. Dental
Restorations and extractions: fillings and removal of decayed teeth.
Dental abscesses: drainage and curettage.

7. Rehabilitation
Botox injections for spastic quadriplegia.

DAY PROCEDURE MEDICAL PROCEDURES (Gwinn *et al.*, 2004)
Immunology: intragram infusions.
Endocrine: testing and pamidronate infusions.
Diagnostic procedures requiring sedation or a general anaesthetic or nitrous oxide
ERG (electroretinogram tests the visual receptors of the eyes)
EEG (electroencephalography records the electrical activity in the brain an investigative test following any
seizure activity).
ABR (auditory brainstem response tests the functioning of the auditory pathway relaying signals to the
brain when a sound is heard) may require a GA or sedation to induce sleep).
CT (computerised tomography records bone and soft tissue anatomy in cross sectional format) may require
sedation or a G–A.
MRI (magnetic resonance imaging provides detailed images of the soft tissue structures of the body
in particular the brain and spinal cord requires a G–A if the child is unable to lie perfectly still for the
45 minutes duration of the scan).

Communication with the child and parent

The staff of day procedure centres play a major role in the child and parental education required for successful day surgery as much of the pain relief and wound care
is required once the child is discharged to home. During the past 25 years, there has
been a transformation in the method of care for children in hospitals. The nurse no
longer provides all the hands on care to the child while the parents simply visit. There
are many generations of parents who have since stated that they felt helpless and
inadequate during their child's hospitalisation (Glasper & Haggarty, 2006). Currently,
nurses have a working partnership with the parents or carer, providing support to
them in the care of their child (Hemphill & Dearmun, 2006).

Depending on the age of the child, it is good practice to be immediately friendly
and welcoming to the parent or carer and to the child concerned. Some younger children who are understandably nervous or shy with strangers may be reassured when
they see the parent and nurse communicating in a friendly manner. Older children
may likewise be shy or bored, but it is good to give them the opportunity to express
themselves, particularly post-operatively when you need their subjective opinion
about pain and nausea. It is useful to be knowledgeable about the developmental stages of children, in particular, their stage of attachment to their parents, their
reactions to strangers, their beliefs about hospitalisation and the considerations that
nurses need to take when communicating with the differing age groups and their parents (Table 6.2).

Table 6.2   Developmental stages of children and nursing considerations (Waterman, 2002)

Age	Infant (Birth to 11 Months)	Toddler (1–3 Years)	Preschool Child (4–5 Years)	School-Age Child (6–12 Years)	Adolescent (13–18 Years)
Stage	Bonded to parents/ immediate family Sensitive to surroundings Very little language	More individual assertive and wilful basic language	Fantasy and magical thinking Good language and cognition, and strong sense of self	Well-developed language with an ability to reason Early self control Basic idea of body functions Beginning concept of death	Independence Peer importance Realistic idea of death
Fears	Mistrust	Any parental separation pain	Pain Disfigurement Frustration Long parental separation	Punishment of pain Disfigurement Death	Loss of autonomy Being trapped Peer pressure Death
Response	Stranger anxiety Crying Withdrawal	Tantrums and loss of control Hyperactive	Withdrawal Fantasy Anger	Withdrawal Demanding behaviour	Stubborness Stoicism Depression Helplessness
Nursing	Enable parent involvement Provide a warm, caring environment and minimise extraneous noises and activity	Enable parent involvement Talk to the child Offer choices as much as possible	Enable parent involvement Talk to the child Use dolls to explain procedures and encourage fantasy or play	Respect the child's privacy Talk with child, be positive about what will happen and encourage them to master the situation	Orientate to and explain what is happening and why Encourage discussion about fears and concerns Enable control and choice Stress peer acceptance

A word about siblings

The siblings of children with chronic illnesses may undergo attitude changes and their self-esteem may also deteriorate (Mathews, 2006). The best way to reduce sibling anxiety is very similar to reducing parental anxiety. Keep them informed, explain any procedures, ask for their opinion and let them feel important. If nurses are able to develop a rapport and trusting relationship with the siblings (Mathews, 2006), this, in turn, improves the rapport with the hospitalised child, increasing the trust in the nursing staff felt by the family as a unit.

Children with special needs

Day procedure centres like other paediatric wards admit children with special needs. These children often have complex care, are frequently hospitalised, and can be known by staff as the 'frequent flyers' of the unit. They may suffer a range of conditions such as cerebral palsy with spastic quadriplegia, in which instance they may be wheel chair bound, and may require percutaneous enteric gastrostomy (PEG) feeds. They may have a long history of seizure disorders or may have acquired brain injuries, metabolic disorders, muscular dystrophy, micro cephalic, and not to mention the large range of congenital malformations, abnormalities and syndromes. Some of these children have been fostered out to care when parents found themselves unable to cope with the complexity of their disabilities and many are cared for by their natural parents. These 'special' children tend to be very much loved by parents and carers alike.

It is particularly important for the nursing staff to establish a collaborative partnership with the parents and carers of special needs children. The parents themselves are to some extent institutionalised and can become very frustrated with the repetitive nature of hospital admissions. Often these parents prefer to provide all the care for these children, whilst others who may well be exhausted see the admission as an opportunity for them to take a break. Either way, particular effort needs to be taken to ensure that their stay is well organised as the child may require review by multiple medical teams.

Pre-admission preparation

The hospital admissions office posts a letter to the parents detailing the date and time of admission, the fasting time required, and an information sheet about their admission.

The pre-admission process is used to reduce the time taken to admit the child on the day of the procedure. It can involve either a phone call to the child's home or a pre-admission attendance at clinic. Both provide the opportunity to gather valuable information such as:

- the child's medical and surgical history;
- medications;
- allergies;
- history of previous anaesthetics and whether they suffered any adverse effects;
- dietary requirements and methods of feeding (such as PEG feeds, normal toddler diet and gluten free);
- provide a record the child's immunisation status;
- check to see if they have had known infectious contact (such as chicken pox or measles) in the previous 2–3 weeks before theatre;
- ensure that the child is otherwise well and therefore suitable for an anaesthetic.

This is all the information that can be collected on the phone. At the pre-admission clinics or on the day of admission, the consent for the procedure can be signed and the child's baseline observations recorded.

Admission to the day procedure centre: preparations for surgery

A registered nurse (RN) admitting the child completes a set of baseline observations, including the child's weight, temperature, pulse, respirations and oxygen saturation (SaO$_2$) preferably before the anaesthetist reviews the child. The weight is required to calculate premedication and anaesthetic doses on a milligram per kilogram ratio, and the observations provide a means of ascertaining if the child is well and fit for theatre. A brief medical and surgical history of the child is recorded, including the child's allergies, immunisation status and a check to see if the child has had any recent contact with infectious diseases (such as chicken pox). The junior doctor of the surgical or medical team may also medically admit them. The majority of surgical cases will be reviewed by the anaesthetist on the ward prior to surgery to ensure they are well enough for a general anaesthetic and to determine if they require any premedication.

Premedication

The majority of children undergoing any type of painful procedure receive a paracetamol premedication. Occasionally, a sedative/hypnotic such as midazolam is also given, usually in cases where the child exhibits excessive anxiety. Children with asthma may need a nebuliser of Ventolin included in their premedication orders. The drugs are ordered on a milligram per kilogram (mg/kg) basis and the paracetamol dose is usually a 6-hour dose. If any sedation premedication is given, the child will require monitoring of pulse, respirations and oxygen saturation whilst awaiting theatre transfer. They will be transported to theatre on a trolley with oxygen and suctioning units available on the trolley and a portable oxygen saturation monitor.

The medical order to give a premedication is prescribed by the anaesthetist and will have either a given time or a stat (immediate) order. In this tertiary paediatric facility, two RNs are required to check the drug and to re-calculate that the prescribed mg/kg dose is correct according to the weight of the child. The two must then check that the child has the correct name band on, that matches the child, the medication sheet and the chart. They need to re-check the allergy status and confirm in the instance of a paracetamol pre-medication, that no other paracetamol has been given in the 6 hours prior to the prescribed dose. Once these checks are complete, the child is given the dose.

Documentation and allergy alerts

The labels recording the child's name, date of birth, hospital record number and address and phone numbers are checked to ensure they are correct for the child and that the correct chart is with the child. Allergy alerts vary from institution to institution. In this tertiary paediatric facility, a red armband is applied to children with allergies, with the child's label on the armband and any allergies and their reactions clearly noted on the band. The allergy is likewise documented on the medication sheet and by the anaesthetist on the anaesthetic record. Children without allergies receive a blue armband.

Fasting status

The fasting time from food required for all general anaesthetics (whether given a gas or an intravenous anaesthetic agent) is 6 hours. They may drink water or clear apple juice only, up to 2 hours prior to surgery. However, if the parent gives their baby a bottle of half milk half water (by not considering the diluted milk as a food), at 6 a.m. for an 8 a.m. case, it is classified as a food and they will not be adequately fasted for a general anaesthetic until 12:00. In this instance, they may be cancelled if the theatre bookings for the afternoon take precedence.

All elective surgery cases must be properly fasted. It is only the emergency surgical admissions, where the child's life or limb will be compromised, that a general anaesthetic will be given when the child is not fasted. In these instances, a rapid sequence induction is given and pressure must be applied to the cricoid to block the oesophagus during intubation to minimise the risk of aspiration of the stomach contents. The risk to the child's life or limb then overrides the risk of aspiration during induction. An explanation of the risks of aspiration, and the policy that only the acute emergency cases will be anaesthetised when not fasted, may reduce some of the anger felt by parents who have misunderstood the fasting instructions and discover that their child may be cancelled as a result.

The theatre checklist

The theatre checklist is completed with a record of fasting status, consent for the procedure, armband on, allergies noted, baseline observations and weight recorded. The premedication (if ordered) has been given and a check of loose teeth, glasses, hearing aid or contact lenses, correct documentation and personal items. Any jewellery or nail polish is removed, and the child is dressed in his or her own or hospital attire providing there is no metal on the garments. The precaution against metal (jewellery or clothing) originates from the use in theatre of electrosurgical cutting and coagulation of tissue (diathermy). A high frequency current passes through the patient from the diathermy forceps and exits the patient via a diathermy plate; a gel covered pad plugged into the diathermy machine (Werder & Thompson, 2002). If the patient comes into contact with any metal, the current may exit via the metal rather than the diathermy plate, which can cause a burn. As a precaution, the policy is no metal in garments and all metal jewellery removed or covered in a protective tape, regardless of the need for diathermy for the procedure. There is some confusion as to the no metal rule and some parents think that they too must remove all metals.

It helps to let the parents know that the pre-operative checklist is repeated in theatre as a safety measure to make absolutely sure that the correct child is going into the correct theatre for the correct procedure. In this tertiary paediatric facility, it is hospital policy for the surgeon to use an indelible pen to mark the limb or side of the body to be operated on prior to surgery and to confirm with the child and parent that it is correct. Mistakes can and have been made, so the more precautions to safeguard against error the better.

The child is then ready and awaiting a call from theatre and will often stay in the large play area equipped with many distractions ranging from computer games to ride on cars. Once the child is admitted, the opportunity is there to educate the parents or carers about what to expect on the child's return from theatre. The timing of the discharge advice prior to surgery is important as the parents are often too tired or stressed after their child's surgery to take on any new information just prior to discharge and may find themselves unable to adequately understand the information provided to them (Kankkunen *et al.*, 2002). The time of discharge is also a busy period as the intravenous access device is removed and discharge medical summaries and follow-up appointments are given at the same time.

Parental and child education

Education is one of the most important aspects of nursing care in a day procedure centre. Verbal information alone is insufficient and needs to be supplemented with well-presented printed material (Jarrett, 2001). Prior to the introduction of day surgery, the post-operative care was performed by nursing staff trained and experienced to watch for signs of post-procedural or post-operative complications such as:

- allergic reactions;
- excessive pain;
- bleeding;
- fevers;
- infection;
- nausea and vomiting.

With the advent of day procedures and day surgery, nurses observe the child and record observations for 1–2 hours (longer for some procedures such as bronchoscopy and adenoidectomy). Once the discharge criteria are met, the nurse discharges the child to home in the care of the parent or carer. Subsequent post-operative care is left up to the parents or carer of the child. Along with an explanation of possible complications and how to recognise them, the parent is given the contact numbers for the day surgery centre and for the hospital's emergency department for after hour's concerns. This ensures that phone help is available and from there the decision can be made to either bring the child back to the hospital or for them to return to their GP. In this paediatric facility, an education brochure is available for the majority of procedures, with generic brochures available for the rest. The brochure outlines a synopsis of the procedure, what to expect following the procedure, how long it is estimated to take and any specific post-operative care. The brochures also discuss analgesia and the protocols for effective relief of pain and/or nausea and any symptoms of possible complications to be aware of. Because the brochure contains the contact numbers for the day procedure centre and the Department of Emergency Medicine, the parents can take their child home knowing that help is available to them should they have any concerns. It is more effective to verbally talk through the information in the brochure with the parents as they tend to be swamped in paperwork and some may never read it or be aware of the phone help available.

Whilst there are specific education requirements for the differing procedures, there are some aspects of post-operative education that are standard for many procedures. These are outlined below.

Pain and day surgery

Pain management is a complex issue and relies on an individualised patient assessment (see Chapter 4 for a detailed account of pain in children). Some of the symptoms of pain can include:

- the child stating they have pain (regardless of what analgesia has been given);
- nausea can be a symptom of unrelieved pain;
- the child is lying still, reluctant to move;
- pyrexia;
- tachycardia;
- hypertension;
- pale and/or clammy.

In the case of the older child, it helps to remind them that our intention is for them to be comfortable, and if they find that they have pain, to tell the nurse or their parent so that we may give them something to take the pain away. If the child is too shy or frightened to speak up, nurses need to rely on the non-verbal cues and the parents own assessment of their child's distress.

The majority of children undergoing any type of painful procedure receive a paracetamol premedication. Occasionally a sedative/hypnotic such as midazolam is also given, usually in cases where the child exhibits excessive anxiety. In theatre local infiltrate anaesthetic is often injected to numb the area of surgery for several hours. Stronger analgesia such as fentanyl or morphine can be given in theatre or recovery. The post-operative analgesia may include oral analgesia such as paracetamol, ibuprofen, oxycodone or codeine phosphate. Nursing staff must be aware that both paracetamol and an intravenous equivalent of ibuprofen can both be administered intravenously by the anaesthetist. It is important for the recovery staff to notate the time given on the medication chart to avoid duplication of such doses orally.

The parents need to know what doses can be given when. For example, a child was given a 6 hourly dose of paracetamol at 09:00 as a premedication, and then given a 6-hour dose of codeine phosphate on return to the ward at 11:00, and was then fit for discharge at 12:30. In this case, the parents had paracetamol and *Painstop* (paediatric paracetamol and codeine mix available over the counter at pharmacies) available at home. They need to know that they can give *either* paracetamol at 3 p.m. (6 hours after the paracetamol premedication) or *Painstop* at 5 p.m. (6 hours after the codeine phosphate dose). Alternatively, the child may be given alternating paracetamol and ibuprofen. For example, if the same 6 hourly dose of paracetamol given at 09:00 as a premedication was followed by an 11 a.m. dose of ibuprofen, then the parents can give Paracetamol at 3 p.m. (6 hours after the Paracetamol premedication) as well as ibuprofen at 5 p.m. (6 hours after the ibuprofen dose). It is good practice to write the times down for the parents to limit confusion.

The discharging nurse needs to stress that analgesia is best given before the effects of the local infiltrate wear off and importantly that pain not covered by such simple analgesia as discussed above may warrant a medical review of the child either at their own GP or by returning to the Emergency Medicine Department at the hospital.

Nausea and vomiting

Some of the typical signs of nausea include the following:

- pallor;
- they can become clammy to touch;
- they may lie still refusing all offers of food and fluids;
- vomiting.

Unfortunately for some children, nausea and vomiting continues to be a post-anaesthetic complication, although the advent of more effective anti-emetics and other drug interventions such as dexamethasone, an anti-inflammatory drug which also aids in the prevention of nausea, has reduced the incidence. If the child has post-operative nausea and vomiting, and has already received anti-emetics during the procedure, an alternative anti-emetic may be given if ordered or the anaesthetist may order a repeat dose of the anti-emetic given in surgery. If the nausea and vomiting is unresolved, the child will need to be reviewed by the anaesthetist if available or the resident medical officer and may require intravenous fluid therapy and an extended stay prior to discharge. In some instances (dental extractions, adenoidectomy), the child may have swallowed some blood during the procedure, if there is a pool of blood sitting in the stomach the child will tend to vomit despite anti-emetics and generally will continue to feel nauseous until they have expelled the blood. If the nausea and vomiting returns at home and remains unresolved, the child may require medical review either at their own GP or by returning to the Emergency Medicine Department at the hospital.

Bleeding

Any surgical incision has a risk of bleeding post-operatively. If the bleeding has not stopped after a pressure dressing is applied to the wound when possible, the child needs review by the surgeons concerned. Tonsillectomy and adenoidectomy is one of the most common surgical procedures performed in the paediatric population (Edler *et al.*, 2007). In this tertiary paediatric facility, it is hospital protocol for the children undergoing a tonsillectomy to be observed overnight prior to discharge, therefore they do not meet the day surgery criteria.

The most at risk group of children for post-operative bleeding in the day surgery centres are the post-operative adenoidectomies. For this reason, post-adenoidectomies are kept on the ward for 4 hours for observation (sometimes 6 hours depending on the surgeons preference), and their vital signs including oxygen saturation are recorded 15 minutely for 1 hour, then half hourly for 2 hours and then hourly for the final hour.

The regime for ward recovery post-adenoidectomy may vary between surgeons and institutions. Regular surgery has the standard half hourly post-operative observations. In the case of bleeding adenoidal beds, the child can suffer a significant bleed over a relatively short period of time before the child's vital signs indicate haemorrhage. Adenoidal bleeds can trickle down the child's throat and be swallowed by the child until a large vomit of blood or a drop in their vital signs indicates the bleed. This is a medical emergency and requires the ear, nose and throat (ENT) surgeon to return to the ward to review and contain the bleed. This can be achieved by the use of a large bore Foleys catheter and balloon, which is inserted into the nose, the balloon is then inflated and the Foleys retracted until the balloon is applying pressure to the post-nasal space (adenoid bed). The bleed may warrant a return to theatre for further cautery or re-scraping of the adenoidal bed. In many cases, the bleed occurs when adenoidal tissue has not been completely removed. Country children and their parents are required to spend one night in accommodation (family or hospital units) near the hospital due to the risk of a bleed. Parents need to be aware that there is a risk of a post-adenoidal bleed for 1–14 days following surgery. The child needs to abstain from excessive physical activity in that time such as school sports, bike riding running and swimming (Gwinn *et al.*, 2004). The symptoms may include:

- excessive swallowing;
- and/or vomiting of undigested blood;
- pallor and lethargy;
- tachycardia.

Post-surgical bleeds leave the child at risk of infections and usually require 24 hours of intravenous antibiotic coverage, followed by a course of oral antibiotics at home.

In the instance of dental extractions, the cavities are often sutured with dissolvable sutures. The parents are reminded that these do not have to be removed later. If bleeding occurs, a rolled pad of cotton gauze is placed over the extraction site and the child bites down for 30 minutes (if unable the parent can hold the child's mouth closed over the gauze). If bleeding continues, the dentist will need to be contacted to return and may pack the cavity to prevent further bleeding. If bleeding occurs at home and is unrelieved by a pressure wad of cotton gauze, the child should have a medical review either at their own GP or by returning to Emergency Medicine Department at the hospital.

If a child commences to bleed from the operative site once at home, they need to be medically reviewed. A return to the hospital emergency department is preferable but if distance is an issue then local GP or health centre. If the parent has phoned the day procedure unit to ask what to do, it is preferable to get the parents to present to a doctor in person for assessment of the bleed, as it is very difficult and can be dangerous to assess over the phone.

Infection

Any surgical wound has a risk of infection. Parents are alerted to keep dressings dry for the first 48 hours, and depending on the length of time before the follow-up appointment in the doctors rooms or clinic, may remove the dressing unless instructed to keep intact until review. It is important that the parents be alert to any signs of infection, such as:

- fevers;
- discharge from the wound site;
- Offensive smell;
- redness and or swelling;
- increased pain.

If any of these signs of infection develop, the child needs to be medically reviewed.

Fevers

Some surgical procedures have a risk of fevers following the procedure; these include flexible bronchoscopies and sometimes simply having a general anaesthetic. If the temperature is unrelieved by an antipyretic such as paracetamol and persist beyond a 24 hour period, it can be an indication of a chest infection and the child will need to return to the hospital or their GP for review.

Fracture care

New fractures require an overnight admission and as such do not meet the criteria for day stay surgery. Even if the fracture was reduced by closed manipulation, the risks of complications such as pain (unrelieved by simple analgesia) and swelling (the plaster cast may need to be split) require overnight monitoring and an orthopaedic review prior to discharge. Orthopaedic day cases include change of plasters, occasional re-manipulation of existing fractures, removal of wires, pins or plates and orthotic castings. Fracture care is an area like adenoidectomies that requires special attention in the detail given to the parents. The observations to the fractured limb completed by the nursing staff needs to be informally continued at home. This includes the peripheral vascular observations such as the following.

- Colour (the extremities need to remain pink with brisk capillary return).
- Warmth (the fingers or toes should be as warm as the opposite hand or foot).
- Movement (should be able to wriggle fingers or toes).
- Sensation (should be normal without any numbness or tingling).
- Pain (which should be relieved by simple analgesia).

If any of these observations deteriorate, such as the colour or sensation, the parents must elevate the limb if not already elevated and if the colour or sensation does not return, or the pain is unrelieved by simple analgesia, the child needs medical review. A fractured leg should remain elevated on pillows whilst the child rests and a fractured arm may need to be elevated either on pillows across the chest or in a 'gallows' sling (may be made from an inverted pillow slip in which the elbow rests in the pocket of the pillow slip and a string or rope is attached to the other end to suspend the arm up off the bed) suspended from above. If the child presents with deterioration in the neuro-vascular observations or an increase in pain disproportionate to the injury, they may be at risk of developing compartments syndrome.

Compartment syndrome

Identification of compartment syndrome can be difficult in children particularly if they are not able to verbalise the signs and symptoms. Assessment of the limb should be done to the unaffected limb first so that a set of baseline observations can be established with which to compare with the affected limb. (Harvey, 2001). There is a risk of compartments syndrome with any fracture or trauma to a limb. The signs to observe for are increased pain unrelieved by simple analgesia, swelling (which is not visible if a plaster covers the limb) pallor and/or numbness to the fingers or toes. If non-invasive treatment such as elevating the limb or the orthopaedic surgeon splitting the cast to release pressure does not relieve these signs, then the child may have compartments syndrome. Compartments syndrome can occur following surgery or injury to a limb. The muscles of the body are covered in a tough membrane called the fascia. If bleeding or swelling of the muscle occurs after surgery or injury, the pressure can build up to the extend that nerves and blood vessels can become damaged. Because the muscle, nerves and blood vessels are contained within the fascia, the whole unit is termed a compartment, hence the name compartments syndrome. Acute compartments syndrome constitutes a medical emergency and if not treated may result in paralysis, the loss of the limb or death (American Academy of Orthopaedic Surgeons, 2005). Treatment involves a return to theatre for a fasciotomy (incision of the fascia) to release the pressure.

Admission to theatre

When the child is called to theatre, a nurse accompanies the child and parent to the theatre reception area. The ward stage theatre checklist is then rechecked by the RN in theatre reception and often checked again by the anaesthetic nurse who takes the child accompanied by their parent into theatre for induction. The parent must leave once the child is induced. After the checks are completed, the ward nurse returns to the ward. Reminding the child that you will see them when they return and then they can have a drink/ice block, and something to eat often reduces their anxiety.

Ward stage recovery: post-operative care

In order to be discharged from the post-anaesthetic care unit (recovery), the child must meet the following criteria:

- Easily roused
- Can maintain and protect (the gag reflex) own airway
- Stable vital signs equivalent to pre-operative values or as specified by anaesthetist (e.g., SaO_2 above 94%)
- No obvious surgical complications
- Pain nausea and vomiting controlled
- Documentation complete
- Child is clean, dry, warm and comfortable (Waterman, 2002).

If a child is anxious or distressed and not ready for return to the ward, the recovery staff will organise for the parent to join them in recovery; once recovered, the parents can return with the child and nurse escort to the ward. The recovery RN provides a bedside handover of the child. This includes the procedure the child has undergone, the post-operative medical orders, the type of anaesthetic and the analgesia given in theatre and recovery and a visual check of any wounds and their dressings. The ward RN then completes a set of observations. Ward observations are repeated half hourly except for adenoidectomies that are completed 15 minutely. These duplicate the ongoing assessments that were recorded in recovery:

- Monitoring of the airway, respirations and oxygen saturations
- Circulation, pulse, blood pressure (where required), colour
- Temperature
- Level of consciousness, rousability or sedation
- Pain
- Wound ooze, dressings, drains
- Intravenous access
- Special observations such as circulation for limb surgery or blood sugar levels.

Post-operative recovery on the ward must be for a minimum of 1 hour, more for certain procedures.

Transport – anaesthetics outside the OR

There are a number of types of diagnostic and therapeutic procedures requiring a general anaesthetic outside of the OR. Many of these children are admitted to day surgery pre- and post-procedure for admission and then post-anaesthetic care. The procedures are generally non-invasive but may require the child to lie motionless for extended periods. The younger child tends to require a GA to ensure they lie still.

Examples of such procedures include total body irradiation (TBI) necessary before a bone marrow transplant, computerised tomography (CT) scans, magnetic resonance imaging (MRI) scans, ultrasound guided fine needle aspirates, bone scans at nuclear medicine and some audiology testing.

When the child receives a general anaesthetic outside the OR, there are some safety issues that need to be addressed. The child may walk or be carried by a parent to the procedure site (such as the X-ray or MRI department) but must be recovered and transported back to the ward on a trolley, which has oxygen and suctioning equipment. The safety measures required for the recovery and transport of a child who has received a general anaesthetic outside the OR include the following personnel and equipment:

- A paediatric anaesthetist to administer the anaesthetic
- A paediatric anaesthetic nurse/technician to assist
- A RN with advanced airway management skills to recover the child
- A patient transport trolley
- Oxygen and suctioning equipment
- A portable SaO$_2$ monitor with an audible pulse and alarm
- An air viva resuscitator with appropriate sized masks and guedell's airways
- Patient chart and recovery observation sheet
- Pillow and warm blanket.

The recovery environment must have wall unit oxygen and suction and an emergency call system. In this tertiary paediatric facility, there is a team of transport nurses who liaise with DPC and the anaesthetic team to transport the patient to the procedure ensuring all the appropriate equipment and personnel are available. In some instances, the anaesthetist will escort the child directly following the general anaesthetic to the ward area. In such cases, the transport nurse is required to remain with the child on the ward until they have met the recovery discharge criteria. They can then handover the patient to the ward staff who will complete the ward post-anaesthetic observations for a minimum of 1 hour prior to discharge (Royal Children's Hospital, 2004).

Drinking and eating

Some procedures such as a flexible bronchoscopy involve the use of an anaesthetic spray to the vocal cords. This prevents the child going into laryngospasm during the passing of the bronchoscope through the larynx. The anaesthetic spray may diminish the gag reflex, leaving the child at risk of aspirating or choking if fed before the local anaesthetic has worn off. Because of this, the child is not to take anything orally until 1 hour after their cords were sprayed. For the majority of day surgery cases, the child may be given a glass of water or cordial on return to the ward or an ice block, which is more readily tolerated. If tolerated, they are offered food, usually a within 15–30 minutes after their return. Some parents seek to feed their child immediately on return, but it is preferable to err on the side of caution and commence on fluids first to determine that they are not nauseous or likely to vomit. Babies can be the exception to the rule, given a bottle of milk or formula on return if they refuse water, as the baby's distress on return may simply be hunger, and it is best to eliminate that from their distress before you can determine if they are actually crying in pain. Breast fed babies may be fed immediately following their return to the ward, and may have already had a feed from their mother in the recovery unit.

Voiding

The child may not necessarily void prior to discharge as they may have consumed only one to two glasses of water or cordial since their original fasting time. This is not a problem unless they have undergone a procedure such as a cystoscopy in which case they are to be encouraged to drink until they have voided, as there is a risk of trauma to the urethra, which may prevent them from voiding.

Pain relief

Older children will tend to acknowledge they have pain when asked. The parents are often the best at recognising if their child is in pain. On the initial return to the ward post-anaesthetic, children can be distressed from the effects of the anaesthetic drugs; some of the gas inductions can result in the child being very irritable on return. If the child is due for analgesia on return and has not received any analgesia in recovery, it is often preferable to give analgesia to rule out pain as a reason for their irritability. It can be difficult to assess the level of pain in the preverbal children. If, for example, a hungry child refuses to drink or eat and cannot settle with the comfort of their parents present and yet continues to be distressed, pain is very likely the cause.

Wound care

The wound should be viewed on return to the ward and included as part of the handover from the recovery nurse. It needs to be checked with each subsequent set of observations. Most dressings need to be kept dry and intact for the first 48 hours following surgery. Parents need to be aware of signs of infection such as:

- reddened and/or inflamed wound site;
- fevers;
- offensive smell and/or discharge from the wound;
- increased pain at the wound site.

The reviewing doctor may remove the dressing if the follow-up appointment is within a week of surgery. If longer, the parents are instructed to either soak off the dressing in the bath/shower or remove it when it begins to fall off.

Preparation for discharge

The child must meet the following criteria (which has been both observed and documented) before they may be safely discharged into the care of the parents:

- Vital signs (pulse, respirations and colour) are within normal limits and have been for longer than 30 minutes.

- The child has been alert and orientated to time and place (age appropriate) for 1 hour prior to discharge.
- There is no wound ooze or active bleeding.
- Pain is assessed and controlled with oral analgesia (which must be available at home).
- The child is not vomiting and has tolerated food/fluid as appropriate to the child.

The parent or legal custodian must accompany the child on discharge from the ward. Discharge instructions must be given to the parent or legal custodian accompanying the child, including the hospital's Department of Emergency Medicine contact number for after hour's assistance if needed. Children undergoing certain procedures (such as adenoidectomy) may be required to stay in the ward 4–6 hours postoperatively, and within vicinity of the hospital overnight, if they live too far from the hospital (Gwinn *et al.*, 2004). Once all these criteria are met and the child has ambulated (if appropriate), the intravenous cannula can be removed and the child is ready to go home.

Going home

In order to go home, the RN caring for the child needs to confirm that the parent or guardian has all necessary documentation and medications/dressings as required, including:

- a discharge script if required (dispensed from the hospital pharmacy unless an outside script has been written);
- discharge letter from the medical officer (if not completed may be posted);
- medical certificate if required for the parent or guardian's employee;
- follow-up appointment (may also be posted if not yet scheduled);
- confirmation that the parent or guardian has the information brochure and the hospital phone numbers for any after hour's concerns;
- travel and accommodation subsidy forms completed by the medical officer if required;.
- appropriate transport home.

Conclusion: support at home

Parents are encouraged to phone the day procedure unit or the hospital emergency department (after hours) with any concerns. From there, they will be instructed either to present to their local GP or to return to the hospital, or may simply have their concerns alleviated.

References

Aantaa, R., Manner, T. (1999). Management of the paediatric patient. *Current Opinion in Anaesthesiology*, 12: 649–655.

American Academy of Orthopaedic Surgeons. (2005). Available from http://orthoinfo. aaos.org/fact/thr_report.cfm?Thread_ID=287&topcategory=About%20Orthopaedics (accessed 11 April 2007).

Anderson, K., Anderson, L., Glanze, W. (1994). *Mosby's medical, nursing and allied health dictionary*, 4th ed. Mosby, St. Louis.

Avitsland, T., Kristensen, C., Emblem, R., Veenstra, M., Mala, T. Bjornland, K. (2006). Percutaneous endoscopic gastrostomy in children: a safe technique with major symptom relief and high parental satisfaction. *Journal of Pediatric Gastroenterology and Nutrition*, 43: 624–628.

Edler, A., Mariano, E., Golianu, B., Kuan, C.M., Pentcheva, K. (2007). An analysis of factors influencing postanesthesia recovery after pediatric ambulatory tonsillectomy and adenoidectomy. *Anesthesia and Analgesia*, 104: 784–789.

Ellsworth, P., Cendron, M., Ritland, D. McCullough, M. (1999). Hypospadius repair in the 1990s. *Association of Operating Room Nurses Journal*, 69: 148–156.

Glasper, E., Haggarty, R. (2006). The psychological preparation of children for hospitalisation. In: Glasper, E., Richardson, J. (eds). *A textbook of children's and young peoples nursing*. Churchill Livingstone, Elsevier, Edinburgh.

Gwinn, J., Sullivan, P., Edwards, S., Cliff, K. (2004). *Day procedure centre orientation manual*. Royal Children's Hospital, Brisbane.

Harvey, C. (2001). Compartment syndrome: When it is least expected. *National Association of Orthopaedic Nurses*, 20: 15–25.

Hemphill, A., Dearmun, A. (2006). Working with children and families. In: Glasper, E., Richardson, J. (eds). *A textbook of children's and young peoples nursing*. Churchill Livingstone, Elsevier, Edinburgh.

Heron, A., Shields, L., Tanner, A., Waterman, L. (2002). Surgical procedures on children. In: Shields, L., Werder, H. (eds). *Perioperative nursing*. Greenwich Medical Media, London.

Jaksic, T., Nigro, J., Hicks, M. (2000). Nevus and melanoma. In: Ashcraft, K., Murphy, J., Sharp, R., Sigalet, D., Snyder, C. (eds). *Paediatric surgery*, 3rd ed. M.T. Saunders, Philadelphia.

Jarrett, P. (2001). Day care surgery. *European Journal of Anaesthesiology*, 18: 32–35.

Kankkunen, P., Vehviläinen-Julkunen, K., Pietilä, A. (2002). Children's postoperative pain at home: Family interview study. *International Journal of Nursing Practice*, 8: 32–41.

Koinig, H. (2002). Preparing parents for their child's surgery: Preoperative parental information and education. *Paediatric Anaesthesia*, 12: 107–109.

Laberge, J., Nguyen, L., Shaw, K. (2000). Teratomas, dermoids and other soft tissue tumours. In: Ashcraft, K., Murphy, J., Sharp, R., Sigalet, D., Snyder, C. (eds). *Paediatric surgery*, 3rd ed. M.T. Saunders, Philadelphia.

Maldonado, S., Nygren, C. (1999). Pediatric surgery. In: Meeker, M., Rothrock, J. (eds). *Alexander's care of the patient in surgery*, 11th ed. Mosby, St Louis.

Mathews, J. (2006). Communicating with children and their families. In: Glasper, E., Medline Plus. (2008). Medical Encyclopedia: Chalazion. Available from http://www.nlm.nih.gov/medlineplus/ency/article/001006.htm (accessed 12 May 2009).

Richardson, J. (eds). *A textbook of children's and young people's nursing*. Churchill Livingstone, Elsevier, Edinburgh.

Palmer, B. (1988). Correction of prominent ears. In: Mustard, J., Jackson, I. (eds). *Plastic Surgery in Infancy and Childhood*, 3rd ed. Churchill Livingstone, Edinburgh.

Prabhu, A., Chung, F. (2001). Anaesthetic strategies towards developments in day care surgery. *European Journal of Anaesthesiology*, 18: 36–42.

Royal Children's Hospital. (2004). *Discharge criteria for assessing recovery following a general anaesthetic. Policy and Procedure Manual, Policy number 17001*. Royal Children's Hospital, Brisbane.

Sprinzl, G., Koebke, J., Wimmers-Klick, J., Eckel, H., Thumfart, W. (2000). Morphology of the human thyroglossal tract: A histologic and macroscopic study in infants and children. *The Annals of Otology, Rhinology & Laryngology*, 109: 1135–1140.

Tanner, A. (2002). Paediatric plastic surgery. In: Shields, L., Werder, H. (eds). *Perioperative nursing*. Greenwich Medical Media, London.

Waterman, L. (2002). Paediatric post anaesthetic recovery. In: Shields, L., Werder, H. (eds). *Perioperative nursing*. Greenwich Medical Media, London.

Werder, H., Thompson, A. (2002). Safety measures. In: Shields, L., Werder, H. (eds). *Perioperative nursing*. Greenwich Medical Media, London.

7 Anaesthesia in children

Wendy McAlister

Introduction: What is anaesthesia?

Anaesthesia means the absence of feeling (from the Greek *an*, without and *aesthesia*, feeling). Anaesthesia has been used since ancient times. Drugs such as alcohol, opium, mandrake and cannabis were used to induce a state of anaesthesia. There were also non-drug methods used such as cold, concussion, nerve compression and hypnosis. It was not until 1846 when anaesthesia was first publicly demonstrated using ether. Anaesthesia was induced with the aim to enable a procedure to be undertaken with the least amount of physiological and psychological changes to the patient. Anaesthesia of early years was not as safe as today; patients were given large doses of single drugs such as ether or chloroform. Today's anaesthesia provides the patient with a safer and more balanced approach using combinations of drugs, which reduces the side effects associated with anaesthesia and surgery.

Providing safe anaesthesia involves maintaining and monitoring the airway, oxygenation, blood pressure, circulating blood volume, temperature and patient comfort. Anaesthesia can be divided into two types: general anaesthesia and regional or local anaesthesia.

The anaesthetic nurse

The anaesthetic nurse plays an important role in the continuing care of the paediatric patient. It is the responsibility of the anaesthetic nurse to provide a safe environment for the patient, both physically and psychologically whilst they are under anaesthetic. During anaesthesia the nurse is the patient's advocate.

Anaesthetic nurses work alongside the anaesthetists to provide the best possible care for their paediatric patients. The role of the anaesthetic nurse also includes the following:

- Be the patient's advocate while they are asleep
- Ensuring the right equipment is ready for each patient
- That the anaesthetic machine and other equipment have been checked and is ready for use
- Checking of the patient into theatre
- Assessment of patient prior to anaesthesia
- Assist with patient transfer
- Assist with regional anaesthesia

- Assisting the anaesthetist with induction, intubation, maintenance and emergence
- Attaching of monitors to patient and assessing data
- Ensure patient is comfortable, positioning of patient is important (they cannot do it for themselves)
- Keep patient documentation up to date
- Preparation and administration of drugs, e.g. antibiotics
- Attach infusions
- Assist with invasive monitoring insertion
- Handover of patient to post-anaesthetic care unit.

This role varies from institution to institution and country to country. Many countries offer post-registration courses for nurses to learn the skills to become anaesthetic nurses. Many institutions have in-house training, with on-the-job training.

Children undergoing anaesthesia

The aim of paediatric anaesthesia is to minimize physical discomfort and emotional distress to the child. Many anaesthetists will allow the parent/carer to accompany the child into the induction/theatre room. This can help with the induction, as the child feels safe because the parent/carer is present. Children can become quite anxious and scared when separated from their parents/carers. Not all parents will be able to be with their children when they are anaesthetised. This can be because of age, or because the procedure is an emergency, or anaesthetist's preference.

Children old enough to understand the difference between intravenous (IV) and gaseous induction should be given the choice. Both methods need to be explained to them. Many hospitals will allow the children to wear their own clothes into the theatre and to take a favourite teddy bear or cuddly blanket. This helps to make the children feel more comfortable and safe in an alien environment.

Pre-anaesthetic assessment

Assessing patients before surgery allows for the formulation of a plan for the anaesthetic and care of the patient during the procedure to be developed. It also allows the anaesthetist and anaesthetic nurse the opportunity to meet the patients, the families or carers. This ensures that the medical history of the child and the family are taken into consideration when formulating the anaesthetic plan. With paediatric patients undergoing procedures, it is very important that they are prepared physically and psychologically according to their age.

Preparing paediatric patients psychologically for a procedure will help reduce their anxiety. This preparation needs to be age appropriate. Parents can be an enormous help in this preparation by providing their children with as much information as the children can tolerate about the procedure. There is plenty of literature available in regards to this topic. When assessing the child, it is important to get down to the child's level and to involve the child and the parent in the discussion about the anaesthetic.

Usually there is little physical preparation needed for a procedure, unless the child is undergoing a major surgery such as cardiac or organ transplant. This preparation may include blood tests, chest X-ray, lung function and an ECG. For a patient not undergoing large procedures, physical preparation may include opening their mouth to check their airway, to ensure that there are no loose teeth or other obvious airway obstructions and listening to their lungs, to ensure that they are clear. Loose teeth may have to be removed before intubation, but after the patient is asleep. If not, they may fall out during intubation and obstruct the airway.

The Mallampati is a scoring system used to indicate if intubation is going to be difficult (Mallampati *et al.*, 1985). This scoring system is used successfully in both adults and children. When the patient opens their mouth and sticks out their tongue, certain anatomical features should be visible. If these anatomical features are not visible, this generally suggests how difficult the intubation is going to be. The higher the grade the more difficult the intubation. This enables a plan to be developed prior to intubation (Figure 7.1).

When assessing the patient prior to the procedure, it is important to find out as much information as possible about them. This should include their past and present medical and surgical history, family medical history, medication they might be taking and why, if they have any allergies, and if anybody in their family, or they themselves, have had any problems with anaesthetics. Since many paediatric patients are unable to answer these questions, you will have to rely on the parents or carers for the information.

Many countries use American Society of Anaesthetists (ASA) status as a way of catergorising patients prior to surgery to describe their physical health and assess their anaesthetic risk. It was developed by the ASA (1941), and is equally applicable to children as to adult patients. Box 7.1 shows the ASA categories. In some instances, if surgery is deemed to be an emergency, then an 'E' is placed after the number; 5 is always an emergency and should, therefore, always include an 'E'.

	Grade I	Grade II	Grade III	Grade IV
Anatomical feature	Faucal pillars, soft palate and uvula are visible	Faucal pillars, soft palate and uvula is obscured by base of tongue	Only the soft palate is visible	Not even the soft palate is visible

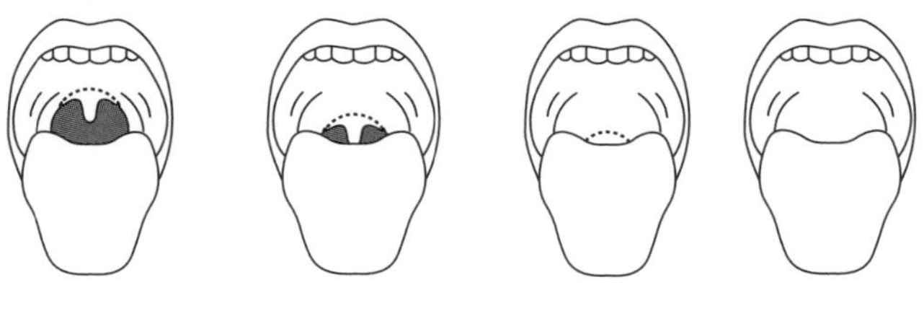

Fig. 7.1   Mallampati scoring system (Mallampati *et al.*, 1985). Illustrations reproduced from Robinson *et al.* (2006), *How to survive in anaesthesia*, with permission from Wiley-Blackwell.

Anaesthetic equipment

The anaesthetic machine is designed to deliver a variable amount of oxygen, air, nitrous oxide and various volatile anaesthetic agents safely to patients, at a continuous

Box 7.1   ASA physical classification system (American Society of Anaesthetists, 2008).

1. A normal healthy patient.
2. A patient with mild systemic disease with no functional impairment.
3. A patient with severe systemic disease with functional impairment.
4. A patient with severe systemic disease that is a constant threat to life.
5. A moribund patient who is not expected to survive without the operation.
6. A declared brain dead patient whose organs are being removed for donor purposes.

constant rate. The machine is also usually the housing for monitors and is used as a workstation. The machine is made up of three main parts:

1. High-pressure system

- *Wall outlets*, where the gas pipelines come out of the wall. Gases under high pressure are delivered through the wall outlets.
- *Gas pipelines* connect the anaesthetic machine to the wall outlets.
- *Cylinders of gases* are included as a back-up system, in case there is a failure of gas from the wall outlets. These gases are also under high pressure.
- *Pressure gauges* indicate the pressure of the gases from the wall outlets or the cylinders to which they are attached.
- *Regulators* reduce the pressure of the gases from the wall outlet or cylinder to allow for better flow control. Gases coming from the wall outlet or cylinder are at too high a pressure to be used without some control of their flow.

2. Low-pressure system

- *Anti-hypoxia device* (if fitted). This prevents gases being delivered with inadequate oxygen content.
- *Oxygen failure alarm* will alarm if there is a drop in pressure or failure of gas in the supply pipeline.
- *Flowmeters* allow for fine control of gas to the patient.
- *Vaporiser* turns liquid into a vapour and enables anaesthetic liquid to be turned into a vapour so that it can be mixed with other gases and delivered to the patient.
- *Common gas outlet* is the opening where the mixed gases come out of the anaesthetic machine.

3. Breathing system

The breathing system consists of two different groups, the circle systems and the T-pieces. They are designed to take gases to the patient from the anaesthetic machine.

- *Circle systems* are so named because of the circular direction of gas flow. The gases flow to the patient, then back through a carbon dioxide absorber and then back to the patient. The gases can flow in one direction only due to one-way valves placed within the circuit. Soda lime is used as the carbon dioxide absorber. This system allows low flow gases to be used.

- *T-piece rebreathing systems* (Figure 7.2). This system allows some rebreathing of gases. High flows of gases are needed to prevent carbon dioxide retention. The T-piece is commonly used in paediatric anaesthesia. The patient can be hand ventilated using a T-piece; usually the patient spontaneously breathes throughout the procedure. There are many variations of the T-piece.

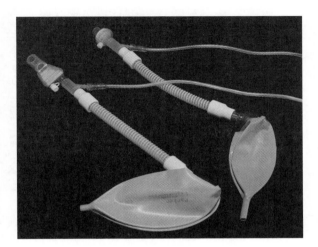

Fig. 7.2 Paediatric T-pieces with gas tubing, filters and rebreathing bags attached.

Both of these breathing systems have infection control measures. These are two viral filters: one positioned between the machine and the breathing circuit and one attached to the breathing device in the patient. These should be disposed of and replaced between each case (Harley *et al.*, 2000).

Scavenging of gases is an important component of the anaesthetic machine. This apparatus, which can be attached to the suction system, removes gases and vapours vented from the breathing system, prevents contamination of the rest of the operating theatre and surrounding environment.

Face masks (Figure 7.3) should be in the appropriate size for each patient. Facemasks come in a variety of sizes from double zero (00) to size five. Double zero masks are

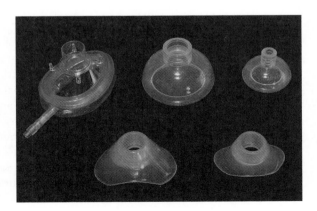

Fig. 7.3 A range of face masks used in paediatrics.

usually used on neonates and size five masks on adults. The appropriate size will depend on the fit, which should ensure that there are no leaks, and the mask covers both the nose and the mouth. The fit is important because in paediatrics gas induction is the most commonly used method for induction. The correct fitting mask also reduces the dead space in the mask.

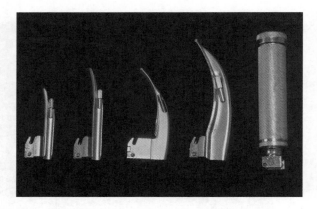

Fig. 7.4 Laryngoscopes – handle, with curved (MacIntosh) and straight blades.

Laryngoscopes (Figure 7.4) are used for the introduction of endotracheal tubes (ETTs) into the trachea. They consist of a handle, which contains the batteries, and a blade, which has a light in it so as the vocal cords can be visualised. Blades come in varying sizes from a zero to a four. They can also be straight or curved (Macintosh). Straight blades are more commonly used in children under 1 year. The handle is held in the left hand and the blade is introduced into the right side of the mouth. The tongue is pushed to the left as the blade is advanced. The light source illuminates the pharyngeal structures. If a curved blade (also called Macintosh blade) is used, the blade is advanced until the epiglottis is visualised. Upward leverage is applied to the handle, lifting the epiglottis and exposing the vocal cords. The ETT is then introduced and passed through cords. Curved blades are used in older children, while a straight-bladed laryngoscope is used in children. The blade is advanced over the epiglottis, trapping it and lifting it when upward leverage is applied, and the ETT inserted. It is always important to have a spare laryngoscope handle and blade ready, just in case of light failure.

Airways

ETTs (Figure 7.5) provide a patent airway in the unconscious patient. Modern tubes are single use and made of clear PVC plastic that softens at body temperature. ETTs are used to ensure gases go straight into the lungs and not into the stomach, therefore protecting the patient's airway. ETTs come in a variety of sizes and styles. Sizes vary from 2.5 to 10 mm in whole and half sizes and the measurement is the internal diameter of the tube. Styles include nasal, oral, cuffed, non-cuffed, reinforced, rae, microlaryngoscopy and double lumen. These are all made from clear plastic so that secretions and condensation can be seen. They contain a radio-opaque thread so that their position can be assured by X-ray if necessary. Tubes also have measurements printed on them

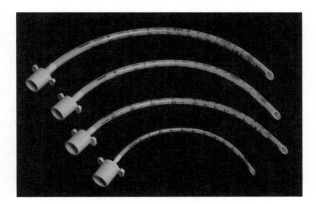

Fig. 7.5 Paediatric ETTs (note absence of cuff).

for insertion length. There is a bevel on the tip of the tube designed to be atraumatic to tissues. The 'Murphy eye' – an extra hole on the side of the tube just above the tip – is a safety feature that allows for ventilation if the tip is occluded. Standard 15-mm connectors on all tracheal tubes fit the 22-mm breathing circuit connectors.

In children, it is important to choose the correct size as too large a tube can cause damage and oedema. Un-cuffed tubes are most commonly used in paediatrics so as to prevent oedema to the cricoid ring. Choosing the appropriate size is important. The following demonstrates formulae that can be used for calculating the appropriate size and length of ETT. These formulae are appropriate only for children over the age of 1 year (Rusy & Usaleva, 1998).

- Internal diameter (mm) = (age/4) + 4
- Insertion length (cm) = (age/2) + 12 for oral tubes
- Insertion length (cm) = (age/2) + 15 for nasal tubes

For example, for a 4-year-old child it would be (4/4) + 4 = 4 mm ETT

oral tube length would be (4/2) + 12 = 14 cm
nasal tube length would be (4/2) + 15 = 17 cm

Once the tube size is chosen, it is important to have a tube one size larger and one size smaller ready for use. The correct size tube is the one that passes through the vocal cords easily and ensures that there is a small, audible leak. Sometimes a malleable introducer may be necessary to facilitate the introduction of the tube through the vocal cords. Once the tube is in place the introducer can be removed.

Laryngeal mask airway (LMA) (Figure 7.6) is an effective airway management device which sits at the distal end of the pharynx above the level of the vocal cords to maintain a patent airway (Anaesthesia UK, 2009). LMAs are widely used throughout paediatric procedures, especially in short duration anaesthetics, and provide an adequate airway without the need for intubation. The LMA can be used in patients with difficult airways as there is no need to visualise the vocal cords. LMAs are most commonly used in spontaneously breathing anaesthetised patients, although positive pressure ventilation may be applied. They are used in operations where muscle relaxation is not required, and where duration is less than 3 hrs. However, the main

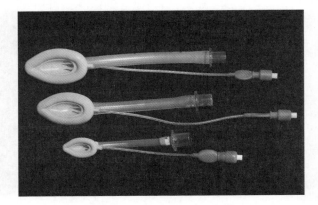

Fig. 7.6 Laryngeal mask airways.

disadvantage with an LMA is that it does not protect against aspiration. They are reusable and can be cleaned and sterilised between uses, and single-use LMAs are now available. When using reusable LMAs, it is important to ensure that the tubing is clear and flexible, that all the connectors are intact, that the LMA inflates properly and has no holes. They come in a range of sizes (Table 7.1) and styles, and these include classic, ProSeal™, Fasttrac™ and reinforced.

Table 7.1 Laryngeal mask sizes

Size	Weight of Patient	Amount of Air in Cuff
1	<5 kg	<4 ml
1.5	5–10 kg	<7 ml
2	10–20 kg	<10 ml
2.5	20–30 kg	<14 ml
3	30–50 kg	<20 ml
4	Small/normal adult	<30 ml
5	Normal/large adult	<40 ml

Oropharyngeal airway (Guedel's) (Figure 7.7) can be used to assist with an airway before intubation and after extubation. Once a patient is unconscious, their tongue can

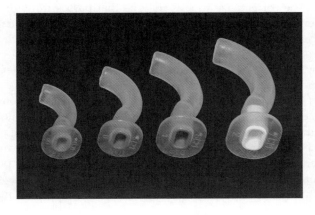

Fig. 7.7 Oropharyngeal (Guedel's) airways in different sizes.

become floppy and collapse backwards, occluding their airway. Insertion of a correct sized airway can reopen the child's airway by pulling the tongue forward. Choosing the correct size is very important, because if an airway is too small it will not pull the tongue out of the way, and if it is too large then the oropharyngeal airway can occlude the airway further back. Correct size is determined by measuring the airway against the patient, from the corner of the mouth to the ear lobe. Guedel airways range in size from 000 to 5, and are inserted upside down into the mouth, with the tip pointing to the hard palate, and then turning it over once it is in the back of the throat.

Nasopharyngeal airway can be used in the conscious patient to maintain a patent airway. It is inserted through the nares and along the curvature of the nasopharynx and into the oropharynx. These come in a variety of sizes. Choose one that will fit through the nares.

Anaesthesia

General anaesthesia is the state when the patient is made reversibly unconscious for the duration of the procedure. General anaesthesia causes loss of reflexes, motor skills and sensation, allowing for controlled balanced hypnosis (sleep), analgesia and amnesia. The induction of general anaesthesia is usually with either gas inhalation or IV drugs.

Gas inhalation is the most common, though by no means the only, method of induction in paediatrics. In adults, monitoring and cannulation prior to induction is usually established; in paediatrics, this generally causes too much physical discomfort and emotional distress. Gas induction can be achieved by using a combination of gases, e.g. oxygen, nitrous oxide and a volatile anaesthetic agent. Sevoflurane is commonly used as the volatile agent as it provokes minimal airway irritation and is very fast acting. Gas induction is provided by using a low dead space facemask of the appropriate size, and usually a T-piece connected to the anaesthetic machine. Once gas induction has been achieved, the anaesthetist, more often than not, will cannulate the child and monitoring can be established.

IV induction is typically used in children who have been cannulated prior to arriving in the operating theatre, in the cooperative child, or when a rapid sequence induction is going to be performed. In the cooperative child, it is usual practice to apply a local anaesthetic cream to the area of cannulation as a premedication. IV induction is achieved usually by a combination of drugs, e.g. analgesics, anaesthetic, plus or minus muscle relaxants. Monitoring can usually be commenced prior to induction, if not then it is commenced immediately after induction.

Drugs that can be used in anaesthesia include but are not limited to premedication, anaesthetic, analgesia and muscle relaxants.

Premedications are commonly used in paediatrics in the form of topically applied local anaesthetics on the area where cannulation will be attempted by the anaesthetist. In some countries, as standard practice, other premedications are generally not used unless the child needs to be sedated or the child is extremely anxious. However, in other countries, it is standard practice to use a sedative such as Midazolam as a premedication.

Anaesthetic used can be either IV or inhalation agents. *IV agents* commonly used in paediatric practice include propofol (MIMSOnline, 2008a) and thiopentone (MIMSOnline, 2008b) (Table 7.2) (*Paediatric pharmacopeia*, 2002).

Table 7.2   IV anaesthetic agents commonly used in children

Drug	Effects	Side Effects	Other	Dose
Propofol	Sedation Hypnosis Anaesthesia Rapid onset Short acting (5 minutes) Analgesia	Hypotension Apnoea Excitatory reactions Cough Pain on injection Flush/rash Shivering (recovery)	Can be used to maintain anaesthesia Can be used for sedation Fast awakening	Induction: 2.5–3.5 mg/kg Maintenance: 7.5–15 mg/kg in children 3 years and over
Thiopentone	Hypnosis Anaesthesia Rapid onset Short acting (5 minutes)	Respiratory depression Myocardial depression Laryngospasm Sneezing, coughing Shivering (recovery)	Slow awakening Anticonvulsant	Neonates: 3–4 mg/kg titrated to effect Infants and children: 5–6 mg/kg titrated to effect

Inhalation agents are liquids that are turned into vapour in an agent-specific vapor-iser and then inhaled (Table 7.3). Volatiles are absorbed into the circulation via the alveoli. Volatile agents have few analgesic properties. The minimum alveolar con-centration (MAC) of the volatile agent is defined as the concentration of the agent that prevents 50% of people reacting to surgical stimulus (Eger, 2001). This measure is used to compare the strength of volatile anaesthetic agents, and the agent's MAC nor-mally determines the dose. The use of analgesia with volatiles will usually reduce the MAC. Table 7.3 shows the various MAC of different volatile agents commonly used in paediatric practice.

Table 7.3   Volatile inhalation agents commonly used in children

Drug	Advantages	Side Effects	MAC
Sevoflurane	Rapid onset Rapid recovery Can be used for induction and maintenance of anaesthesia	Airway obstruction Laryngospasm Bradycardia Nausea and vomiting Agitation (recovery) Dizziness (recovery) Malignant hyperthermia	2.5–3.5% in children without analgesia
Isoflurane	Rapid onset Can be used for induction but has a pungent smell Can be used for maintenance of anaesthesia	Hypotension Shivering (recovery) Nausea and Vomiting	1.6–1.8% in children without analgesia
Desflurane	Can be used for maintenance of anaesthesia Rapid recovery	Coughing, breath holding, apnoea and laryngospasm if used as induction agent Nausea and vomiting	5.75–10.65% in children without analgesia

Along with these volatile agents other gases are used. Oxygen or air is used in conjunction with the volatiles, and nitrous oxide can be added. Nitrous oxide and oxygen can be used prior to induction. Nitrous oxide has the added benefit of being an analgesic. Today's anaesthetic machines prevent nitrous oxide being given without adequate oxygen or air, which is potentially dangerous.

Patients are usually paralysed prior to intubation with an ETT, as paralysing the vocal cords and the muscles that control respiration allows intubation and ventilation to occur without resistance. Also, some forms of surgery require the patient's muscles to be relaxed. Such paralysation requires the use of muscle relaxants. These drugs are divided into two types: depolarising and non-depolarising (Table 7.4). The only *depolarising muscle relaxant* available is suxamethonium (MIMSOnline, 2008c). Paralysis occurs in less than 30 seconds, after the patient fasciculates (twitches). Its duration of action is 3–5 minutes and it is broken down by plasma pseudo-cholinesterase. Suxamethonium is used when there is a need for rapid onset of paralysis for intubation, e.g. in emergencies, when the patient has a full stomach, or when there is a

Table 7.4 Paralysing agents

Drug	Effects	Side Effects	Other	Dose
Suxamethonium (depolarising)	Very rapid acting approximately 30 seconds Effects lasts 3–5 minutes	Bradycardia Malignant hyperthermia Excessive salivation	Non-reversible Can be used IM Used in rapid sequence intubation	IV 1–2 mg/kg/dose IM 2.5 mg/kg/dose
Non-depolarising				
Mivacurium	Onset slow 3–4 minutes Effects last 14–16 minutes	Histamine release Hypotension Bradycardia Bronchospasm	Does not need to be reversed Reversed by neostigmine	IV 0.1–0.2 mg/kg
Atracurium	Onset 2–2.5 minutes Effects last 20–25 minutes	Histamine release Hypotension	Reversed by neostigmine	IV 0.1–0.6 mg/kg
Cisatracurium	Onset 2 minutes Effects last 45 minutes	Hypotension Bradycardia Bronchospasm	Reversed by neostigmine	IV 0.1 mg/kg
Rocuronium	Onset 1 minute Effects last 30–40 minutes	Histamine reaction Tachycardia Prolonged paralysis	Increasing the dose decreases the onset time. Can be used in modified rapid sequence Reversed by neostigmine Can be used IM	IV 0.6–1.2 mg/kg
Vecuronium	Onset 2–3 minutes Effects last about 20–40 minutes	Tachycardia Hypotension	Reversed by neostigmine	IV 0.1 mg/kg

need for rapid offset of paralysis, such as difficult intubations, and in short cases. Suxamethonium has some side effects, which include the following:

- In a small percentage of the population, suxamethonium causes prolonged paralysis, as they have altered or deficient plasma pseudocholinesterase.
- It releases potassium from cells and hyperkalaemia can result, especially in patients with extensive burns or muscle damage, spinal injury or neuropathy, or renal failure.
- It raises intracranial and intraocular pressures.
- It causes postoperative muscle pains, especially in children.
- It can be a trigger for malignant hyperthermia.

Non-depolarising muscle relaxants block impulse receptor sites on the muscle, and paralysis occurs when more than 70% of these sites are occupied (MIMSOnline, 2008d). This usually occurs within 3 minutes. Repeated boluses may be given intraoperatively to maintain paralysis, or an infusion may be run. The drug is metabolised by the liver, and as it clears, muscle movement returns. Reversal of block can be increased by the use of an antagonist anticholinesterase drug (neostigmine). Atropine or glycopyrrolate are given with the anticholinesterase to prevent bradycardia.

Analgesia

Analgesia can be used in conjunction with the other drugs of anaesthesia. Analgesia can be given pre-, intra- and postoperatively. They can be administered intravenously, intramuscularly, intranasally, orally, topically and per rectum. A detailed explanation of analgesia in children's surgery is given in Chapter 4.

Patient preparation

It is important to ensure that the child is prepared as completely as possible. This preparation begins before the child comes to hospital. It is important that parents/carers talk to their children about their admission to hospital and to answer their questions truthfully. There are videos, books and brochures from most hospitals available for parents/carers and children to help them understand about their admission. Some hospitals encourage the family to visit the hospital prior to the procedure to help facilitate a less stressful hospital admission. Pre-admission visiting will also go some way to ensuring that the family understands the procedure, that any investigations that have been done are satisfactory, that the documentation is up to date, consent is obtained and an anaesthetic plan commenced. It is an opportunity for the staff to inform the child and family about fasting times and whether regular medications should be taken prior to arriving at hospital. Most regular medications should be given prior to the anaesthetic, although the anaesthetist will make that final decision. Anxiety is very common in children attending hospital and everything that can be done to help reduce this is beneficial to the child, the parents/carers and hospital staff.

Fasting

Fasting is thought to reduce the risk of aspiration of stomach contents during induction and at emergence. Fasting times for children depend on their age, health status and, if infants, whether they are breastfed. Too long a fasting time can cause dehydration and hypoglycaemia, especially in infants. In many hospitals, fasting times for elective surgery are 6 hrs for food and 2 hrs for clear fluids prior to surgery, though evidence suggests that a shorter period may be more beneficial in providing comfort to the child, while there is little evidence that the longer period reduces the risk of aspiration (Brady *et al.*, 2005). Research has shown that clear fluids up to 2 hrs prior to surgery (in healthy children) does not increase the risk of aspiration, and existing literature supports shortened fasting periods for breast milk (3 hrs) and formula (4 hrs) (Cook-Stather & Litman, 2006).

Fasting may not always be possible due to emergency surgery and if there is any doubt about the patients' fasting a rapid or modified rapid induction is used.

Premedication

Because of the short procedure times common in children's surgery, and the types of procedures performed, many anaesthetists will not prescribe premedications for children, although there is much debate on this issue, and it changes from country to country. Some of the drugs that are used for premedication include:

- topical local anaesthetic cream, placed at the cannula insertion site;
- paracetamol, given prophylactically for pain relief;
- midazolam, for the reduction of anxiety and its amnesic properties;
- temazepam, for its sedative and amnesic properties;
- salbutamol for its bronco dilating properties.

Debate around the use of midazolam discusses the long time of impairment of cognitive function and memory loss in children (up to 48 hrs) (Millar *et al.*, 2007); while others discuss the potential for other drugs such as clonidine (Bergendahl *et al.*, 2005). However, the most commonly used premedication in paediatrics is topical anaesthetic creams to possible IV sites. Its effectiveness in reducing the pain of venous cannulation is well described (Maunuksela & Korpela, 1986; Lander *et al.*, 2006), and if it is the sole premedication, it has no long-term after-effects, so the child is awake and alert once the anaesthetic has worn off.

Loose teeth and nail polish

Children aged between about 6 and 12 years may have loose teeth, which need to be identified prior to induction. If these fall out during induction, they can cause an airway obstruction. Such teeth may need to be extracted by the anaesthetist prior to induction (and after the child has become unconscious). It is important that the teeth be given to the parents after the procedure, and that the child and parents be informed that this is going to happen prior to the anaesthetic. While such procedures would be covered legally by the consent form and clauses within it which describe events which are part of the anaesthetic administration, the child needs to know that their tooth may have to be removed.

Nail polish inhibits the infrared light of oxygen saturation monitors from passing through blood vessels in the fingers and also masks any colour change that could be seen by the eye. Nurses and anaesthetists need to be able to observe for cyanosis in the nail bed as an indicator of respiratory insufficiency, and so nail polish needs to be removed before the child comes to the theatre. Most theatre checklists will have a checkpoint to be completed about removal of nail polish and also that loose teeth have been identified.

Hearing aids and glasses

Hearing aids are helpful for communication prior to induction. If the child cannot hear, then his or her anxiety levels increase. However, it is also important to ensure that hearing aids are removed after induction as they can be damaged or lost. They may also cause trauma to the patient if diathermy is used during the procedure. Spectacles should be removed just prior to induction. Ensure glasses and hearing aids are placed in a container with the child's name on it and that they are sent to the PPACU with the patient. Being able to see and hear while waking up can reduce the child's anxiety and fear.

Jewellery

All jewellery should be removed prior to entrance to the operating theatre for infection control reasons, and to prevent it from getting lost. However, it may be less stressful for some children and parents if the jewellery is removed after induction. If jewellery cannot be removed, then it should be taped, but it is important to note that some jewellery may cause traumatic injury to the patient if diathermy is used during the procedure.

Preparation prior to patient arrival

Discussing the list with the anaesthetist prior to its commencement will allow the anaesthetic nurse time to prepare and gather all necessary equipment.

- The anaesthetic machine needs to be thoroughly checked prior to the child's arrival to ensure that the machine is functioning correctly. The Australian and New Zealand College of Anaesthetists (2003) has comprehensive checklists for checking the anaesthetic machine, at three levels. The first, the Level 1 check, is done by technicians on a regular basis. The Level 2 check is done at the start of every operation list and the Level 3 check must be done before every case. Any qualified health professional who is accredited in anaesthetic care can undertake the Level 2 and 3 checks, but the responsibility lies with the anaesthetist.
- Ensure that all monitoring equipment is ready, the necessary cables, leads and accessories are present, appropriate sizes are available and that everything is functional.
- Have all the airway equipment for the child available and ensure that sizes are correct. Ensure that alternative sizes are available if they are needed.
- Cannulation equipment is organised and ready for use.
- IV fluids and giving set are prepared. IV fluid pump available if needed.
- Warming equipment is ready and appropriate sizes are available.
- Regional equipment is ready and available.

- Invasive monitoring equipment needs to be available if needed.
- Patient positioning equipment needs to be in the theatre. Ensure adequate pressure relieving devices are available.
- Documentation is accessible.
- There may also be patient-specific equipment required.

Patient arrival in theatre

On arrival in the theatre complex the patient needs to be checked in. Most hospitals have a preoperative checklist. This list should include patient's details, patient identification, the operation they are having, fasting times, allergies, consent, what premedication and whether it has been given, whether the patient has had X-rays or other investigations, where parents will be waiting and if the child is bringing a favourite toy or security object with them (this should be labelled with the child's name). The preoperative checklist should have been filled out by the ward staff and then completed by the theatre staff.

If the parent/carer is coming into the theatre or induction room with the child, they need to be dressed in theatre clothes, e.g. theatre gown, theatre cap and boots. Many anaesthetists will allow a parent/carer to accompany the child into the theatre or induction room. Having a parent/carer in the induction/theatre room whilst the child is being anaesthetised can relieve anxiety and stress in the child. The use of a warm blanket can also help relieve anxiety in the patient. The child should be allowed to bring their doll, teddy bear or other comforter with them until they are unconscious, and it should be placed alongside them in the PPACU while they are regaining consciousness.

Induction

This is the process by which the patient is rendered unconscious, by either gas inhalation or IV drug. Some anaesthetists may allow the child to sit on their parent/carer's lap while they are induced. It is optimal to provide a quiet, relaxed environment for this process. This is the time when the parent/carer can provide comfort and support for their child. They can tell their child their favourite story or may sing their favourite song to them. Once the child is unconscious, the parent/carer should be escorted from the room. It is important to reassure the parent/carer that hospital staff will provide the best care possible for their child.

Parents/carers who are coming into the induction/theatre room need to be informed about what the child will look like and how they might behave as they are becoming unconscious. Their eyes might roll backwards and the child may wriggle around. As they go through the excitation phase and they will become very floppy. Parents/carers need reassurance that all this is normal.

Once the parent/carer has been escorted from the room, the child will have an IV cannula inserted and the necessary anaesthetic drugs given. The appropriate monitoring is applied; the minimal monitoring consists of being able to monitor circulation, ventilation and oxygenation (Australian and New Zealand College of Anaesthetists 2006 PS18). This can be accomplished by using pulse oximetry, capnography, ECG (normally three leads in children) and non-invasive blood pressure (NIBP).

If the child is being intubated, then muscle relaxants may be given preceding intubation. Spraying the vocal cords with local anaesthetic can also paralyse them and enable intubation without muscle relaxants. The child is ventilated via a facemask until the muscle relaxants have taken effect, then the ETT is passed through the vocal cords. The vocal cords are visualised using a laryngoscope with the appropriate blade. The placement of the tube is then checked and when the anaesthetist is happy with its position the tube is secured in place. The decision whether or not to intubate will be made on several criteria, and there are advantages and disadvantages with this approach (Table 7.5).

Table 7.5   Advantages and disadvantages of intubation in children

Advantages of Intubation	Disadvantages of Intubation
Allows for positive pressure ventilation	Can cause trauma to airway
Helps prevent aspiration of gastric contents	Patient vocal cords needs to be paralysed
Direct ventilation of lungs	Correct placement of tube can be difficult
	Teeth can be damaged

Indications for intubation include:

- the position that the child will be placed in during the procedure; some positions make it difficult to maintain an airway;
- where controlled ventilation is necessary for the procedure;
- in patients with unknown fasting times;
- when an airway cannot be maintained by other means.

Often a decision is made to use an LMA instead of intubation with an ETT. An LMA can be inserted without the use of a laryngoscope. In paediatrics, the LMA is inserted upside down and then rotated 90° once it reaches the tonsils. The LMA needs to be inflated and secured into place once the anaesthetist is happy with the placement. Table 7.6 shows the advantages and disadvantages of using an LMA, and these will help guide the anaesthetist's decision (Black & McEwan, 2004).

Table 7.6   Advantages and disadvantages of LMA insertion in children

LMA Advantages	LMA Disadvantages
No trauma to the vocal cords	Gastric inflation
Not effected by the shape of the patient's face	Cannot be used with high-pressure gases
Can be used in difficult intubation patients	Does not prevent aspiration
Easy to insert	

The child's eyelids should be taped shut to prevent any damage to the cornea. The child should be made as comfortable as possible as he or she is unable to adjust his or her own position under anaesthesia. Pressure should be alleviated from all nerves, bony prominences and vessels. Pressure relief devices should be used wherever possible, e.g. an evacuatable mattress (Wadsworth *et al.*, 1996). Ensure that surgical staff do not lean on the operating table or on the child patient, as this can change positioning, or may result in occluding tubes, etc. which are under drapes. Anaesthesia is maintained throughout the procedure by either the use of volatiles, which are continually added to the breathing circuit, or by the use of total intravenous anaesthesia (TIVA), which, as the name suggests, is a continuous infusion of an anaesthetic agent such as propofol IV. Other drugs are also given as required.

Rapid sequence induction

Rapid sequence induction reduces the risk of aspiration during induction. The anaesthetic nurses' role is very important throughout this procedure. Before a rapid sequence induction, there needs to be a plan set in place. All drugs need to be at hand and drawn in well-labelled syringes, under strict protocols. Monitoring needs to be placed on the patient prior to induction, IV access is mandatory. Patient should be pre-oxygenated for at least 5 minutes.

When the anaesthetist has given the anaesthetic agents and the muscle relaxant (usually suxamethonium) and the patient is losing consciousness, the anaesthetic nurse places pressure on the cricoid cartilage usually with the thumb and index finger; in very small children and infants, one finger applying pressure across the cricoid cartilage is sufficient. This pressure is not released until the ETT is in position and the anaesthetist instructs that cricoid pressure can be released (Padley, 2004).

Fluids

Fluids are regularly given throughout procedures to replace losses due to surgery and fasting. There are three different types of fluids used – crystalloids, colloids, blood and its components. Crystalloids contain sodium in concentrations similar to those of plasma. Hartmann's solution, sodium chloride solutions and glucose solutions are all crystalloids. Colloids are solutions that expand blood volume. These include Hemacel™, Albumex 4™ and Gelofusine™. In paediatrics, it is most important to accurately document all fluid infusion volumes to ensure that fluid overload does not occur. A controlled infusion pump or syringe driver should always be used. For long cases, urine output should be measured hourly (Harley *et al.*, 2000).

Monitoring

Monitoring of paediatric patients should include ECG, pulse oximetry, capnography and NIBP. Additionally, temperature, invasive blood pressure measurement, central venous pressure monitoring, neuromuscular monitoring and heart and breath sounds monitoring can be used.

- ECG shows the electrical activity of the heart, the heart rate, and shows the cardiac rhythm.
- Pulse oximetry gives a reading of the blood oxygen levels expressed as a percentage. The appropriate probe should be used. The percentages should be kept above 95 to prevent hypoxia, although it should always be remembered that visualising your patient may provide early indications of hypoxia, as there can be a time lapse in electronic monitoring.

- Capnography measures the concentration of carbon dioxide during expiration. Capnography is used as an indication of adequate ventilation.
- NIBP gives a reading of the child's blood pressure. Most modern monitors allow for NIBP to be taken automatically at specified time intervals.
- Temperature probes are used to continuously measure temperatures. Children are particularly prone to developing hypothermia. There are a range of thermometers used in paediatric anaesthesia, including skin, rectal, tympanic, oral and other thermometers (Bissonnette *et al.*, 1989), though a reliable, non-invasive method of measuring core temperature is elusive (Hooper, 2006).
- Invasive blood pressure measuring may be necessary in some cases, e.g. cardiac, spinal surgery or in very sick children. Invasive blood pressure measures blood pressure from inside the artery, and is the most accurate way of measuring blood pressure.
- Central venous pressure monitoring reflects the pressure in the right atria. Inotropes and other potent drugs can be given via this access.
- Neuromuscular monitoring, using peripheral nerve stimulation, should be used whenever a neuromuscular block has been used.
- Heart and breath sounds are monitored by the use of a precordial or oesophageal stethoscope. This type of monitoring can give useful information about heart rate and rhythm, cardiac output, presence of air in the heart, ventilation and bronchospasm.

Documentation

It is important to ensure that all documentation is up to date, that all fluids given, all drugs given and all observations are recorded in the child's chart. This chart must accompany the child to the PPACU.

Anaesthetic emergencies

Airway

- Laryngospasm
- Bronchospasm
- Difficult airway
- Aspiration.

LARYNGOSPASM is the most common airway emergency in children. Laryngospasm occurs when the vocal cords close or spasm, and cause a partial or complete obstruction of the airway. This can be caused by intubating (without the use of muscle relaxants) or extubating the patient when the anaesthetic is very light, or by some form of irritant touching the vocal cords, e.g. blood, mucous or a foreign body (Black & McEwan, 2004). The following are characteristics of, and treatment for, laryngospasm:

- In a partial obstruction there may be some noise, but in a complete obstruction there is no noise.
- Oxygen saturations will drop.
- Increased respiratory effort, use of axillary muscles.

- Tracheal tug.
- In a complete obstruction the chest rises and falls, but there is no air movement.
- The child may be difficult or impossible to ventilate.

Treatment:

- 100% oxygen
- Continuous positive pressure ventilation
- Deepen anaesthesia
- Suxamethonium may be needed to paralyse the vocal cords and to establish ventilation.

BRONCHOSPASM occurs when the bronchi constrict making it difficult to ventilate the patient (Thompson, 2002). An audible wheeze may be heard. Bronchospasm can be caused by:

- asthma;
- anaphylaxis;
- ETT touching the carina;
- secretions.

Treatment:

- Increase oxygen flow
- Light suction
- Consider retracting ETT slightly
- Deepen anaesthesia
- Administer bronchodilator
- Administer adrenaline for anaphylaxis.

ASPIRATION occurs when foreign material enters the lung. This is usually gastric contents. If aspiration occurs:

- place the child on her or his left side;
- suction the ETT or LMA;
- suction the oropharynx;
- apply cricoid pressure;
- ensure a chest X-ray is taken to check the lung fields.

DIFFICULT AIRWAYS can be caused by:

- congenital abnormalities;
- high arched palate;
- short jaw;
- restricted mouth opening;
- restricted neck movement.

Management:

- If identified prior to induction, a plan which involves the whole surgical and anaesthetic team is necessary.
- Ensure help is available.
- Difficult airway trolley and equipment ready and to hand.

- Inhalation induction, then the airway is assessed.
  - Can the patient be hand ventilated easily? If not, the child may need to be woken.
  - Oxygenate patient.
  - Oropharyngeal airway.
  - LMA may be used if appropriate (have at hand).
  - ETT may be needed with an introducer (have at hand).
- Unexpected difficult airway.
  - Call for help.
  - Get the trolley containing equipment for rapid intubation.
  - Oxygenate child.
  - Anaesthetist will decide whether to continue with anaesthetic or wake up the child.

Anaphylaxis

This is a life-threatening emergency. Anaphylaxis is the immune system's exaggerated response to a stimulus. In anaesthetic practice, the stimulus is normally a drug but can be latex or blood/blood product (Padley, 2004). Clinical signs of anaphylaxis include:

- rash, erythema;
- soft tissue swelling of face and upper airway, which can progress to generalised swelling;
- bronchospasm;
- hypotension;
- tachycardia;
- cardiac arrest.

Treatment:

- Discontinue all agents that could have caused anaphylaxis
- Call for help
- Remove all latex
- Give adrenaline (in repeated doses if necessary)
- 100% oxygen
- Maintain airway
- Monitor vital signs
- Support circulation with fluids
- Document anaphylaxis
- Identify stimulus (this will need to be done post-anaesthetic).

Suxamethonium apnoea

Plasma cholinesterase breaks down suxamethonium, thus reversing it (Padley, 2004). Some people have a deficiency in plasma cholinesterase which inhibits the breakdown of suxamethonium, resulting in prolonged paralysis. This is normally diagnosed when the patient fails to spontaneously breathe once the suxamethonium effects should have worn off. Treatment for suxamethonium apnoea is continued ventilation and anaesthesia until the child begins to breathe and move. Anaesthesia is continued to prevent anxiety and stress in the patient. Suxamethonium apnoea should be documented and the patient should wear a medical alert bracelet.

Malignant hyperthermia

Malignant hyperthermia is a rare inherited hypermetabolic disorder causing massive acceleration of cellular metabolism and uncontrolled muscle spasm (Padley, 2004). Malignant hyperthermia causes increases in carbon dioxide, heat and lactic acid production and increased oxygen requirements. It is caused by suxamethonium and anaesthetic volatiles. If untreated, malignant hyperthermia causes death. Signs and symptoms can occur at any time throughout the anaesthetic, even in recovery. Malignant hyperthermia is diagnosed by:

- muscle rigidity post-anaesthetic;
- unexplained hypercapneoa;
- unexplained tachycardia and hypertension;
- unexplained desaturation and cyanosis;
- increase in temperature (this may be a late sign).

Treatment:

- Cease administration of all volatile agents.
- Hyperventilate via a clean circuit.
- 100% oxygen.
- Administer reversal for hypermetabolism (Dantrolene).
- Cool patient with cool fluids.
- Correct metabolic disorders (acidosis, hyperkalaemia).
- Administer diuretics and increase fluids to prevent renal failure.
- As this condition is genetically determined. All family members should undergo testing.

Malignant hyperthermia should be documented and the patient should wear a medical alert bracelet.

Emergence

Once the procedure is finished, the child needs to be returned to consciousness and woken up. All volatiles and anaesthetic agents are ceased and 100% oxygen is administered. Neuromuscular function needs to be tested if muscle relaxants were given. Reversal may be necessary.

Before removal of the ETT, the oropharynx should be suctioned to remove excess secretions, the patient should be breathing spontaneously and be able to respond to commands (appropriate to age), e.g. 'open your eyes'. When the child is maintaining his or her airway, he or she can be transferred to the PPACU. If the patient has an LMA *in situ* it either needs to be removed when the child is deep under anaesthetic or when the patient is awake. If the patient is 'in between', there is an increased risk of laryngospasm. The LMA is not deflated prior to removal, as this prevents secretions from irritating the larynx. The patient may be transferred to the PPACU with the LMA *in situ*.

Regional anaesthesia

Regional or local anaesthesia is used for some surgical procedures and for postoperative pain relief. Regional anaesthetics can be used individually or as an adjunct to general anaesthesia (Black & McEwan, 2004).

Administration

- Topical anaesthetics can be used for biopsies and cannulation sites.
- Local anaesthesia is obtained by infiltrating the area prior to or after surgery.
- Peripheral nerve block is obtained by infiltrating local anaesthetic around the nerve proximal to the surgical site.
- Central nerve block is obtained by injecting local anaesthetic in the epidural space or the subarachnoid space. Insertion of epidural and spinal anaesthesia is done under sterile conditions.

Epidural anaesthesia

For epidural anaesthesia, a large bore 'tuohy' needle is inserted and guided between the vertebrae and into the epidural space (Thompson, 2002). Once in the epidural space, a fine catheter is inserted through the needle and the needle removed, while the catheter is left *in situ*. This allows for top-up anaesthesia to be given intraoperatively and can be left *in situ* for postoperative pain relief. This method of anaesthesia will anaesthetise the nerves as they pass through the epidural space, and will provide anaesthesia all along the selected nerves. An epidural anaesthetic can be used at any level of the spinal column. If being used for postoperative pain relief, an infusion pump is usually attached, and this delivers a continuous and constant amount of local anaesthetic. A narcotic may be added to improve control of postoperative pain. Side effects of epidural anaesthesia include the following:

- Hypotension.
- Nausea due to the hypotension.
- Dural puncture occurs if the needle is advanced into the dura causing CSF leak. This results in headache. If local anaesthetic is injected into the dural space, it can cause a high spinal anaesthesia.
- Urinary retention may occur and the insertion of an indwelling catheter may be necessary.
- Close and specific monitoring, assessment and documentation are required.

Spinal anaesthesia

Spinal anaesthesia is achieved when a fine needle is passed through the dura and into the subarachnoid space below the spinal cord, usually at L4–5 (Thompson, 2002). A small amount of local anaesthetic is injected into this space where it comes into contact with spinal nerves. This produces a complete block of sensory and motor nerves. It is important to ensure that the patient's legs are not raised as this will force the local anaesthetic higher up the spinal column, causing high spinal anaesthesia to occur.

In this case, the child may stop breathing and ventilation will be necessary until he or she begins to breathe. Side effects of spinal anaesthesia include:

- hypotension (IV fluids should be given to increase circulating fluid volumes);
- nausea due to hypotension;
- urinary retention may occur and the insertion of an indwelling catheter may be necessary;
- high spinal anaesthesia.

Caudal blocks

Caudal blocks are often used instead of epidural blocks in young children as the epidural space offers little resistance to the spread of local anaesthetic (Mather & Hughes, 1996). Local anaesthetic is injected into the caudal canal with an 18-gauge needle which can be replaced with a fine catheter if it is to be used for continuous postoperative pain management. It is important to ensure that the recommended dose of the drug is not exceeded. It is also important to monitor for side effects until the effects of the local anaesthesia have completely worn off (Table 7.7).

Table 7.7   Regional anaesthetic drugs and their effects and side effects

Drug	Used for	Side Effect	Dose	Duration
Emla™	Topical	Allergic reaction Mild local irritation	Thick layer	
Amethocaine	Topical	Allergic reaction Local irritation	Thick layer	
Bupivacaine with or without adrenaline	Local infiltration, peripheral nerve block, spinal, caudal, epidural, regional	Rare	2 mg/kg	>3 hrs
Lignocaine with or without adrenaline	Local infiltration	Cardiovascular	5 mg/kg	60–90 minutes with adrenaline 90–120 minutes
Ropivacaine	Local infiltration, peripheral nerve block, epidural, caudal in neonates	Hypo-, hyperten-sion bradycardia	2.5 mg/kg	Long

References

American Society of Anaesthesiologists. (2008). *ASA physical status classification system. American Society of Anaesthesiologists.* Available from http://www.asahq.org/clinical/physicalstatus.htm (accessed 25 January 2008).

Anaesthesia UK. (2009). Primary FRCA Syllabus: The laryngeal mask. Anaesthesia UK. Available from http://www.anaesthesiauk.com/article.aspx?articleid=238(accessed 12 May 2009).

Bergendahl, H., Lönnqvist, P.A., Eksborg, S. (2005). Clonidine: An alternative to benzodiazepines for premedication in children. *Current Opinion in Anaesthesiology*, 18: 608–613.

Bissonnette, B., Sessler, D.I., LaFlamme, P. (1989). Intraoperative temperature monitoring sites in infants and children and the effect of inspired gas warming on esophageal temperature. *Anesthesia & Analgesia*, 69: 192–196.

Black, A., McEwan, A. (2004). *Paediatric and neonatal anaesthesia: Anaesthesia in a nutshell*. Butterworth Heinemann, Edinburgh.

Brady, M., Kinn, S., O'Rourke, K., Randhawa, N., Stuart, P. (2005). Preoperative fasting for preventing perioperative complications in children. *Cochrane Database of Systematic Reviews*, Issue 2. Art. No.: CD005285. DOI: 10.1002/14651858.CD005285.

Cook-Stather, S.D., Litman, R.S. (2006). Modern fasting guidelines in children. *Best Practice & Research Clinical Anaesthesiology*, 20(3): 471–481.

Eger, E.I. (2001). Age, minimum alveolar anesthetic concentration, and minimum alveolar anesthetic concentration-awake. *Anesthesia & Analgesia*, 93: 947–953.

Harley, I., Hore, P., Rosewarne, F. (2000). *An introduction to anaesthesia*, 4th ed., Heidelberg, Vic.

Hooper, V.D. (2006). Accuracy of noninvasive core temperature measurement in acutely ill adults: The state of the science. *Biological Research for Nursing*, 8: 24–34.

Kemp, C., McDowell, J.M., Bogovic, A., Lilley, B.J., Cranswick, N., Tibballs, J. (eds). (2002). *Paediatric pharmacopeia*. Royal Children's Hospital, Pharmacy Department, Melbourne, Vic.

Lander, J.A., Weltman, B.J., So, S.S. (2006). EMLA and Amethocaine for reduction of children's pain associated with needle insertion. *Cochrane Database of Systematic Reviews*, Issue 3. Art. No.: CD004236. DOI: 10.1002/14651858.CD004236.pub2.

Mallampati, S.R., Gatt, S.P., Gugino, L.D., Desai, S.P., Waraksa, B., Freiberger, D., Liu, P.L.b (1985). A clinical sign to predict difficult tracheal intubation: A prospective study. *Canadian Anaesthetic Society Journal*, 32: 429–434.

Mather, S., Hughes, D. (1996). *A handbook of paediatric anaesthesia*, 2nd ed. Oxford Medical Publications, Oxford.

Maunuksela, E.L., Korpela, R. (1986). Double-blind evaluation of a lignocaine–prilocaine cream (*EMLA*) in children. Effect on the pain associated with venous cannulation. *British Journal of Anaesthesia*, 58: 1242–1245.

Millar, K., Asbury, A.J., Bowman, A.W. *et al.* (2007). A randomised placebo-controlled trial of the effects of midazolam premedication on children's postoperative cognition. *Anaesthesia*, 62: 923–930.

MIMSOnline. (2008a). Prescribing information. *Propofol injection*. MIMS Abbreviated Prescribing Information, Section: 16(a) Anaesthetics – local and general. Available from http://mims.hcn.net.au.ezproxy.library.uq.edu.au/ifmx-nsapi/mims-data/?MIval=2MIMS_abbr_pi&product_code=5822&product_name=Propofol+Injection (accessed 1 February 2008).

MIMSOnline. (2008b). Prescribing information. *Thiopentone sodium*. MIMS Abbreviated Prescribing Information, Section: 16(a) Anaesthetics – local and general. Available from http://mims.hcn.net.au.ezproxy.library.uq.edu.au/ifmx-nsapi/mims-data/?MIval=2MIMS_abbr_pi&product_code=1918&product_name=Pentothal (accessed 1 February 2008).

MIMSOnline. (2008c). Prescribing information. *Suxamethonium chloride injection BP*. MIMS Abbreviated Prescribing Information, Section: 16(b) Neuromuscular blocking agents. Available from http://mims.hcn.net.au.ezproxy.library.uq.edu.au/ifmx-nsapi/mims-data/?MIval=2MIMS_abbr_pi&product_code=1937&product_name=Suxamethonium+Chloride+Injection+BP (accessed 28 January 2008).

MIMSOnline. (2008d). Prescribing information. *Pancuronium bromide injection BP*. MIMS Abbreviated Prescribing Information. Section: 16(b) Neuromuscular blocking agents.

Available from http://mims.hcn.net.au.ezproxy.library.uq.edu.au/ifmx-nsapi/mims-data/?MIval=2MIMS_abbr_pi&product_code=1933&product_name=Pancuronium+Bromide+Injection+BP (accessed 28 January 2008).

Padley, A.P. (2004). *Westmead pocket anaesthetic manual*, 2nd ed. McGraw Hill Medical, North Ryde.

Rusy, L., Usaleva, E. (1998). Anaesthesia breathing systems. Update in anesthesia: Practical procedures. *Paediatric Anaesthesia Review*. Available from http://www.nda.ox.ac.uk/wfsa/html/u08/u08_003.htm (accessed 1 February 2008).

The Australian and New Zealand College of Anaesthetists. (2003). *PS31 – Recommendations on checking anaesthesia delivery systems – 2003*. Available from http://www.anzca.edu.au/resources/professional-documents/professional-standards/ps31.html (accessed 28 January 2008).

Thompson, A.M. (2002). In: Shields, L., Werder, H. *Perioperative nursing*. Greenwich Medical Media, London.

Wadsworth, R., Anderton, J.M., Vohra, A. (1996). The effect of four different surgical prone positions on cardiovascular parameters in healthy volunteers. *Anaesthesia*, 51: 819–822. DOI: 10.1111/j.1365-2044.1996.tb12608.x.

8 The paediatric post-anaesthetic care unit

Eunice Hanisch

Introduction

The paediatric post-anaesthetic care unit (PPACU) is a strange environment within a strange environment (the operating theatre suite). The emotional needs of children require special consideration in such a place, as do the needs of their parents. The PPACU nurse should realise that the perioperative experience can be frightening for children and that they require one-to-one care. In addition, the practicalities of IV lines, drains and the like necessitate extra security and monitoring (Queensland Health, 2005). The children's ability to metabolise drugs used for anaesthesia, and regain consciousness quickly, means that if left unattended during the wake-up period, the children may be put at risk of falls and accidental injury.

The PPACU recovery nurse is part of the multidisciplinary perioperative team. As a team member, the nurse should utilise effective interpersonal skills with patients, family members and colleagues (doctors, nurses, allied health professionals and clerical staff).

In the PPACU

The PPACU nurse must apply pharmacological and physiological knowledge of the anaesthetic and surgical process, and should prepare and maintain equipment that must be readily available for emergencies. Knowledge of post-anaesthetic emergencies is imperative, and so the nurse must have the requisite skills. These include:

- management of a compromised airway (bronchospasm and laryngospasm);
- management of post-operative nausea and vomiting (PONV);
- management of hypothermia;
- management of respiratory and cardiac arrest.

The PPACU nurse must have the ability to assess and manage post-operative pain (Queensland Health, 2005a,b). The short and extremely vulnerable period of time that the nurse spends with the child is critical to the post-operative outcome. The child is closely monitored and only when stable is he or she discharged to the ward area.

The paediatric patients are not little adults – obviously, size, age and weight demand different treatment (Advanced Life Support Group, 2001). Anatomical and physiological differences change with age; therefore, the nurse must have full knowledge of this. The main differences between adults and children reside in the respiratory and cardiovascular systems, and in thermoregulation (Johnson, 2003; Advanced Life Support Group, 2001). The Advanced Life Support Group (2001), which educates health professionals about resuscitation, uses specific categories of ages when talking of children (Box 8.1), and these are relevant internationally. This saves confusion when describing such things as rates for cardiac compression, and are used in most countries.

Box 8.1 Age categories as used by the Advanced Life Support Group (2001, p. 10)

Newborn:	<72 hr old
Neonate:	first 28 days of life
Infant:	from 1–12 months
Child:	<13 years old

The main anatomical differences between children and adults are:

- Children have a proportionately larger head (can result in increased heat loss) and short neck.
- Children have narrow nostrils.
- Children have a large tongue (may obstruct airway in an unconscious child).
- Children may have loose teeth (e.g. foreign body).
- Children have compressible floor of mouth (requires care in the positioning of the fingers when holding the child's airway).
- Children have a horseshoe-shaped epiglottis (projects posteriorly at 45°, making tracheal intubation difficult (Queensland Health, 2005a).

The anatomical differences change with age, for instance, infants less than 6 months old are obligate nasal breathers. The nasal passages are easily obstructed by the presence of mucous secretions, and upper respiratory infections are common.

Figures 8.1–8.3 and Box 8.2 demonstrate the different positions and techniques used for manual airway support in children, related to age. These are important for PPACU nurses to learn and practice, as airway support in all its forms is at the core of what nurses in post-operative recovery do, and is an essential life-saving technique.

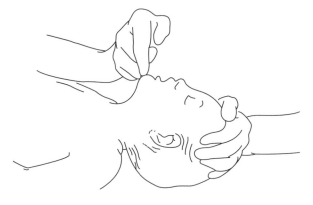

Fig. 8.1 Manual airway support in a child: neutral position. Reprinted from Advanced Life Support Group (2001), by kind permission of Wiley-Blackwell.

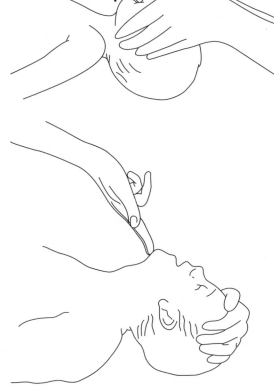

Fig. 8.2 Manual airway support in a child: sniffing position. Reprinted from Advanced Life Support Group (2001), by kind permission of Wiley-Blackwell.

Fig. 8.3 Manual airway support in a child: jaw support. Reprinted from Advanced Life Support Group (2001), by kind permission of Wiley-Blackwell.

Box 8.2   Manual airway support in a child

Age	Airway Management
Infant	Head tilt and chin lift (neutral position)
Small child	Sniffing position
Large child	(>8 years) semi-extension to full neck extension

Source: Queensland Health (2005a, p. 65).

Box 8.3   Mnemonic for airway management in children

Looking	for chest and/or abdominal movement
Listening	for breath sounds
Feeling	for breath

Source: Queensland Health (2005a, p. 64).

The mnemonic '*ABC*' is a simple way to remember the basics of resuscitation – *Airway, Breathing* and *Circulation*. These form the basis of all the knowledge and skills required for a PPACU nurse. It is vitally important that advanced life-support skills are kept up to date and assessed yearly. Box 8.3 shows another mnemonic – used to remind one what to do with a post-operative and unconscious child.

The post-operative environment

In the post-operative environment, Australia and New Zealand follow guidelines of both the ANZCA (Australia & New Zealand College of Anaesthesists) (2006) and ACORN (Australian College of Operating Room Nurses) (2006), while the UK look to the Royal College of Anesthetists Guidelines for Anaesthetic Care (Simpson, 2004). In the USA, the American Society of Anesthesiologists (2008) publishes such guidelines, while in Canada, the Canadian Society of Anesthesiologists (2007) has similar standards. There is a range of other such guidelines from the non-English-speaking world. Box 8.4 shows the recommended equipment for a PPACU.

The first recovery rooms were established to centralise patients and personnel. Today, the PPACU must be flexible to cater for a diversity of procedural activities. When designing, one must consider the type of population it will serve. There are many factors that are crucial for the planning/functionality of the PPACU:

- How many operating theatres the PPACU serves
- Number of procedures per day
- Type of procedures
- Patient's acuity.

For an in-patient hospital, the ratio of 1.5:2 PPACU base per operating room (OR) is important for safety of care and also to prevent backup of the OR (Drain, 2003). Paediatric patients require one-to-one nursing care (Shields & Waterman, 2002; Simpson, 2004; Australian College of Operating Room Nurses, 2006; Australian and New Zealand College of Anaesthetists, 2006).

Children's privacy must be taken into consideration. Typically, the PPACU bays are open spaces surrounded by curtains that can be pulled for privacy. The open-floor plan maximises patient safety and staff efficiency. Similar to the authors and guidelines listed above, the American Society of PeriAneasthesia Nurses (ASPAN) (DeFazio Quinn & Schick, 2004) and ACORN (Australian College of Operating Room Nurses, 2004; Drain, 2003) recommend 1:1 ratio for paediatric care.

The ANZCA (2006) recommends the following for the recovery room, regardless of the type of anaesthesia or sedation used:

- An area designed for that specific purpose
- Close to the OR
- Staff trained for the role
- Ability to contact medical staff immediately.

The physical area should use a ventilation system that complies with usual OR standards and the bay space should be a minimum area of $9\,m^2$, with easy access to the patient's head. The layout of bed spaces should provide an uninterrupted view of the total area for each bed space. Oxygen outlet, suction, power outlets, lighting and emergency light must be provided. The walls must be painted in a way that will allow accurate skin colour assessment (Australian College of Operating Room Nurses, 2004b; Australian and New Zealand College of Anaesthetists, 2006).

The equipment and drugs required for each bed space include oxygen flow meter and delivery systems, suction and different sizes and types of suction catheters, pulse

Box 8.4 Recommended equipment for Phase 1 PPACU (adapted from American Society of Post Anesthesia Nursing (ASPAN)

1. One-and-a-half beds will be available in the PPACU for every operating room.
2. Each care unit will be equipped with:
   - A variety of oxygen delivery systems
   - Suction
   - Blood pressure monitor
   - Lighting
   - Means to ensure patient privacy
   - ECG monitor
   - Oxymeter
3. Means to monitor patient temperature and a variety of methods to warm the patient. Supplies to manage malignant hyperthermia.
4. Portable oxygen, suction and cardiac monitoring equipment for transport.
5. Emergency call system.
6. Emergency trolley.
7. Stock medication:
   - Antibiotics
   - Medications for control of blood pressure, hart rate and respiratory drugs
   - Antiemetics
   - Anaesthesia reversal agents
   - Analgesics, narcotic and non-narcotic
   - Muscle relaxants
   - Steroids
   - Sedatives
8. Intravenous supplies.
9. Patient restraints.
10. Stock supplies:
    - Dressings
    - Facial tissues
    - Gloves, goggles, aprons, facial shields and other personal protective equipment
    - Bedpans and urinals
    - Syringes and needles
    - Emesis basin
    - Linen
    - Swabs
    - Ice bags
    - Tongue blades
    - Irrigation trays
    - Several sizes oral and nasal airways
    - Several sizes endotracheal tubes
    - Defibrillator with adult and paediatric sizes

Source: Drain (2003, pp. 48–49).

oxymeter, blood pressure machine with a range of cuff sizes, stethoscope and thermometer. The Australian College of Operating Room Nurses (2004a) includes personal protective equipment for the health care personnel, as well as receptacles for disposal of contaminated waste.

The recovery area must have emergency and other drugs, intravenous equipment and fluids, drugs for pain management, syringes and needles, warming devices for the patient, prompt access to a defibrillator, 12-lead electrocardiogram machine, refrigerator for drugs and blood, a basic surgical tray, blood gas and electrolyte measurement, blood glucose monitoring equipment, a call system to obtain emergency assistance, waste baskets for disposal of infected/dirty materials and sharps containers (Australian College of Operating Room Nurses, 2004; Queensland Health, 2005b).

Drain (2003) recommends immediate access to an 'MH (Malignant Hyperthermia) Kit' and supplies (more details in normothermia, hypothermia, in the section on Malignant Hyperthermia, which follows below). This condition is caused by the drug suxamethonium (see Chapter 7) and occurs in children as well as adults.

The Australian College of Operating Room Nurses Guideline Statement 4 (2004b, p. 4) states that 'a planned and safe environment for both patient and employee' must be ensured. Regular inspections and maintenance of equipment must occur, as well as documentation of unsafe situations and its management. The immediate time after surgery brings the child to extreme vulnerability. In order to maintain safety in readiness for this short and unpredictable time, the PPACU nurse must prepare the environment to receive the child and provide for his or her care.

Oxygen delivery

In the PPACU, the O_2 gas is delivered in litres/min. The more common devices for its delivery to the child include Hudson face masks (see Figure 8.4), nasal cannula, T-circuits and manual ventilation systems (resuscitation bag, Mapleson circuits) (see Figure 8.3) (Queensland Health, 2005b). An important point about the use of these devices: the PPACU nurse must ensure that the mask fits firmly on the child's face to facilitate delivery of O_2; in other words, there should be no leak of gas at the edges of the mask.

Guedel and oropharyngeal airways (see Figure 8.4) are commonly used in PPACU. They prevent airway obstruction by the tongue, and are used for patients who have poor/low gag reflex. Determine the correct size by measuring the distance between the corners of the patient's mouth to the base of the patient's ear (Advanced Life Support Group, 2001). If the gag reflex is present, avoid the use of an oropharyngeal tube or other airway, because it may cause choking, laryngospasm or vomiting. To insert a Guedel's airway, select the appropriate size airway, open the airway using the chin lift, insert the airway concave upwards until the tip reaches the soft palate, rotate it through 180° (convex side upwards) and slide it back over the tongue. Recheck airway patency, provide O_2 and consider ventilation (Figure 8.4).

A nasopharyngeal airway (Figure 8.5) is used in a child who has a gag reflex, but it is not recommended for nasal obstruction, epistaxis, children with a base of skull fracture, or who are on anticoagulants, or abnormal clotting conditions such as haemophilia (Advanced Life Support Group, 2001). Determine the correct size by measuring from the nostril to the tragus of the ear and add 25 mm. Before insertion, assess if any contraindications are present (e.g. base of skull fracture), select an appropriate size, lubricate the airway with a water-soluble lubricant, insert the tip into the nostril and direct it posteriorly along the floor of the nose. Gently pass the turbinates with a slight rotating motion and continue until the flange rests on the nose. If there is difficulty inserting the airway, consider using the other nostril or a smaller size. Recheck airway patency, provide O_2 and consider ventilation (Advanced Life Support Group, 2001).

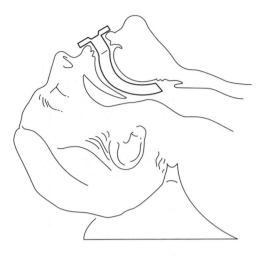

Fig. 8.4 Inserting a Guedel's airway. Reprinted from Advanced Life Support Group (2001), by kind permission of Wiley-Blackwell.

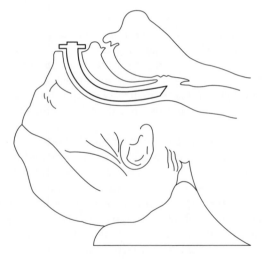

Fig. 8.5 Inserting a nasopharyngeal airway. Reprinted from Advanced Life Support Group (2001), by kind permission of Wiley-Blackwell.

Endotracheal tubes and intubation are explained in detail in Chapter 7, but it is important to note that ETTs must be on hand in the PPACU in case a child needs to be reintubated post-anaesthetic. This occurs if the child does not breathe effectively, perhaps as a result of incomplete reversal of the anaesthetic, or if he or she has severe, irresolvable laryngospasm, or various other causes. The anaesthetist must be called immediately, as this is an emergency (all PPACU nurses must know, from the very start of their employment in the unit, where the emergency call buttons are in each recovery bay).

Size selection of ETTs is shown in Chapter 7. In the PPACU, when reintubating, always have one size bigger and one size smaller of the ETT selected. While ETTs in children are usually uncuffed, always have both cuffed and uncuffed, of a range of sizes, to hand. As a general rule, cuffed ETTs are used only for children aged 8 years and above because of the possible risk of tracheal stenosis and ulceration. These occur because high cuff pressure decreases the blood supply in the tracheal mucosa (Drain, 2003; De Fazio Quinn & Schick, 2004; Queensland Health, 2005a).

Some children come to the PPACU with a laryngeal mask airway (LMA) *in situ* (see Chapter 7). These have to be removed by the PPACU nurse as the child awakes. Often, a child will, as part of the waking process, pull the LMA out by him or herself; alternatively, the nurse can remove it as the child regains consciousness. It is important to have suction to hand as one of the main complications of LMA removal is laryngospasm, caused by saliva and/or mucus that has pooled around the inflated cuff of the LMA dropping onto the vocal cords. Rapid suction is needed if it looks like there is fluid in the mouth or larynx (Queensland Health, 2005b).

Suction

Suction is often required to remove secretions from nose and mouth. Tracheal suction is a more advanced skill, and nurses in the PPACU must follow the policies on this provided by the organisation for which they work, and which can vary from hospital to hospital.

Physiological assessment and management of the paediatric post-anaesthesia patient

The primary purpose of the PPACU nurse is the evaluation and stabilisation of the post-operative patient. The emphasis during this critical period is on anticipation and prevention of complications deriving from anaesthesia or surgery. The PPACU nurse has the obligation to consider the child's physical and psychological status. Upon admission to the PPACU, the patient is accompanied by the anaesthetist who reports the child's history, type of surgery, anaesthetic agents and any problems or complications in the OR. A rapid (but thorough) assessment of airway patency, breathing and circulation is performed. Oxygen saturation, respiratory rate, temperature, inspection of the surgical site, dressings, drains and bleeding are also checked and recorded. After the initial assessment and observations, the PPACU nurse must systematically assess the child's total condition (Johnson, 2003; McGaffigan & Christoph, 2003).

A – Airway management and B – Breathing

In children, the respiratory assessment has high priority because of the effects of ineffective ventilation on cardiac function. The majority of cardiac arrhythmias and arrests are the result of respiratory failure. Airway problems are common during emergency and in the immediate post-operative period. In children, their anatomical differences to adults mean that a different approach is required. Hence, all nurses who come to work in PPACU, who may be experienced in post-operative care but who are not specialist paediatric nurses, must be trained in the care of children in this area. As mentioned in other chapters, the anatomical differences of children to adults that pertain to the post-anaesthetic period include a large tongue in proportion to mouth size, which is a potential for airway obstruction. A short neck is a potential for compromised airway and difficult intubation, as is the normal narrowing of trachea at cricoid cartilage ring. A small airway opening causes a potential increase in airflow resistance and any small amount of mucus, oedema or foreign body may cause airway obstruction. Infants, in particular, breathe through their noses (Bergeson & Shaw, 2001), and they and small children use abdominal muscles to inhale. The cartilage of the larynx is easily compressed, causing a risk of narrowing airway. This happens when neck is flexed or extended. The larynx is very susceptible to spasm, and the epiglottis is short, stiff and U-shaped, causing difficult intubation and if swelling is present, it narrows the airway, causing potential airway obstruction. The tonsils are usually enlarged, the intercostal muscles are poorly developed, accessory muscles are not used to help inspiration and the diaphragm is used for ventilation (De Fazio Quinn & Schick, 2004; Queensland Health, 2005a,b; Stow, 2007).

The PPACU nurse must assess the child's skin colour, respiratory rate, pattern of breathing, depth of respirations and quality of breath sounds. Measure respirations by observing respiratory rate over 1 min, evaluate quality and symmetry of chest movements, allow child to cry before employing comfort measures and observe for respiratory distress.

Respiratory distress is marked by:

- increased heart rate
- increased respiratory rate
- grunting
- inspiratory and/or expiratory wheezing
- intercostal recession
- cough
- nasal flaring
- sternal retractions
- tracheal tug
- increased work of breathing
- cyanosis
- apnoeic episodes.

Some or all of these may be present. The increased respiratory rate is a response to respiratory distress. The potential causes are related to the respiratory distress itself, excess fluid volume, pain, hypothermia and/or fever. In the instance of decreased respiratory rate, the potential causes may be the anaesthetic agents, administration of opioids and pain (De Fazio Quinn & Schick, 2004). Cardiovascular changes in children post-anaesthesia are shown in Table 8.1.

Respiratory complications and nursing interventions

Airway obstruction

The first priority of the PPACU nurse is to establish a patent airway. A common cause of airway obstruction is the tongue, which is relaxed because of muscle relaxants and anaesthetic agents. Other causes include soft tissue oedema and foreign body such as sponges or packs. Signs and symptoms of obstruction are use of accessory muscles, nasal flaring, abdominal and diaphragmatic contractions, decreased O_2 saturation, snoring, retraction of intercostals muscles and decreased inhaled air.

Table 8.1 Cardiovascular changes in children in the post-anaesthetic period

Age	Respiratory Rate (per minute)	Heart Rate Awake (bpm)	Heart Rate Asleep	Heart Rate Exercise/ Fever	Blood Pressure
Newborn	45–60	100–180	80–160	<220	65/40
12 months	40	80–160	70–120	<200	95/65
3 years	30	80–120	60–90	<200	100/70
6 years	25	70–115	60–90	<200	90/60
12 years	20	65–90	50–90	<200	110/60

Source: De Fazio Quinn & Schick (2004, pp. 162–164).

Nursing interventions include repositioning of the child to its side, affecting a chin lift, suction, O_2 administration, insertion of oral or nasal airway and notification of the anaesthetist (Johnson, 2003; De Fazio Quinn & Schick, 2004; Queensland Health, 2005b; Odom-Forren, 2007).

Laryngospasm

Laryngospasm is prevalent at the ages 1–3 months and with a history of recent respiratory infection. It is the result of exaggerated reflex of the glottic closure causing the approximation of the vocal cords. It can be caused by inadequate depth of anaesthesia with sensory stimulation by secretions, manipulation of the airway and surgical stimulation. Prolonged laryngospasm causes respiratory failure and arrest. The length of time it takes for this to occur is often dependent on the individual child. In some children, particularly infants, the time period is a matter of seconds; in older children, minutes, but every episode of laryngospasm is potentially fatal if not dealt with effectively. *Laryngospasm is always an emergency situation, so call for help.*

Signs and symptoms are the use of accessory muscles, partial to complete obstruction, and respiratory sounds may vary from high-pitched squeaks to total absence of sounds.

Nursing interventions include administration of 100% O_2 and Positive Pressure Ventilation by mask, removal of stimulus and jaw trust. The anaesthetist may administer muscle relaxant, and reintubation may be required. If this happens, it will have to be done speedily, so being prepared to reintubate is vital (De Fazio Quinn & Schick, 2004; Queensland Health, 2005b; Odom-Forren, 2007).

Bronchospasm

Bronchospasm is a lower airway obstruction caused by spasm of the bronchial tubes. It is caused by pre-existing airway disease such as asthma, allergy, anaphylaxis, histamine release, aspiration, mucous plug, foreign body and pulmonary oedema. Signs and symptoms are increased respiratory rate, mild to severe dyspnoea, intercostal retractions, inspiratory and expiratory wheezing and cough.

Nursing interventions demand O_2 therapy, making the child sit upright, reassuring him or her (and the parents), suction secretions, notifying the anaesthetist and administering bronchodilators as ordered.

In some cases, epinephrine, methylprednisolone, antihistamine or dexamethasone may be given. It is also important to have the equipment to hand for ventilation and reintubation should they be ordered by the anaesthetist (De Fazio Quinn & Schick, 2004; Queensland Health, 2005b; Odom-Forren, 2007).

Apnoea or decreased respiratory rate

Apnoea and decreased respiratory rate have varying causes, but both can be relatively common in post-anaesthetic premature babies and neonates. They can be caused by anaesthesia, narcotics, barbiturates, sedative administration and hypothermia. Signs and symptoms range from shallow, slow to absent respirations.

Nursing interventions will depend on the cause, and will include patient stimulation, O_2 and airway support by bag and mask, chin lift, insertion of oral airway and suction. If unresolved after stimulating the baby or child, an *emergency* exists and the anaesthetist must be called, or, if necessary, a respiratory arrest code. Treatment can include administration of naloxone if the child is narcotised and active heating if hypothermic. Reintubation and ventilation may be needed (De Fazio Quinn & Schick, 2004; Queensland Health, 2005b).

Stridor

Stridor is a shrill, harsh sound heard during inspiration and/or expiration. It is produced by air flowing through a narrowed respiratory tract, and can be caused by tracheal irritation and oedema. Signs and symptoms are crowing respiration, tachypnoea and the use of accessory muscles for respiration.

Nursing interventions include administering humidified O_2, elevating the head of the bed and notifying the anaesthetist, who may prescribe epinephrine (De Fazio Quinn & Schick, 2004; Queensland Health, 2005b).

Croup

Croup is a term used to describe a group of conditions characterised by inspiratory stridor, a crowing cough, hoarseness and a variable degree of respiratory distress. Its causes include irritation caused by intubation, an ETT that is too large for the child's trachea, traumatic and repeated intubations, coughing with the ETT in place, a change of the child's position while intubated, a long surgical procedure and consequent prolonged anaesthetic, surgical trauma and pre-existing infection. Signs and symptoms usually appear within 1 hr after extubation and may intensify in the next 4 hr, and are usually completely resolved within 24 hr. The child will present with stridor, intercostal and sternal retractions, hoarseness, crowing cough and a variable degree of obstruction that will cause varying degree of distress.

Nursing interventions include administering humidified O_2, elevating the bed head and notifying the anaesthetist, who may prescribe epinephrine, dexamethasone, hydration and reintubation if airway is too compromised (De Fazio Quinn & Schick, 2004).

C – Circulation

Multiple factors influence the myocardial function in association with age. Normally, the respiratory and heart rate decreases with increasing age. The newborn heart function has little cardiac reserve because it is at near-peak ventricular function. The paediatric patient, in general, shows the usual signs of impending shock or airway obstruction (Table 8.1). If the problem is not corrected promptly, the child's physiological status will deteriorate (Johnson, 2003). The PPACU nurse must assess heart rate, character and volume of the pulse, colour and warmth of the skin and peripheries, and check peripheral perfusion by checking capillary the nurse must observe O_2 saturation and check the ECG waveform, which should be even and uniform (Queensland Health, 2005b).

The young child has a high percentage of water in relation to his or her body weight. Consequently, younger children have an increased risk and speed of dehydration than older children. The infant has immature cardiac function and an immature sympathetic nervous system. These factors result in a cardiac output reliant on the heart rate rather than on stroke volume. The stroke volume increases as the child grows and the heart augments in size, leading to a greater cardiac output. Tachycardia and bradycardia are the main forms of dysrrhythmias amongst infants and children. Tachycardia results in decreased ventricular filling time that will compromise cardiac output and lead to cardiac collapse. Bradycardia leads to physiologic dysfunction such as hypoventilation and hypoxia, and can result in myocardial hypoxia and acidosis, leading to cardiac arrest. Children have a higher circulating blood volume per kilogram than adults. Any blood loss greater than 10% will have a severe impact on the total blood volume and can result in shock. Blood loss of more than 15% must be replaced, and children may come into the PPACU with blood transfusions *in situ* (Queensland Health, 2005a,b; Stow, 2007).

Cardiovascular assessment

Vital signs vary depending on the age and state of the child (Table 8.2). Assess circulation and perfusion by evaluating heart rate, blood pressure, skin colour and distal perfusion (palpate peripheral pulses) (De Fazio Quinn & Schick, 2004). Cyanosis and tachypnoea are signs of impending respiratory failure and an indication of positive haemodynamic instability.

Tachycardia is a normal way of increasing cardiac output. Possible causes are decreased perfusion caused by impending shock, hyperthermia, pain, early respiratory distress and medications (atropine, morphine, epinephrine).

Bradycardia is of great danger in paediatric patients. Possible causes are respiratory distress (of which bradycardia is a late sign), hypoxia, vagal response and increased intracranial pressure (ICP).

Hypertension can occur in children, though it is much rarer than in adults, and is almost always from some extraneous cause rather than an intrinsic disease process (except in, e.g. conditions such as renal disease and cardiac abnormalities). Possible causes are excess of intravascular fluids, carbon dioxide retention, pain, increased ICP and medications such as ketamine and epinephrine.

Hypotension in post-anaesthetic children is usually caused by anaesthetic agents (halothane, isoflurane, enflurane), opioids and, importantly, it can be a late sign of shock (De Fazio Quinn & Schick, 2004).

Table 8.2   Children's normal ranges for vital signs

| | Normal Vital Signs By Age | | | |
Age	Temperature (°C)	Pulse Rate (beats/min)	Respiratory Rate (breaths/min)	Blood Pressure (mmHg)
Newborn	36–37.2	120–160	30–60	Systolic 46–92 Diastolic 38–71
3 years	36.4–37	80–125	20–30	Systolic 72–110 Diastolic 40–73
10 years	36.4–37	70–110	16–22	Systolic 83–121 Diastolic 45–79
16 years	36.4–37	55–90	15–20	Systolic 93–131 Diastolic 49–85

The normal range of the child's temperature will depend on the method used. Temperatures exhibit circadian rhythms at all ages.
Source: Adapted from James *et al.* (2002, p. 235).

Thermoregulation and temperature abnormalities

The body maintains its temperature between 36°C and 38°C by thermoregulatory mechanisms in the central nervous system (CNS). Input is received from thermoreceptors in the skin, nose, oral cavity, thoracic viscera and spinal cord (Drain, 2003).

Normothermia is defined as a condition of normal body temperature and a condition where an environmental temperature does not cause more or less activity of body cells (Stedman, 2006). The body temperature is regulated by the hypothalamus, which controls the regulatory centre. The major sites of heat production are muscles (5%), liver (50%) and glands (15%) (Ferrara-Love *et al.*, 2004).

The central temperature controls two primary responses: (a) physiological thermoregulation (sweating, shivering, peripheral vasomotor tone). These responses fine-control the regulatory process of body temperature. As a result, sweating, shivering and alteration in the peripheral vasomotor tone occur. They also reduce heat production, lowering the metabolic rate, and increasing muscle tone and shivering to enhance heat production. (b) Behavioural thermoregulation conveys the subjective feelings of comfort and discomfort (Drain, 2003). Body temperature has a circadian cycle, and temperatures are lower in the morning than in the afternoon (Litwack, 1997; Drain, 2003). Body heat is removed by four methods of heat transfer: (i) radiation, (ii) conduction, (iii) convection and (iv) evaporation. Radiation is the major way of heat transfer (Drain, 2003).

Hyperthermia, or a body temperature above 39.4°C, is suggestive of intracranial pathology, e.g. meningitis, pancreatitis or urinary tract infection, especially if accompanied by shaking chills. A mild fever suggests upper respiratory infection.

Fever combined with shivering, peripheral vasoconstriction, weakness, hypotension, tachycardia and tachypnoea should be evaluated. High fever without symptoms suggests viral etiology. Shaking chills are indicative of bacteraemia (Litwack, 1997). Newborns and infants have a decreased ability to produce heat. In order to maintain body temperature within normal limits, they metabolise brown fat, cry and move vigorously. Thus, newborns and infants respond to a cold environment (such as an operating theatre) by increasing their metabolism, which leads to increased O_2 consumption and production of organic acids (Johnson, 2003).

Operating theatres are usually cold places, and children (especially infants) admitted to PPACU often experience some thermal imbalance, i.e. body core temperature outside the normothermic range of 36–38°C (Litwack, 1997; Drain, 2003).

Hypothermia is defined as a core body temperature of less than 35°C (Abelha *et al.*, 2005). The American College of Surgeons classifies hypothermia into three stages:

(1) Mild: 32–35°C
(2) Moderate: 30–32°C
(3) Severe: below 30°C (Bellamy, 2007).

Hypothermia causes impairment and abnormalities in different organs and systems. It can lead to a decrease in O_2 release to the tissues and with concomitant depression in myocardial contractility, peripheral vasoconstriction, ventilation–perfusion mismatch, increased blood viscosity and shifts to the left in the oxyhaemoglobin-dissociation curve. Hypothermia decreases platelet function and diminishes the activation of the coagulation cascade.

Inadvertent core hypothermia is often a characteristic of the immediate post-operative period. Anaesthesia impairs central thermal regulation, while the cool ambient temperature of the OR, and large administration of fluids to the patient contributes to heat loss. The initial response to cold is to generate and conserve temperature. Post-operatively, hypothermia is complicated by shivering and peripheral vasoconstriction. Post-anaesthesia shivering (PAS) increases cardiac and energy demand, raising O_2 production and an increase in cardiac work (Abelha *et al.*, 2005). PAS can also cause airway obstruction and increased somnolence post-operatively (Drain, 2003). Apart from causing discomfort and increased post-operative pain, PAS augments blood pressure and intraocular pressure, and interferes with monitoring (English, 2002). Hypothermia can cause decreased drug metabolism and clearance, and delay wound healing (Berthal, 1999). Other complications include prolonged post-anaesthetic recovery and hospitalisation (Sessler, 2001; Suleman *et al.*, 2002; Abelha *et al.*, 2005).

Rewarming the child is a priority in the PPACU, following the ABC assessment. Any wet and cold gowns and linen should be removed and dry gowns and warm blankets applied (Odom-Forren, 2007). If an infant or small child arrives in the PPACU with hypothermia, the nurse should assess for:

(1) vital signs (core temperature, pulse, respiratory rate);
(2) pulse oxymetry wave form and saturation;
(3) the degree of emergence from anaesthesia.

The hypothermic child should remain intubated and sedated. Continuous ECG monitoring is necessary until core temperature reaches 35°C. In order to avoid excess O_2 demand and acidosis associated with hypothermia, newborns and infants should be maintained in a neutral thermal environment in the PPACU by use of incubators, warmed blankets, infrared heating lamps, warm-air blankets or elevated room temperature. The head should be covered and minimal exposure to the environment should be maintained when physical assessment is performed (Johnson, 2003).

During routine assessment in the PPACU, observe for:

(1) cyanosis of extremities;
(2) dysrrhythmias secondary to hypothermia;

(3) Reparalysis (dose of reversal agents in the hypothermic child is no longer effective when the metabolic rate increases in response to warmer temperature).

Institute warming measures such as heated blankets, forced air heat, radiant heat, warmed IV fluids, cover head and torso, humidify and warm gases and monitor temperature until normothermia is achieved (De Fazio Quinn & Schick, 2004; Ferrara-Love, 2004).

Safety precautions should be kept in mind. If a water mattress is used, the temperature should not exceed 37°C, and layers of sheets between the mattress and child should be used to prevent burns. If using a warm-air heating device, follow the manufacturer's guidelines. Never put the warm-heating tube between two blankets or it may result in burns. Monitor the device temperature to prevent overwarming or injury. Keep records of the core body temperature and device temperature (Johnson, 2003).

The expected outcome for the hypothermic child or infant should be:

(1) a core temperature of 36°C or higher;
(2) all signs and symptoms related to hypothermia should be resolved;
(3) The child should verbalise an acceptable level of warmth (age related) (De Fazio Quinn & Schick, 2004).

Hyperthermia may be an indication of an infectious process or it may indicate a hypermetabolic process, malignant hyperthermia (MH) (Odom-Forren, 2007). Fever usually refers to temperatures of 37.8–40°C. Hyperthermia refers to temperatures above 40°C. Fever occurs because heat production is quicker than heat loss, from a disease process, inflammatory response, drug reactions and allergic responses. Sometimes, the child may have been covered with drapes or plastic on the operating theatre and is unable to lose heat (Hatfield & Tronson, 2002).

Malignant Hyperthermia (MH) is an emergency that has genetic origin and is triggered by volatile anaesthetic agents and the depolarising muscle relaxant succinylcholine (suxamethonium). Death can result from MH if it is not immediately recognised and treated (De Fazio Quinn & Schick, 2004; Ferrara-Love, 2004; Odom-Forren, 2007). The incidence of MH in children is 1:15,000. Many cases are undetected owing to people never having been anaesthetised, or having a short anaesthetic period or because many cases are mild and therefore not diagnosed (Hatfield & Tronson, 2002; Drain, 2003). The onset of MH usually occurs during induction of anaesthesia, though reports of MH recurring in the PPACU exist. Successful management depends on early assessment and intervention (Drain, 2003). Mortality has been reduced since the availability of dantrolene in the late 1970s and has remained at 6–7% since the late 1980s (Redmond, 2001; Odom-Forren, 2007).

MH triggering agents are:

(1) *Pharmacological* – succinylcholine (suxamethonium), volatile inhalation agents (halothane, enflurane, sevoflurane, desflurane), IV potassium when given rapidly. Other possible triggers are Chlopromazine, Prochlorperazine and Haloperidol.
(2) *Non-pharmacological* – stress, trauma, heat, pain, mental agitation, shivering (Redmond, 2001; Hommertzheim & Steinke, 2006; Odom-Forren, 2007).

MH signs, symptoms and diagnosis

- Symptoms are non-specific. One early sign of MH is muscle rigidity.
- Masseter muscle spasm may be seen by the anaesthetist, making intubation difficult after administration of succinnylcholine (suxamethonium).
- Unanticipated doubling or tripling of end-tidal carbon dioxide, resulting in tachypnoea.
- Early, generalised erythematous flush that causes skin to feel warm, but the core temperature may be normal.
- Later, mottled skin followed by cyanosis.
- Increased PCO_2, acidosis and dysrrhythmias.
- Tachycardia.
- Temperature elevation is often a late sign. Temperature rate increases 1°C every 3–5 minutes up to 42°C.
- Rhabdomyolysis as a result of skeletal muscle breakdown, which shows by brown or cola-coloured urine.
- Elevated levels of myoglobin in the urine.
- Elevated CK (creatinine kinase).
- Left ventricular failure is a terminal event.
- Pulmonary oedema, rales and frothy sputum.
- DIC (disseminated intravascular coagulation) noted when venipuncture sites begin to bleed (Litwack, 1997; Redmond, 2001; Smith & O'Brien, 2003; De Fazio Quinn & Schick, 2004).

Treatment is aimed at reversing the physiological effects of the trigger, support and symptom management (Table 8.3). The reversal drug of choice, dantrolene sodium, prevents ongoing release of Ca+, but may cause muscle weakness in patients with history of neuromuscular disease and can create a sense of respiratory inadequacy, fatigue, dizziness, blurred vision, nausea and thrombophlebitis. MH requires the use of monitoring devices such as temperature probe, electrocardiogram, arterial O_2 saturation, central venous line, pulmonary artery catheter and IDC. To cool the child, use chilled

Table 8.3 Treatment for malignant hypothermia

Intervention	Rationale
Stop all anaesthetic agents	Remove triggers
Hyperventilate with 100% O_2	Correct hypoxaemia and acidosis
Dantrolene 2.5–10 mg/kg IV	Inhibits release of Ca+
Bicarbonate IV 2–4 mEq/kg	Corrects acidosis
Active cooling	Decrease fever and O_2 demands
Monitor urine output	Evaluate acute tubular necrosis and myoglobinuria
Treat dysrrhythmias, observe blood gasses, temperature, muscle tone, Urine output	Individualise therapy
Monitor laboratory tests (electrolytes, liver enzymes, renal function FBC, coagulation profile)	Assess organ system and physiological functioning

Source: Redmond (2001), Malignant Hyperthermia Association of the United States-MHAUS (2006), Hommertzheim and Steinke (2006).

IV normal saline 0.9% and, if necessary, stomach lavage, bladder and rectum with cold normal saline. However, it is important not to cool the child to less than 38°C to avoid additional problems. Monitor urine output (it should be greater than 2 ml/kg/hr) and test arterial blood gasses every 15 mins to check for acidosis. MH may reoccur within several hours to several days in 25% of the patients. The prescribing doctor, usually the attendant anaesthetist, will order administration of dantrolene 1 mg/kg q 4–6 hr IV for up to 48 hr (Hommertzheim & Steinke, 2006; Malignant Hyperthermia Association of the United States-MHAUS, 2006).

The PPACU nurse inherits the management of the patient with MH. A child with MH may present in the PPACU within the first hour (and up to 12 hr post-operatively). Once the MH is under control, nursing interventions will focus on cardiac output, thermoregulation, ventilation and fluid and electrolyte management. The child with MH will require ICU admission for 24–48 hr (Redmond, 2001). *MH is an emergency*, and PPACU staff should be prepared for the crisis. The PPACU must maintain an MH kit of all drugs and fluids required for its treatment (Box 8.5). Keep clear instructions and develop a crisis response plan. Make sure that MH treatment protocol is posted in a highly visible place. Monitor and update staff education. Have dantrolene (36 vials) readily available (De Fazio Quinn & Schick, 2004).

In summary, be prepared to recognise, intervene effectively and manage the MH patient.

Post-operative nausea and vomiting

Post-operative nausea and vomiting (PONV) is a common and potentially serious complication amongst the paediatric population. The incidence of PONV increases after the age of 3 years and peaks up in children aged 11–14 years (Culy *et al.*, 2001). It is also influenced by factors such as gender, body weight, previous history of PONV, type of anaesthetic agent, ventilation techniques, post-operative analgesics and surgical procedure. As examples, strabismus surgery has a 50–80% incidence of PONV, while adenotonsillectomy has 50–70% (Culy *et al.*, 2001). Other types of surgery associated with PONV include ear surgery, dental surgery, laparotomy and orchidopexy (Munro, 2000; Ferrara-Love, 2004). The results of PONV in children range from extensive discomfort and prolonged recovery-room stay to unscheduled hospital admission. A myriad of pharmacological agents have been used for the prophylaxis of PONV in children. Some examples are:

- butyrophenones – of which droperidol showed the greatest benefit;
- phenothiazines – prochlorperazine, perpherazine;
- benzamines – metoclopramide was the most effective, and antihistamines.

The adverse side effects (sedation, restlessness, hypotension, dry mouth, dysphoria, hallucinations and extrapyramidal symptoms) have limited the use of these drugs. Droperidol has been withdrawn in the UK because of its potential side effects on cardiac QT interval (Culy *et al.*, 2001; News in brief, 2001). A new class of antiemetics used for prevention of the PONV are the 5-HT3 receptor antagonists ondansetron, granisetron, tropisetron and dolasetron. Ondansetron was the first 5-HT3 receptor antagonist to be introduced for the management of chemotherapy and radiation-induced emesis in children. Intravenous and oral ondansetron 0.1 mg/kg up to 4 mg given immediately before or after induction of general anaesthesia is a very effective

Box 8.5 Malignant hyperthermia kit

Malignant Hyperthermia Kit Supplies
   An MH kit should be immediately accessible to operating rooms.

Drugs
1. Dantrolene sodium IV, 36 vials
2. Sterile water for injection (without bacteriostatic) to reconstitute Dandrolene, 1000 mls × 2
3. Sodium bicarbonate (8.4%), 50 mls × 5
4. Furosemide, 40 mg/ampules × 4 ampules
5. D50, 50 mls vials × 2
6. Calcium chloride (10%) × 2
7. Regular insulin, 100 units/ml × 1 (refrigerated)
8. Lidocaine HCl (2%), 1 box = 2 g or 20 mls vials × 5

General equipment
1. Syringes (60 mls × 5) to dilute dandrolene
2. Mini spike IV additive pins × 2 and multiAd fluid transfer sets × 2 (to reconstitute dandrolene)
3. Angiocaths: 20G, 22G, 24G (4 each) for IV access and arterial line
4. NG tubes (variety of sizes)
5. Blood pump
6. Irrigation tray with piston syringe (× 1) for NG irrigation
7. Toomy irrigation syringes (60 mls × 2) for NG irrigation
8. Large clear plastic bags for ice
9. Bucket for ice
10. Disposable cold packs × 4

Monitoring equipment
1. Oesophageal temperature probes
2. CVP kits (variety of sizes)
3. Transducer kit

Drip supplies
1. D5W, 250 mls ×1
2. Microdrip IV set × 1

Nursing supplies
1. Large sterile drape (for rapid drape of wound)
2. Three-way irrigating Foley catheters (variety of sizes)
3. Urine meter × 1
4. Toomy irrigation syringe (60 mls) × 2
5. Rectal tubes: 14F, 16F, 32F, 34F
6. Large clear plastic bags for ice × 4
7. Small plastic bags for ice × 4
8. Tray for ice

Laboratory testing supplies
1. Syringes (3 mls) or ABG kits × 6
2. Blood specimen tubes (2 paediatric and 2 large tubes) for CK, myoglobin, SMA 19 (LDH, electrolytes, thyroid studies)
   PT/PTT, fibrinogen, fibrin split products, CBC, platelets, blood gas syringe (lactic acid level)
3. Urine cup × 2: myoglobin level
4. Urine dipstick: Haemoglobin

Forms
1. Laboratory requests
2. Adverse Metabolic Reaction to Anaesthesia Report form
3. Consult form
(Adapted from Malignant Hyperthermia Association of United States)

antiemetic (Culy *et al.*, 2001). The management of nausea and vomiting starts preoperatively and continues into the intraoperative period. There is no single method of prevention or treatment of PONV. It is paramount not to oversedate the patient when medicating for nausea and vomiting. Ondansetron has become popular because of the lack of side effects and dexamethasone also has been proved useful (Odom-Forren, 2007).

The PPACU nurse must protect the airway of an unconscious or semi-conscious patient to prevent possible aspiration of gastric contents. Children can be placed in the recovery position and have his or her mouth and pharynx suctioned (Hatfield & Tronson, 2002). Signs and symptoms of aspiration include:

- tachypnoea and hypoxaemia related to a decrease in lung compliance;
- wheezing;
- coughing;
- dyspnoea;
- hypotension;
- apnoea;
- bradycardia.

The treatment revolves around promoting tissue oxygenation. O_2 is given via positive pressure by mask or ETT to maintain arterial oxygenation. If the child is intubated, the trachea can be suctioned. X-ray and, if necessary, bronchoscopy is performed to remove any particles causing obstruction (Drain, 2003; Odom-Forren, 2007).

However, no single intervention is effective to prevent or treat PONV. The PPACU nurse should avoid sights, smells or conversations near the patient that could stimulate nausea and vomiting. When moving children, move them slowly and turn their trolley from the foot end, so as not to swing the head in a wide arc (Hatfield & Tronson, 2002; Ferrara-Love, 2004).

Opioids act on the brain stem centres and cause nausea and vomiting, and all the inhalants and induction agents can cause vomiting. Propofol is the least likely of the induction agents to cause nausea and vomiting, while neostigmine at the end of surgery contracts the stomach and may cause vomiting upon ambulation. In the PPACU, nausea and vomiting also may be induced by pain, hypotension, hypoxia, hypovolaemia, anxiety and swallowed blood. Nausea and vomiting after epidural or spinal anaesthesia may be a sign of hypotension and needs immediate intervention. The conscious patient usually dry retches before vomiting, and so it is easier to sit them up so vomiting is easier and less risky (Hatfield & Tronson, 2002).

Antiemetic drugs

Antihistamines block H1 receptors. Their antiemetic effect is due to their anticholinergic muscarinic blocking activity.

Cyclizine is effective against opioid-induced vomiting (Oldman *et al.*, 2003), though some debate exists over its efficacy when compared with more modern drugs such as ondansetron (O'Brien *et al.*, 2003).

Promethazine (Phenergan®) can be used as a pre-anaesthetic medication for prevention and control of post-operative vomiting. This acts as antiemetic, hypnotic, tranquilliser and a potentiator of anaesthetics, hypnotics, sedatives and analgesics. It should be avoided in children with signs and symptoms suggestive of Reye's Syndrome. There is potential for central and obstructive apnoea and reduced arousal. Excessive dosages may cause hallucinations, convulsions and sudden death. Promethazine should not be used in children younger than 2 years (MIMS Online, 2006).

> *Reye's Syndrome – A combination of acute encephalopathy and fatty tissue infiltration of the internal organs that may follow acute viral infections. The cause is unknown; however, there appears to be an association with the administration of aspirin. Usually affects people under 18 years of age. Signs and symptoms include exanthematous rash, vomiting and confusion. In the late stage extreme disorientation, coma seizures and respiratory arrest. Mortality ranges from 20–80%* (Mosby's Medical, Nursing, & Allied Health Dictionary, 1994, p. 1366).

Prochlorperazine (Stemetil®) is an antiemetic and antipsychotic. It is not recommended for children under 10 kg or under 2 years. It delays emergence from anaesthesia, causes acute dystonic reactions, leading to cyanosis to laryngospasm, apnoea requiring ventilation, and life-threatening tetanus-like syndromes, coma and even death (MIMS Online, 2007a).

Metoclopramide (Maxolon®, Raglan®) is useful for symptoms induced by handling of the abdominal organs (bowel, uterus, ovaries), or when blood is swallowed (MIMS Online, 2007b). It is ineffective against opioids-induced vomiting and motion sickness. Metoclopramide can cause unpredictable 'Extrapyramidal Syndrome' in children.

> *Extrapyramidal syndrome – Children, young adults, and debilitated elderly patients are susceptible to extrapyramidal syndrome (dystonia and nystagmus). The patient develops muscle rigidity, and marked oscillations of the eyes (nystagmus) known as an occulogyric crisis* (Mosby's Medical, Nursing, & Allied Health Dictionary, 1994, p. 228).

Droperidol is used as premedication and anaesthetic, though it cannot be given to children under 2 years. It can cause impaired alertness, extrapyramidal reactions, tardive dyskenesia and ventricular arrhythmias (MIMS Online, 2007c). This drug is one of the butyrophenones, which have strong antidopaminergic activity. They are also alpha-blockers, and in large doses cause postural hypotension.

5-HT3 antagonists

Ondansetron (Zofran®, Zantron®) is a specific antagonist of 5-HT3 receptor in the vomiting centre. It is an anti-nauseant and antiemetic, may cause headache, has few side effects and does not cause Extrapyramidal syndrome. Children are more likely to benefit from prophylaxis. Ondansetron increases large bowel transient time (MIMS Online, 2007d).

Granisetron (Kytril®) is largely used for the prevention of cytotoxic-induced nausea and vomiting. It can cause headache, constipation, diarrhoea, asthenia (weakness), hypertension, rash, taste disturbances and somnolence. There is no experience in the use of Kytril® in the prevention and treatment of PONV in children (MIMS Online, 2005).

Catecholamines

Ephedrine is a common drug sometimes used for PONV, but causes pallor, fever, headache and dry nose, mouth and throat (MIMS Online, 2004).

Pain management in the PPACU (see also Chapter 4)

Upon the child's arrival in the PPACU, immediate assessment of the ABC (airway, breathing and circulation) is imperative. The airway is assessed for patency, O_2 is administered, respirations counted and pulse oxymetry applied. After checking and documenting the vital signs, level of consciousness, IV line functioning and security and wound ooze, an extensive report is given by the anaesthetist or anaesthetic nurse. This report should contain, first, the type of surgery or procedure and the anaesthesia technique and anaesthetic agents used. The presence of tubes, drains and catheters should be noted, and the estimated fluid loss and replacements given during the surgery. Also, it is important to know any complications that occurred during anaesthesia and the procedure. All perioperative information should be checked – vital signs, temperature, laboratory results, radiology findings, allergies, disabilities, mobility status, prostheses, birth history and developmental stages. It is important to be told where the parents are waiting for the child, and any problems they may have. Also, the child's emotional status upon arrival at the operating theatre suite is important as it may have a bearing on his or her behaviour and emotional state when he or she awakes (Odom-Forren, 2007).

Pain can play a large part in the child's experience of surgery and hospital admission. Chapter 4 deals with pain and pain relief in depth. The PPACU nurse should be aware of the myths surrounding pain in children, including that children do not feel pain; that they will not remember having pain; that a child is not in pain if he or she can be distracted or is sleeping; that children can tolerate pain better than adults; that medication can only be given when the patient exhibits obvious signs of pain; that a child cannot tell where he or she hurts and that addiction is a side effect of pain management (DeFazio Quinn & Schick, 2004; Odom-Forren, 2007). It is vital to remember that patients respond to pain in different ways. The child's self-report is the most important data. Other data includes having what is known to be a painful procedure, the presence of behavioural signs such as crying and restlessness and psychological changes (Odom-Forren, 2007). When assessing the child in PPACU, look for physiological changes such as increased blood pressure, increased respiratory rate, decreased O_2 saturation, flushed skin, restlessness, sweating or dilated pupils and assess the child according to his or her developmental level, and use tools appropriate for the child's age (DeFazio Quinn & Schick, 2004).

While assessing for pain in the PPACU, consider:

- the child's previous pain experiences;
- the child's normal response to pain;
- the child's vocabulary to communicate pain;
- the inclusion of parents or caregiver in assessing the pain;
- environmental factors such as cold or crowded rooms, alarms and noises from other patients (Merckel & Malviya, 2000; DeFazio Quinn & Schick, 2004).

Ideally, the post-operative pain treatment should be commenced preoperatively. For instance, the use of age-related education preoperatively, inclusion of the patient and parents in care planning and pre-admission hands-on play with hospital equipment (DeFazio Quinn & Schick, 2004). The anaesthetist may decide to give intraoperative treatment such as regional block and administration of analgesics, and they are administered in the PPACU. Also, analgesics and opioids can be given orally, intravenously (intermittent/continuous infusions) or as in combination therapy of opioids with acetaminophen or NSAIDs. PCAs and NCAs should be used for timely administration of drugs. The PPACU nurse should give analgesics as prescribed and avoid waiting for severe pain before medicating the child (see Chapter 4).

The PPACU nurse observes and documents behavioural and physiological signs of pain. Note verbal and non-verbal responses, assess vital signs and assess for other factors that might affect the child: separation, fear, anxiety and loss of control, and cultural beliefs related to pain. Keep in mind the child's developmental stage when monitoring pain and use an appropriate pain tool. Implement non-pharmacological strategies such as distraction, relaxation techniques, massage, warm blankets, positioning. Provide a quiet and calm environment, and if possible, reduce environmental noise and light (DeFazio Quinn & Schick, 2004) (though the latter can be very difficult in the post-operative recovery environment). In the PPACU, prevention of pain is begun. The PCA (Patient Controlled Analgesia) and NCA (Nurse Controlled Analgesia) are recommended ways of drug administration that prevent delays in analgesia. However, the paediatric patient with a PCA must be able to understand the concept of self-administering analgesia, and the stages of development and cognitive processes should be considered as well as the principle of dose titration. Most importantly, parents/caregivers must be educated/instructed not to press the PCA button for the child (Queensland Health, 2006). While this must be part of the preoperative education for both children and parents, it is in the PPACU that they first encounter the PCA, so the PPACU nurse must be able to explain and describe the equipment and techniques to them. The PPACU nurse must follow and comply with the policy pertinent to the health care facility (Ewing & Long, 2003; DeFazio Quinn & Schick, 2004). The drug classes that are the most important in the PPACU setting are local anaesthetics, anti-inflammatories and opioids (see Chapters 4 and 7).

Infection control

Infection control has always been important during the perioperative period. Nowadays, it is even more relevant because of multi-resistant organisms, e.g. MRSA, blood-borne diseases that are infectious to hospital staff, e.g. HIV, and the range of blood-borne hepatitis organisms, and those carried by droplet, e.g. tuberculosis and H5N1. Standard precautions should be applied to blood and all body fluids for all patients (Odom-Forren, 2007).

Standard precautions in PPACU include:

- hand washing after patient contact;
- wear gloves if anticipating contact with blood and body fluids;
- wear gown, plastic apron and goggles if any chance of splashing;
- place soiled linen in leak-proof bags and label as infectious;

- use tightly sealed specimen containers to prevent leakage;
- wipe up spills immediately;
- routine cleaning with neutral detergent;
- avoid injury from contaminated sharps (do not recap needles, and dispose of sharps in correct sharps containers) (Hatfield & Tronson, 2002).

Transmission-based precautions must be implemented when a patient is known or is suspected of being infected. These are based on the model of transmission shown in Box 8.6.

Box 8.6 Transmission model

Contact	Transmission is host-to-host or host-to-inanimate object
Droplet	Contact with microorganisms that travel 1.5 m or less from cough, sneeze or suction
Airborn	Transmission from particles dispersed by air currents, air handling and ventilation

Source: Odom (2003, p. 40).

It is important to remember that all patients, i.e. children, are potentially infectious. Also, while working in PPACU, if staff have an infection, they should not come to work. The children are particularly vulnerable post-anaesthetic, and are likely to acquire airborne viruses that can cause major complications.

> *Germs don't fly – they hitch hike. Wash your hands properly before and after touching a patient (Hatfield & Tronson, 2002, p. 38).*

Principles for preventing cross infection in PPACU:

- Wear proper protective clothing
- Do not wear wedding rings or any jewellery
- Keep the PPACU tidy, do not use it as storage area
- Place contaminated material in leak-proof containers and remove them at regular intervals
- Wash hands
- Wear disposable gloves and eye protection when there is any possible contact with the child's body fluids (Hatfield & Tronson, 2002).

Fluid and electrolyte balance

Infants and young children are vulnerable to changes in their fluid and electrolyte balance. Dehydration causes disturbances in the acid–base balance. The causes of dehydration are a decrease in fluid intake or fluid loss that will result in rapid extracellular fluid loss. The resulting electrolyte imbalance will subsequently become intracellular fluid loss, which causes cellular dysfunction, and can lead to hypovolaemic shock and death.

There are three degrees of dehydration:

(1) Mild: 3–5% loss of body weight
(2) Moderate: 6–9% loss of body weight
(3) Severe: 10% or more loss of body weight (DeFazio Quinn & Schick, 2004).

Box 8.7   Maintenance fluid requirements and expected minimum urine output in children, by weight and age group

Daily fluid requirement by body weight	
≤10 kg	100 mls/kg
10–20 kg	1000 mls + 50 mls for each kg between 10 and 20 kg
>20 kg	1500 mls + 20 mls/kg for each kg over 20 kg
Minimum urine output by age/group	
Infants and toddlers	>2–3 mls/kg/hr
Pre-schoolers and young school-age children	>1–2 mls/kg/hr
School-age children and adolescents	0.5–1 mls/kg/hr

DeFazio Quinn & Schick (2004, p. 157)

Box 8.7 shows the fluid requirements and expected urine output for children, by body weight and by age group.

Physiologically, children (and infants) have special needs when it comes to fluid and electrolyte balance. Because of the higher percentage of water in the extra cellular fluid (ECF), infants can lose equal to their ECF within 2–3 days. Infants have an immature renal function, therefore they are less able to concentrate urine. They have a higher peristalsis rate in their gut, with an immature lower oesophageal sphincter, making them more prone to gastroesophageal reflux, which can lead to dehydration and electrolyte imbalances. Infants have a harder time compensating for acidosis than older children (or adults) because of their decreased ability to acidify urine. Young children and infants have a higher metabolic turnover of water relative to adults because of a higher metabolic rate, and often are unable to verbalise or communicate thirst. When compared with adults, infants and children have a greater body surface area in relation to body mass, resulting in a greater potential for fluid loss via the skin and gastrointestinal tract. In premature infants, water content is 90%, in full-term infants 75–80%, in pre-school children 60–65% and in adolescents and adults it is 55–60%, with a larger proportion of fluid in the extra cellular space. The immune system of an infant or child is not as strong as an adult's, so the young are more susceptible to infections, fever, gastroenteritis and respiratory infections, all of which can result in fluid and electrolyte disturbances and fluid-volume deficit. In addition, some infants and children are at higher risk of infection because of increased exposure to infections in day care and nursery environment (DeFazio Quinn & Schick, 2004). All these factors have significance for the nurse in PPACU, who must be able to recognise the patient at risk of either fluid deficit or overload.

PPACU nursing assessment includes skin colour and turgor, perfusion and vital signs related to fluid imbalance (rapid, weak, thready pulse, increased respiratory rate, decreased blood pressure). The child may be irritable, lethargic, confused, and infant cry may be high pitched and weak. Check the operation and anaesthetic sheets, and blood loss, to ascertain the management of intake and output during the surgical procedure, and also the fluid chart to determine fluid intake both during and prior to surgery and anaesthetic administration. Nursing interventions include correction of the imbalance and treatment of the underlying cause (DeFazio Quinn & Schick, 2004).

Hypervolaemia is caused by an excess of fluid in the body. Infants and young children are at risk of hypervolaemia because of excessive fluid administration and an increase in levels of antidiuretic hormone and aldosterone production in response to stress due to surgery (DeFazio Quinn & Schick, 2004). Signs and symptoms of hypervolaemia include restlessness, increased activity, periorbital oedema, tachycardia, dyspnoea and oedema of extremities. Nursing interventions comprise strict observation of vital signs, highly regulated administration of fluids by infusion pump, strict monitoring of intake and output and notification of the doctor if any signs or symptoms of hypervolaemia worsen.

Wounds and dressings

IV lines, catheters and drains

Immediately upon arrival in the PPACU, immediately following the ABC assessment, and as an integral part of the initial check of the child, the nurse must observe and record wound status in terms of blood loss or discharge, swelling, dressing integrity, drainage systems – type, patency, estimated loss. The nurse must notify the surgeon of intense bleeding and reinforce dressings if necessary. IV lines, catheters and drains must be safely anchored (Queensland Health, 2005a,b).

Patient positioning

Management of the unconscious patient

Refer to the section on 'Airway Management and Breathing'.

Safety and comfort

Intraoperative positioning and effects of anaesthetics have implications upon recovery, and because of this, combined with the anaesthetic, the child will experience changes in the respiratory system. These can include alteration to pulmonary blood flow volume, which affects the volume of blood available for oxygenation; reduced lung expansion due to the reduced ability of the diaphragm to increase abdominal pressure and post-operative pain. Positioning and anaesthesia cause mismatch of ventilation of lung tissues and perfusion, resulting in increased risk of hypoxia.

Cardiovascular changes include hypotension related to positioning and anaesthetic agents; pooling of blood caused by dilated vascular beds; pressure and obstruction of vessels. Neurological changes comprise peripheral and superficial nerve damage from mechanical pressure, obstruction and stretching. Finally, integumentary and musculoskeletal system changes can lead to pressure ulcers from compression, friction, shearing and maceration. Nursing interventions to avoid damage of the above systems include correct positioning, cushioning of bony areas, use of gel pads, skin inspection while assessing the patient and documentation of any abnormalities or discrepancies. Side rails and brakes should be applied at all times, and the child positioned in accordance with the surgical procedure. Rewarm the child if necessary, assess pain levels and keep the child clean and dry (Queensland Health, 2005b).

Latex allergy

With the use of rubberised products such as surgical gloves, the incidence of latex allergy has meant that many practices in the OR have to be changed to accommodate both patients and staff with this condition. The incidence is 8–17% of health care workers and up to 68% of children with spina bifida (related to multiple routine procedures in which they are exposed on a regular basis to latex, e.g. catheterisation with a rubber-based urinary catheter). These can be compared with an incidence of less than 1% of the general population in the USA (Palosuo, 1998; American Latex Allergy Association, 2008).

Type I (immediate) is IgE mediated and anaphylactic. This reaction is systemic, the onset of symptoms occurs within minutes and is life threatening.

Type IV (delayed) is a T cell–mediated reaction that occurs 48–96 hr after exposure. In general, it is localised to the area of contact. This is also known as 'allergic dermatitis', 'T cell–mediated allergy' or 'chemical allergy' (American Latex Allergy Association, 2008).

Type I symptoms range from mild to severe. They include:

- hives or welts;
- reddened, itchy or teary eyes;
- swelling of the affected area;
- sore throat, hoarse voice;
- runny nose;
- abdominal cramps;
- headaches;
- chest tightness, wheezing or shortness of breath.

In the PPACU, management is based upon (Queensland Health, 2002):

- checking for identification of allergy in notes, bed/trolley, armband;
- notification of all departments and services involved (medical, nursing, catering, cleaning services, allied health);
- provision of synthetic gloves;
- damping-dusting furniture and equipment to remove traces of latex and contaminated powder, and letting them dry;
- acquiring latex-free kit, listing and identifying all latex products and alternative products;
- planning of procedures accordingly, for instance some hospitals have implemented systems to treat latex-sensitive patients by allocating them first on daily surgical lists;
- always be prepared to treat anaphylactic shock.

Various organisations in many countries provide guidelines for wards, operating rooms, recovery, birthing suites and other procedural areas. The most important objective is to attempt to provide a latex-free environment by reducing contact with latex equipment and diminishing the possibility of an allergic reaction. Identification of such patients and staff is a must. Question individuals at risk, for instance, children with spina bifida. Label the patient's records and remove all latex gloves.

In the PPACU, use synthetic gloves and recover the child in the theatre in order to reduce possible contamination with latex powder from nearby rooms. At handover of the child to the collecting ward staff, PPACU staff must ensure that ward staff are aware of the patient's allergy. Check surgical drains, urinary catheters and any other equipment used in surgery to ensure that rubber items have not been used inadvertently. Cover limbs with linen to protect skin from contact with rubber cuffs when checking blood pressure. Check oxymeter probes for rubber (they can be used over clear dressings) and do not draw up drugs through rubber bungs, nor give drugs where there is a rubber stopper within the vial (Queensland Health, 2002). It is important to always ensure that the latex allergy information about the patient is passed on to other health care professionals.

Children with epilepsy

The child with epilepsy may fit in the PPACU due to their daily medication being withheld, and agents and drugs such as propofol, enflurane, methohexitone and pethidine can cause fitting. Other causes include hypoxia, hypoglycaemia, local anaesthetic toxicity, hypocarbia, pyrexia, hypocalcaemia, water intoxication and malignant hypertension (Hatfield & Tronson, 2002).

Management of a fitting child

- Turn the child into recovery position
- Suction the airway
- Give 100% O_2 via mask
- Support breathing
- Get help, ask for resuscitation trolley
- Do not force anything into the child's mouth
- Protect the child, so that he/she does not harm self
- Record vital signs
- Attach pulse oxymeter, ECG and BP monitor
- Secure IV access
- Further management may include IV thiopentone, diazepam or phenytoin
- Consider possible aspiration (Hatfield & Tronson, 2002).

Delayed emergence

Delayed emergence is uncommon in children, but it does occur. In the advent of delayed emergence, three main questions should be answered:

(1) Is there evidence of a life-threatening condition?
(2) Is there evidence that anaesthetic agents could be the reason for delayed emergence?
(3) Are there medical/surgical reasons for delayed emergence?

After ruling out any of the above, observe the patient. Children respond to anaesthetic agents in a variety of ways. Some may nap for the rest of the day, while others return to their baseline quickly. It should be emphasised that the paediatric patient responds to the stress of surgery and anaesthesia by sleeping and resting. Efforts made by PPACU staff and parents should be aimed at arousal (Hatfield & Tronson, 2002).

Emergence delirium

Sometimes the paediatric patient experiences agitation during emergence. The child will appear to have perceptual difficulties, not knowing where he or she is or what is happening. Hazardous and treatable conditions should be excluded before assuming anxiety, unfamiliar surroundings and other reasons. Common causes of emergence delirium include:

- hypoxia;
- pain;
- hypercapnia;
- full bladder;
- hypoventilation;
- premedication (ketamine, hyoscine);
- acidosis;
- volatile anaesthetics;
- hypoglycaemia;
- hypothermia;
- increased ICP (Hatfield & Tronson, 2002).

Factors predisposing to emergence delirium are:

- young age;
- alcohol or drug abuse;
- inadequate psychological preparation;
- intraoperative hypoxia;
- intraoperative hypotension;
- intraoperative cholinergic drugs;
- intraoperative awareness.

Management of emergence delirium comprises:

- O_2 therapy at 100%;
- pulse oximetry and ensuring saturations are adequate;
- restraining the child if necessary;
- parents to help with wakening the child (Hatfield & Tronson, 2002).

Discharge of the patient from the PPACU

Criteria for discharging patients from the PPACU are related to where the patient is being transferred, the type of surgery, physiological status and level of wakefullness and activity. In 1970, Aldrete and Kroulik introduced a scoring system for discharge from PPACU based on clinical assessment. Observations regarding the wound, drains, catheters, bleeding, urinary and gastrointestinal output must be included, as should the child's haemodynamic status, temperature, pain level, IV administration and general comfort (Odom, 2003). Box 8.8 shows the PARS system.

The PPACU nurse must ensure that the patient is stable before discharging them from the unit. Each hospital will have guidelines and policies for this, where the criteria for discharge are described. To provide continuity of care, the time spent and care

Box 8.8   Post-anaesthesia recovery score (PARS)

Activity
0 = Unable to lift head or move extremities voluntarily or on command.
1 = Can lift head or move extremities voluntarily or on command.
2 = Able to move four extremities voluntarily or on command. Can lift head and has controlled
    movement.

Respiration
0 = Apnoeic, needs ventilator or assisted respiration.
1 = Laboured/limited respirations. Breathes by self but has shallow, slow respirations. May have
    an oral airway.
2 = Can take a deep breath and cough well. Has normal respiratory rate and depth.

Circulation
0 = Has abnormal high/low blood pressure; BP 50 mmHg or pre-anaesthetic level.
1 = BP 20–50 mmHg of pre-anaesthetic level.
2 = Stable BP and pulse. BP 2 mmHg of pre-anaesthetic level (minimum 90 mmHg systolic).

Neurologic status
0 = Not responding or responding only to painful stimuli.
1 = Responds to verbal stimuli but drifts off to sleep easily.
2 = Awake and alert.

Oxygen saturation
0 = O_2 saturation <90% even with O_2 supplement.
1 = Needs O_2 inhalation to maintain O_2 saturation >90%.
2 = Able to maintain O_2 saturation >92% on room air.

Source: Odom (2007, p. 38).

given in the PPACU must be recorded. A verbal report of the child's status must be provided to the next nurse responsible for post-operative management (Little, 1996).

Some factors that will delay post-operative recovery in children include residual anaesthetic or neuromuscular blockade, hypothermia, hypoxaemia, acid–base imbalance, hypercarbia, hypovolaemia and elevated ICP. The PPACU nurse should avoid giving early oral fluid intake, which may cause vomiting. It is advisable to wait until the child asks for a drink (Johnson, 2003).

Psychological assessment

Parents in the PPACU

Increasingly, parents are requesting more involvement in relation to the care of their children in surgery. The desire to participate in their child's care and to be present during procedures is growing. However, permission to participate in paediatric patient anaesthetic management has not always been given by anaesthetists and surgeons (Munro & D'Erico, 2000). The surgical experience creates anxiety for parents and children. For the young, the reason and necessity for surgery may be concepts difficult to grasp. The unfamiliar environment, loss of control and emergency of the situation are all anxiety provoking, and the child's temperament has been shown to influence his or her behaviour in response to stressful situations (Voepel-Lewis *et al.*, 2000). Pre-anaesthetic sedatives have been shown to reduce anxiety, easing separation and promote smooth anaesthetic induction (Munro & D'Erico, 2000). However, the use of premedication may have disadvantages such as increased pharmaceutical cost, increased demands on perioperative staff and equipment and possibly prolonged recovery (Voepel-Lewis *et al.*, 2000). Studies have shown that parental presence minimises anxiety, reduces the need for premedication, avoids distress of separation and possibly decreases post-operative anxiety (Munro & D'Erico, 2000). A complex relationship exists between parental and child anxiety, previous hospitalisation, preoperative preparation and the child's temperament. Voepel-Lewis *et al.* (2000) found that parents were the best predictors of their children's separation behaviour. In the PPACU, the same involvement is wanted and/or required by parents as that in the pre-anaesthetic phase, as they believe that they are able to help their child. It is widely recognised that parental presence is helpful to both children and staff. In some hospitals, it is a standard of care. Benefits of family involvement in the child's recovery include diminished anxiety for both parent and child, rapid orientation after emergence and increased satisfaction. However, as with parent-present induction of anaesthesia, parents should be prepared with what to expect in the PPACU. The hospital/institution should establish guidelines as to when it is appropriate to involve the parents. Parameters such as ability to maintain airway and to be haemodynamically stable should be considered before parents join their recovering child in the PPACU (Voepel-Lewis *et al.*, 2000). Parental presence should be permitted if staffing and the physical structure of the unit permit. Restrictions for parental presence might include lack of privacy, the child's acuity and the fast turnover of the PPACU. However, some children may have a prolonged stay in the PPACU, waiting for a bed in the wards, waiting for another procedure or the lack of post-operative bed. The PPACU may have to establish criteria that will accommodate a variety of situations such as when death of a patient may be imminent in the receiving ward; when the patient must return to surgery; when the child's well-being depends on the presence of his or her parents and when the child requires an interpreter (Odom-Forren, 2007).

Parental presence is often based on hospital policy or tradition rather than on family needs, though policies vary among institutions. Often, the PPACU nurses determine when, and if, parents are able to come into the unit (Jackson *et al.*, 1997). In this study, family members reported that the reason they wanted to come into PPACU was 'to see the patient', while nurses did not see this as such an important need for the parents (Jackson *et al.*, 1997) (Figure 8.6).

The Royal Children's Hospital in Brisbane, Australia undertook a study entitled 'Evaluation of Parental Visitation in the Post Anaesthetic Care Unit' in 2002 (which is currently under revision). Nevertheless, the study showed that 35% of staff agreed that parents should routinely visit their children in PACU. The staff identified that information about PACU should be provided to parents and it should contain:

- the way to behave during an emergency;
- the need for confidentiality and privacy;
- a warning that parents would see procedures performed on other children;
- an explanation of the behaviours that children exhibit post-anaesthesia.

Unlike an earlier study, which found that parents' being in PPACU did not relieve the children's anxiety levels, but did reduce those of the parents (Bru *et al.*, 1993), they found that visiting the PPACU did not reduce parental anxiety to a greater extent than not visiting the PPACU. However, positive outcomes were made regarding the

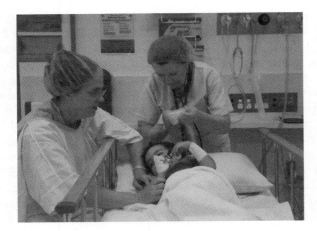

Fig. 8.6   A child with his mother in PPACU.

PPACU visit experience, including that parents wish to be given the opportunity to visit PPACU; that staff determine if parents can be invited into PPACU without negatively impacting on the safety of the children or the work of the PACU staff; that criteria for visitation must take into account the staff and parental needs and that some modifications of the physical environment were needed in order to provide an aesthetically pleasing PPACU for children and parents. These modifications should consider staff and parents' concerns about privacy and confidentiality.

Psychological considerations

Above all, by addressing parental needs, the PPACU nurse will help to diminish the stress on the child (Johnson, 2003). The PPACU is a strange environment, with strange people wearing strange clothing (hats, masks, goggles, gloves). Allowing the child to bring a special toy to help with the environmental change will help, especially during emergence. Johnson advocates that parents should be allowed to be with the child as soon as practical and before his or her awakening. During the emergence stage, the PPACU nurse should meet the emotional needs of the child according to his or her stage of development. For instance, a baby likes to be held and or rocked, cuddled in a warm blanket, having head or back rubbed, taking into consideration the type of surgery and level of emergence from anaesthesia. From ages 2 to 3 years, the children need reassurance. They are at the stage of autonomy versus self-doubt, and too young to reason. Their greatest fear is related to separation from parents, pain, physical harm, strange environment and the unknown. The pre-schooler, ages 3–6 years, is more independent but in the PPACU, dependency happens because of pain or immobilisation. The nurse should provide opportunities for independence by allowing alternative ways of care, e.g. allowing the child to determine whether or not to have their favourite toy beside them (Johnson, 2003). The school-age child (6–12 years) seeks approval and usually does not tolerate failure. This is the time to encourage self-care as much as possible, promote self-expression and acknowledge achievements (e.g. compliment him or her on accomplishments during recovery from anaesthesia).

Table 8.4 Types of communication with children

Types of Communication		
Verbal	Spoken words	• May be some language barriers • Misunderstanding
Non-verbal	Most reliable	• Child's natural way of expression
Communication Skills		
Listening		• Understand level of language development and child's • Developmental level • Explain procedures
Observation		• Gives cues about child • Observe eyes, facial expression, tone of voice, body language, movement, cry, whining, silence, parental interaction with child
Silence		• Child is afraid or shy, angry, busy

Source: De Fazio Quinn & Shick (2004).

At this age, the child has a colourful imagination and could easily distort reality. The adolescent (12–18 years) vacillates between dependence and independence, idealism and realism, confidence and uncertainty. To this age group, privacy is paramount, therefore keep him or her covered and screened from other patients in the PPACU (Johnson, 2003). The PPACU nurse, by addressing the developmental needs of the child and promoting parental involvement will lead the family to a positive experience for them all.

Always, when nursing children, effective communication is one of the core factors in the care experience, for children and parents and staff. This is as true in PPACU as in any other care context. De Fazio Quinn and Shick (2004), using Eriksson's and Piaget's development theories when referring to the communication and educational needs of the paediatric patient, recommend that the PPACU nurse should, when dealing with children, consider the types of communication shown in Table 8.4.

References

Abelha, F.J., Castro, M.A., Neves, A.M., Landeiro, N.M., Santos, C.C. (2005). Hypothermia in a surgical intensive care unit. *BMC Anesthesiology*, 5. Available from http://www.biomedcentral.com/content/pdf/1471-2253-5-7.pdf (accessed 4 February 2008).

Advanced Life Support Group. (2001). *Advanced paediatric life support. The practical approach*, 3rd ed. BMJ Books, BMA Publishing Group, London.

American Latex Allergy Association (2008). *Latex allergy statistics*. American Latex Allergy Association, Slinger, Wisconsin. Available from http://www.latexallergyresources.org/topics/LatexAllergyStatistics.cfm (accessed 4 February 2008).

American Society of Anesthesiologists. (2008). *Guidelines for patient care in anesthesiology*. Available from http://www.asahq.org/publicationsAndServices/standards/13.pdf (accessed 1 February 2008).

Anderson, K.N. (1994). *Mosby's medical, nursing, and allied health dictionary*, 4th ed. Mosby, St. Louis.

Australian and New Zealand College of Anaesthetists. (2006). *PS4 recommendations for the post-anaesthesia recovery room – 2006.* Available from http://www.anzca.edu.au/resources/professional-documents/professional-standards/ps4.html (accessed 1 February 2008).

Australian College of Operating Room Nurses. (2004a). *Staffing Requirements – Standard Statement 5.* Australian College of Operating Room Nurses, Adelaide.

Australian College of Operating Room Nurses. (2004b). *Standards: G4 Management of Postanaesthesia Recovery (PAR) Unit.* Australian College of Operating Room Nurses, Adelaide.

Australian College of Operating Room Nurses. (2006). *2006 ACORN standards for perioperative nurses including nursing roles, guidelines, position statements and competency standards.* Available from http://www.acorn.org.au/index.php/content/view/60/62/ (accessed 1 February 2008).

Bellamy, C. (2007). Inadvertent hypothermia in the operating theatre: An examination. *Journal of Perioperative Practice*, 17(1): 18–25.

Bergeson, P.S., Shaw, C.J. (2001). Are infants really obligatory nasal breathers? *Clinical Pediatrics*, 40: 567–569.

Berthal, E.M.M. (1999). Inadvertent hypothermia prevention, the anesthetic nurse's role. *British Journal of Nursing*, 8: 17–25.

Bru, G., Carmody, S., Donohue-Sword, B., Bookbinder, M. (1993). Parental visitation in the post-anesthesia care unit: A means to lessen anxiety. *Children's Health Care*, 22: 217–226.

Canadian Society of Anesthesiologists. (2007). *Guidelines to the practice of anesthesia: Revised edition 2007.* Available from http://www.cas.ca/members/sign_in/guidelines/practice_of_anesthesia/ (accessed 1 February 2008).

Culy, C.R., Bhana, N., Plosker, G.L. (2001). Ondansetron: A review of its use as an antiemetic in children. *Paediatric Drugs*, 3: 441–449.

De Fazio Quinn, D.M., Schick, L. (2004). *Perianesthesia nursing core curriculum: Preoperative Phase I & Phase II PACU Nursing.* Saunders, St. Louis.

Drain, C.B. (2003). *Perianesthesia nursing: A critical approach*, 4th ed. W.B. Saunders, Philadelphia.

English, W. (2002). Post-operative shivering, causes, prevention and treatment. *Update in Anaesthesia*, 15: Article 3.

Ewing, P.H., Long, S.P. (2003). In: Drain, C.B. (ed.). *Perianesthesia nursing: A critical care approach*, 4th ed. W.B. Saunders, Philadelphia.

Ferrara-Love, R. (2004). In: De Fazio Quinn, D.M., Schick, L. (eds). *Perianesthesia nursing core curriculum: Preoperative Phase I and Phase II PACU Nursing.* W.B. Saunders, St. Louis.

Hatfield, A., Tronson, M., 2002. *The complete recovery room book*, 2nd ed. Oxford University Press, Oxford.

Hommertzheim, R., Steinke, R. (2006). Malignant hyperthermia – The perioperative nurse's role. *Association of Operating room Nurses Journal*, 83: 149–171.

Inpharma. (2001). News in brief: Droperidol to be discontinued in the UK. *Inpharma*, 1: 20.

Jackson, L.B., Marcell, J., Benedict, S. (1997). Nurse's attitudes toward parental visitation on the postanesthesia care unit. *Journal of Perianesthesia Nursing*, 12: 2–6.

Johnson, D.L. (2003). In: Drain, C.B. (ed.). *Perianesthesia nursing: A critical approach*, 4th ed. W.B. Saunders, Philadelphia.

Little, D.J. (1996). In: Fairchild, S.S. (ed.). *Perioperative nursing: Principles and practice*, 2nd ed. Lippincott, Philadelphia.

Litwack, K. (1997). Practical points in the evaluation of postoperative fever. *Journal of Perianesthesia Nursing*, 12: 100–104.

Malignant Hyperthermia Association of the United States-MHAUS. Online Brochure. (2006). *ABCs of Malignant Hyperthermia, Anesthetic List for MH – Susceptible patients, Mixing Dantrolene.* Available from http://medical.mhaus.og/index.cfm/fuseaction/OnlineBrochures.Display/BrochurePK/BCD9151D-3048-709E-5A445BC0808B4767.cfm (accessed 2 September 2008).

Mater Children's Hospital (2006). Post anaesthetic care phase, observations & documentation. Policy No. MHS, WCH-MCH –091. Mater Children's Hospital, Brisbane.

McGaffigan, P.A. Christoph, S.B. (2003). In: Drain, C.B. (ed.). *Perianesthesia nursing: A critical approach*, 4th ed. W.B. Saunders, Philadelphia.

Merckel, S., Malviya, S. (2000). Pediatric pain, tools and assessment. *Journal of Perianesthesia Nursing*, 15: 408–414.

MIMS Online. (2004). Ephedrine sulfate. MIMS Abbreviated Prescribing Information. Section: 2(h) Adrenergic stimulants, vasopressor agents. Available from http://mims.hcn.net.au.ezproxy.library.uq.edu.au/ifmx-nsapi/mims-data/?MIval=2MIMS_abbr_pi&product_code=1274&product_name=Ephedrine+Sulfate+Injection+%28DBL%29 (accessed 3 February 2008).

MIMS Online. (2005). Kytril, Granisetron. MIMS Abbreviated Prescribing Information Section: 9(g) Noncytotoxic and supportive therapy. Available from http://mims.hcn.net.au.ezproxy.library.uq.edu.au/ifmx-nsapi/mims-data/?MIval=2MIMS_abbr_pi&product_code=6893&product_name=Kytril (accessed 3 February 2008).

MIMS Online. (2006). *Promethazine hydrochloride.* Prescribing information. Available from http://mims.hcn.net.au.ezproxy.library.uq.edu.au/ifmx-nsapi/mims-data/?MIval=2MIMS_abbr_pi&product_code=1311&product_name=Phenergan (accessed 3 February 2008).

MIMS Online. (2007a). Stemetil: MIMS Abbreviated Prescribing Information Section: 3(h) Antiemetics, antinauseants. Available from http://mims.hcn.net.au.ezproxy.library.uq.edu.au/ifmx-nsapi/mims-data/?MIval=2MIMS_abbr_pi&product_code=553&product_name=Stemetil (accessed 3 February 2008).

MIMS Online. (2007b). Maxolon. MIMS Abbreviated Prescribing Information. Section: 3(h) Antiemetics, antinauseants. Available from http://mims.hcn.net.au.ezproxy.library.uq.edu.au/ifmx-nsapi/mims-data/?MIval=2MIMS_abbr_pi&product_code=547&product_name=Maxolon (accessed 3 February 2008).

MIMS Online. (2007c). Droperidol. MIMS Abbreviated Prescribing Information. Section: 3(c) Antipsychotic agents. Available from http://mims.hcn.net.au.ezproxy.library.uq.edu.au/ifmx-nsapi/mims-data/?MIval=2MIMS_abbr_pi&product_code=473&product_name=Droleptan+Injection (accessed 3 February 2008).

MIMS Online. (2007d). Ondansetron Injection. MIMS Abbreviated Prescribing Information. Section: 9(g) Noncytotoxic and supportive therapy. Available from http://mims.hcn.net.au.ezproxy.library.uq.edu.au/ifmx-nsapi/mims-data/?MIval=2MIMS_abbr_pi&product_code=7827&product_name=Ondansetron+Injection (accessed 3 February 2008).

Munro, H. (2000). Postoperative nausea and vomiting in children. *Journal of Perianesthesia Nursing*, 15: 401–407.

Munro, H., D'Erico, C. (2000). Parental involvement in perioperative anesthetic management. *Journal of Perianesthesia Nursing*, 15: 397–400.

O'Brien, C.M., Titley, G., Whitehurst, P. (2003). A comparison of cyclizine, ondansetron and placebo as prophylaxis against postoperative nausea and vomiting in children. *Anaesthesia*, 58: 707–711.

Odom, J. (2003). In: Drain, C.B. (ed.). *Perianesthesia nursing: A critical approach*, 4th ed. W.B. Saunders, Philadelphia.

Odom-Forren, J. (2007). In: Rothrock, J.C. (ed.). *Alexander's care of the patient in surgery*, 13th ed). Mosby/Elsevier, St. Louis.

Oldman, M., Youngs, P., Johnson, A. (2003). A response to 'A comparison of cyclizine, ondansetron and placebo as prophylaxis against postoperative nausea and vomiting in children' O'Brien CM, Titley G, Whitehurst P, Anaesthesia 2003; 58: 707–11. *Anaesthesia*, 58: 1151.

Palosuo, T. (1998). Which came first – food allergy or natural rubber latex allergy? Are there any studies to support your reply? *Source to Surgery, the Newsletter of the Ansell Cares Scientific Advisory Board*, 6: 3.

Queensland Health. (2002). *Latex guidelines for health care facilities*. Queensland Organisational Development, Employment Relations and Strategies, Employment Work Practices, Brisbane.

Queensland Health. (2005a). *Transition to Practice – Nurse Education Program – Perioperative. Module 2 – Anaesthetic Nursing Care*. Queensland Government, Brisbane.

Queensland Health. (2005b). *Transition to Practice – Nurse Education Program – Perioperative. Module 4 – Postanaesthetic Nursing Care*. Queensland Government, Brisbane.

Queensland Health. (2006). *Acute pain management workbook*. Queensland Health, Brisbane.

Redmond, M.C. (2001). Malignant hyperthermia: Perianesthesia recognition, treatment and care. *Journal of Perianesthesia Nursing*, 6: 259–270.

Sessler, D.F. (2001). Complications and treatment of mild hypothermia. *Anesthesiology*, 95: 531–543.

Shields, L., Waterman, L. (2002). In: Shields, L., Werder, H. (eds). *Perioperative nursing*. Greenwich Medical Media, London.

Simpson, P. (2004). *Guidance on the provision of anaesthetic services for post-operative care guidelines for the provision of anaesthetic services (July 2004)*. Royal College of Anaesthetists. Available from http://www.rcoa.ac.uk/index.asp?PageID=477 (accessed 1 February 2008).

Smith, B., O'Brien T. In: Drain, C.B. (ed.). *Perianesthesia nursing: A critical approach*, 4th ed. W.B. Saunders, Philadelphia.

Stedman, T.L. (2006). *Stedman's medical dictionary*, 28th ed. Lippincott, Williams & Wilkins, Philadelphia.

Stow, J. (2007). In: Rothrock, J.C. *Alexander's care of the patient in surgery*, 13th ed. Mosby/Elsevier, St. Louis.

Suleman, M.I., Doufas, A.G., Akca, D., Ducharme, M., Sessler, D.F. (2002). Insufficiency in a new temporal-artery thermometer for adults and pediatric patients. *Anesthesia and Analgesia*, 95: 67–71.

Voepel-Lewis, T., Tait, A.R., Malviya, S. (2000). Separation and induction behaviors in children: Are parents good predictors? *Journal of Perianesthesia Nursing*, 5: 6–11.

9   Fetal surgery

Roy Kimble

Introduction

This chapter provides an overview of fetal surgery. Fetal surgery is a relatively new specialty and should be regarded as mainly experimental. Fetal surgery should only be undertaken in the few centres in the world where a full fetal surgical programme exists.

Fetal surgery is undertaken either to:

(1) Correct a congenital abnormality before birth to improve post-natal outcome. These abnormalities must carry a very high incidence of major morbidity or mortality to justify correction.
  • Spina bifida
  • Twin–twin transfusion
  • Congenital cystic adenomatoid malformation (CCAM) with hydrops
  • Amniotic bands
(2) Intervene to alter the sequence of events resulting from an abnormality in order to prevent death or major morbidity. The causative abnormality itself is not removed and will require definitive surgery post-natally:
  • Bladder neck obstruction
  • Congenital diaphragmatic hernia
(3) Secure tracheal intubation or perform another procedure at the time of a planned Caesarean section prior to division of the umbilical cord. This is known as *ex utero* intrapartum treatment (EXIT).

History

Fetal surgical techniques using animal models were first developed at the University of California, San Francisco, during the 1970s and 1980s. In 1981, the first human open fetal surgery in the world was performed in this centre under the direction of Dr. Michael Harrison. The fetus had a bladder neck obstruction causing hydronephrosis. A vesico-amniotic shunt was placed to relieve the obstruction. The fetus survived and the defect was corrected post-natally. Since that time, many procedures for several different fetal conditions have been developed, and a shift has occurred away from open procedures to relatively safer minimally invasive techniques. Animal models have provided much of the evidence needed to progress to human fetal surgery. The problems with this approach are twofold. First, these models are created surgically at a gestational age well after the abnormality arises in the human fetus, and so the full spectrum of consequences of the abnormality is not reproduced. Second, the main animal model used is the pregnant sheep. Favoured by researchers because of the long gestation and fetal size comparable to humans, the ovine uterus is very non-reactive and much more amenable to manipulation and surgery. It is very easy to progress the ovine pregnancy to term after fetal intervention, whereas the human pregnancy in similar circumstances invariably ends with a preterm delivery. These two factors gave rise to much world enthusiasm in the 1990s where it was thought that fetal surgery would make a great impact on post-natal outcomes. Unfortunately, this has not been the case and most human trials have been disappointing at best. However, the research into this field has allowed us to have a much better understanding of the pathophysiology of congenital abnormalities. The other factor to consider is the improvements made in post-natal care, which has taken away much of the need for antenatal intervention. This has been most true for the fetus with congenital diaphragmatic hernia.

The risks of fetal surgery

It is important to understand that when operating on the fetus there are two patients: mother and fetus. Fetal surgery can result in major morbidity or mortality for either and this needs special consideration. Open fetal surgery involves opening the abdomen of the mother, and through a hysterotomy deliver the fetal part requiring surgery. This carries very high risks for both the fetus and the mother, with preterm labour being the almost universal result. Maternal complications include pulmonary oedema from tocolytics, amniotic fluid leaks and the usual possible complications from an abdominal wound (Adzick & Harrison, 1997). The hysterotomy in fetal surgery is invariably in the upper segment of the uterine corpus and thus is comparable to a classical Caesarean section. This puts the pregnancy into a high-risk group for uterine disruption during labour, and delivery after open fetal surgery and all future deliveries should be by Caesarean section (Adzick & Harrison, 1997). Fetoscopy allows for fetal repair without a large hysterotomy incision. The fetoscope is either inserted through both maternal abdominal wall and uterus or directly through the uterus after exposure of the uterus through an abdominal incision. This fetoscopic surgical approach has the potential to expand the indications for *in utero* surgery by decreasing fetal risks, facilitating intervention earlier in gestation and reducing preterm labour. Percutaneous ultrasound-guided procedures, if possible, offer a further reduction in potential complications.

Morbidity can be kept to a minimum if fetal surgery is confined to tertiary centres of excellence that have a well-established fetal surgical programme (Golombeck *et al.*, 2006). A 24-year review of fetal surgery was carried out at the Fetal Treatment Center at the University of California, San Francisco of 187 pregnant women who underwent fetal intervention for a congenital abnormality either by open surgery, fetoscopy or percutaneous ultrasound-guided procedures (Golombeck *et al.*, 2006). There were no maternal deaths, but significant short-term morbidity was observed in all groups. Open surgery carried most morbidity with significantly increased rates of intensive care, prolonged hospitalisation and blood transfusion. There were no significant differences between endoscopic procedures and open surgery in the incidence of premature rupture of membranes, pulmonary oedema, placental abruption, post-operative vaginal bleeding, preterm delivery, or interval from maternal-fetal surgery to delivery. Chorion-amnion membrane separation was seen more often in the endoscopy group. Complications were significantly less in the percutaneous ultrasound-guided procedures (Golombeck *et al.*, 2006).

Fetal conditions amenable to fetal surgery

Twin–twin transfusion syndrome

Twin–twin transfusion syndrome (TTTS) occurs in approximately 15% of monochorionic pregnancies and results from shunting of blood from one twin, the donor, to the other twin, the recipient, through placental vascular anastomoses. Untreated, TTTS is associated with high perinatal mortality and morbidity (mainly neurological). The two current treatment options in TTTS are serial amnioreduction and fetoscopic laser occlusion of vascular anastomoses (Lopriore *et al.*, 2007). There is now good evidence from several centres that endoscopic laser ablation can reduce fetal mortality and post-natal neurological impairment. However, even with selective antenatal laser ablation, mortality is still around 23–30%, and 17% of the survivors have significant neurological impairment (Lopriore *et al.*, 2007; Gray *et al.*, 2006).

Congenital diaphragmatic hernia

Congenital diaphragmatic hernia (CDH) carries an overall mortality of around 50% despite optimal planned tertiary care. This substantial mortality is attributed to pulmonary hypoplasia caused by the presence of abdominal viscera in the chest during intrauterine life. There are several ultrasound findings that help in predicting mortality in affected fetuses, and include: liver or stomach in the chest, polyhydramnios, an unfavourable head-lung ratio and an early diagnosis. Much effort has gone into developing an antenatal intervention that will achieve better lung growth. It was originally thought that repair of the actual diaphragmatic hernia defect *in utero* was the answer, as this had been performed successfully on fetal sheep. In San Francisco, a human trial was commenced in the late 1980s but had to be discontinued after it was shown that the only survivors were those that could have been predicted to survive without intervention (Harrison *et al.*, 1993). All the fetuses with liver in the chest died owing to kinking of the umbilical vein on return of the liver to the abdomen. A fundamental problem was that the animal model that they used never had liver in the chest. Later it was shown that tracheal occlusion *in utero* causes lungs to expand greatly owing to the fetal lungs being net producers of fluid (Hedrich *et al.*, 1994). Unfortunately, although large, these lungs lack compliance and have a paucity of surfactant production, vital for normally functioning lungs. Several techniques of tracheal occlusion have been perfected, the least invasive being endoscopic balloon insertion. A prospective randomised trial in human using this technique was discontinued when it was noted that the survival rate in fetuses treated with tracheal occlusion was no better than if antenatal intervention had not taken place (73% versus 77% survival respectively) (Harrison *et al.*, 2003). The results showed not a failure in the technique but instead highlighted the significant improvements that have occurred in the post-natal management in babies with CDH. Research is now underway to determine if there is any group of fetuses with CDH that may benefit from antenatal intervention.

Urinary tract obstruction

Bladder neck obstruction, if severe, will affect the fetus in two ways. First, the obstructive uropathy will cause secondary damage to kidneys, resulting in renal impairment. Second, oligohydramnios due to decreased urine outflow causes pulmonary hypoplasia. Prenatal intervention for obstructive uropathy has the potential to increase pulmonary survival and improve renal outcomes. The least invasive way to intervene is to bypass the obstruction by inserting a vesico-amniotic shunt under ultrasound guidance. There has also been some success with fetal cystoscopy and ablation of posterior urethral valves either by laser, diathermy or with a saline jet. Strict criteria are essential prior to intervention including presence of oligohydramnios and favourable urine electrolytes as measured by serial bladder aspiration. Results from several centres performing these procedures are fairly disappointing with a high rate of renal insufficiency in survivors (Biard *et al.*, 2005). The poor results are almost certainly due to much of the damage having already occurred prior to intervention. Future success may well depend on determining which fetuses are in the poor prognostic group earlier in pregnancy prior to the development of oligohydramnios.

Congenital cystic adenomatoid malformation

Congenital cystic adenomatoid malformation (CCAM) is a developmental abnormality of the lung, usually affecting a single lobe where there is disorganised growth of bronchial tissue and cysts of variable size. The majority of babies with this lung abnormality go through pregnancy uneventfully. In a few, however, the mass effect caused by the lesion causes cardiovascular embarrassment and fetal hydrops. Fetal hydrops is defined by having two or more of the following: subcutaneous oedema, ascites, pleural effusion or pericardial effusion. When associated with hydrops, untreated fetuses with a CCAM universally have a fatal outcome. Without hydrops, the vast majority will survive. It has been shown that open fetal surgery and lobectomy on these fetuses with CCAM and hydrops can offer a 50% survival rate (Grethel *et al.*, 2007). More importantly, there is some good evidence that appropriately timed maternal steroid administration may result in a resolution of the hydrops, and a good outcome without the need for surgery (Peranteau *et al.*, 2007; Johnson *et al.*, 2006). Trials on this latter approach are awaited.

Spina bifida

Despite encouraging results from fetal animal model studies, prenatal closure of spina bifida defects have not been shown to significantly change outcomes in terms of bladder or neurological function. There is evidence however that the need for ventriculoperitoneal shunting is reduced, which may have long-term neurological benefits (Johnson *et al.*, 2006).

Sacrococcygeal teratoma

Sacrococcygeal teratoma is a rare tumour found in approximately 1:40,000 pregnancies. Most affected fetuses will have an uneventful pregnancy and can await surgery post-delivery. However, the occasional fetus will develop high-output cardiac failure, resulting in hydrops due to a high blood flow to the lesion. Like hydrops affecting the fetus with a CCAM, hydrops in this situation is fatal. Several successful attempts at debulking or excision of sacrococcygeal teratomas complicated by hydrops have been reported (Grethel *et al.*, 2007).

Amniotic bands

Amniotic bands sometimes cause constriction of a fetal limb. In situations where blood flow is impaired and the limb is at risk, division of the band can be performed fetoscopically.

Skin biopsy

Several inherited rare, but lethal skin conditions exist that can only be diagnosed by fetal skin biopsy. A biopsy can be successfully taken in these situations with a pair of biopsy forceps passed through a needle under ultrasound control.

Ex utero intrapartum treatment (EXIT)

Large neck masses, usually teratomas, can cause airway compression. These neonates can often be very difficult to intubate at the time of delivery, and a tracheostomy is sometimes necessary. When a fetus with a neck mass and a potential airway obstruction is diagnosed antenatally, an EXIT procedure can be planned. At the time of Caesarean section, only the head and neck are delivered, leaving the baby on its placental blood flow. This buys valuable minutes where the airway can be assessed and either endotracheal intubation or tracheostomy performed (Figure 9.1). All neonates

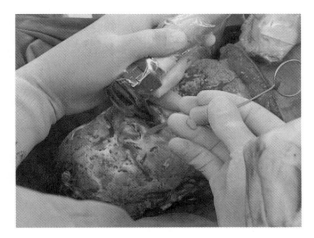

Fig. 9.1 Fetus with neck mass undergoing EXIT procedure

with CDH and an artificial tracheal occlusion (see above) need to be delivered this way, and have the occlusion device removed prior to intubation.

The future

The future for fetal surgery is not certain. Better tocolytics are certainly required to stabilise the uterus and allow for a longer gestation. However, some treatments are proving their worth, including endoscopic treatment for twin–twin transfusion, which is the main indication for fetal intervention in most centres. The trend generally is to move away from invasive open procedures, and to a move towards minimally invasive techniques. Improvements with post-natal care have removed much of the need for fetal intervention, and this has certainly been the case with the fetus with CDH.

References

Adzick, N.S., Harrison, M.R. (1997). The fetus as a patient. In: Oldham, K.T., Colombani, P.M., Foglia, R.P. (eds). *Surgery of infants and children*. Lippincott-Ravin Publishers, Philadelphia.

Biard, J.M., Johnson, M.P., Carr, M.C., Wilson, R.D., Hedrick, H.L., Pavlock, C., Adzick, N.S. (2005). Long-term outcomes in children treated by prenatal vesicoamniotic shunting for lower urinary tract obstruction. *Obstetrics and Gynecology*, 106: 503–508.

Golombeck, K., Ball, R.H., Lee, H. (2006). Maternal morbidity after maternal–fetal surgery. *American Journal of Obstetrics and Gynecology*, 194: 834–839.

Gray, P.H., Cincotta, R., Chan, F.Y., Soong, B. (2006). Perinatal outcomes with laser surgery for twin–twin transfusion syndrome. *Twin research and human genetics: the official journal of the International Society for Twin Studies*, 9: 438–443.

Grethel, E.J., Wagner, A.J., Clifton, M.S., Cortes, R.A., Farmer, D.L., Harrison, M.R., Nobuhara, K.K., Lee, H. (2007). Fetal intervention for mass lesions and hydrops improves outcome: A 15-year experience. *Journal of Pediatric Surgery*, 42: 117–123.

Harrison, M.R., Adzick, N.S., Flake, A.W., Jennings, R., Estes, J., MacGillivray, T., Chueh, J., Goldberg, J., Filly, R., Goldstein R. (1993). Correction of congenital diaphragmatic hernia *in utero* VI. Hard earned lessons. *Journal of Pediatric Surgery*, 28: 1411–1417.

Harrison, M.R., Keller, R.L., Hawgood, S.B., Kitterman, J.A., Sandberg, D.L., Lee, H., Filly, R.A., Farrell, J.A., Albanese, C.T. (2003). A randomized trial of fetal endoscopic tracheal occlusion for severe fetal congenital diaphragmatic hernia. *New England Journal of Medicine*, 13: 1916–1924.

Hedrich, M.H., Estes, J.M., Sullivan, K.M., Bealer, J.F., Kitterman, J.A., Adzick, N.S., Harrison, M.R. (1994). Plug the lung until it grows (PLUG): A new method to treat congenital diaphragmatic hernia *in utero*. *Journal of Pediatric Surgery*, 29: 612–617.

Johnson, M.P., Gerdes, M., Rintoul, N. (2006). Maternal–fetal surgery for myelomeningocele: Neurodevelopmental outcomes at 2 years of age. *American Journal of Obstetrics and Gynecology*, 194: 1145–1152.

Lopriore, E., Middeldorp, J.M., Sueters, M., Oepkes, D., Vandenbussche, F.P.H.A., Walther, F.J. (2007). Long-term neurodevelopmental outcome in twin-to-twin transfusion syndrome treated with fetoscopic laser surgery. *American Journal of Obstetrics and Gynecology*, 196: 231.e1–231.e4.

Peranteau, W.H., Wilson, R.D., Liechty, K.W., Johnson, M.P., Bebbington, M.W., Hedrick, H.L., Flake, A.W., Adzick, N.S. (2007). Effect of maternal betamethasone administration on prenatal congenital cystic adenomatoid malformation growth and fetal survival. *Fetal Diagnosis and Therapy*, 5: 365–371.

10 Perioperative care of children with burns

Roy Kimble and Julie Mill

Introduction

This chapter is intended to give an in-depth account of the nursing management of the burned child in hospital. Acute management and inpatient care are discussed including definitive procedures, post-operative care and discharge planning. Throughout this chapter, the multidisciplinary team approach is emphasised as the best model of care. As the different care providers within the burns team work together, their boundaries merge and it is vital that all have a full understanding of each other's role.

History

Nurses have been caring for children with burns for millennia. However, paediatrics as a separate specialty only came about in the early part of the 20th century, and burn units only started to appear at the time of the Second World War. In the first quarter of the 20th century, hot paraffin wax was often used to coat burns after cleaning. Tanning agents became a popular treatment between the world wars. The effect of both of these treatments was to seal off the burn wound until the eschar separated revealing a granulating surface, which could then be grafted. During this several-week waiting period, many patients succumbed to sepsis, and those who survived inevitably developed unsightly hypertrophic scars and severe contractures. However, as early as 1947, it was recognised that early excision of burn eschar and grafting resulted in better survival (Cope *et al.*, 1947). Progress however was hampered by unacceptable blood loss and sepsis. The 1960s saw the advent of topical antimicrobial agents containing silver such as silver nitrate and silver sulphadiazine, with a resulting dramatic increase in survival rate. It has been estimated that burn wound sepsis at this time was reduced from 60% to 28% (Pruit *et al.*, 1968). In an attempt to improve survival rates and reduce scarring, Janzekovic in 1970 introduced tangential excision and early grafting (Janzekovic, 1970). Trials over the next few years showed that healing time, hospital stay and overall mortality can be reduced by following this technique (Burke *et al.*, 1974; Engrav *et al.*, 1983), with the greatest improvements in survival rates for patients with large burns (Cryer *et al.*, 1991; Demling *et al.*, 1983; Herndon *et al.*, 1989). It was also realised that morbidity was reduced if occupational therapists, physiotherapists, dieticians, psychologists and social workers became an integral part of the burns centre, thus the advent of the first true multidisciplinary burns team. Now in the 21st century, we have entire hospitals devoted to burns mainly in China and USA with bed numbers as many as 3–400, and staffed by highly skilled and specialised personnel. It is from these centres that we can expect the treatments of the future to emerge.

Epidemiology of burns in children

It is estimated that over half a million children are hospitalised with burn injuries per year in the world, with the majority occurring in low- to middle-income countries in Asia and Africa (Burd & Yuen, 2005). Low socio-economic status of the family and low educational level of the mother are the main demographic factors associated with a high risk of burn injury (Ahuja & Bhattacharya, 2004; Van Niekerk *et al.*, 2004). Other factors associated are: high population density, high levels of household crowding and psychological stress within the family. Worldwide burns in the under-5 age group account for a quarter to a half of all burn injuries attending burn centres (Laloe, 2002; Ansari-Lari & Askarin, 2003; Komolafe *et al.*, 2003). The majority of burns to young children occur as accidents in the home environment (Van Niekerk *et al.*, 2004; Laloe, 2002; Ansari-Lari & Askarin, 2003; Bangdiwala *et al.*, 1990; Hemeda *et al.*, 2003) (Figure 10.1). Most regions, however, report scalds as causing the majority of burns to young children (Van Niekerk *et al.*, 2004; Laloe, 2002; Ansari-Lari & Askarin, 2003; Tarim *et al.*, 2005; Belba & Belba, 2004; Al-Shehri, 2004; Ramakrishnan *et al.*, 2005; Dewar *et al.*, 2004; Davies *et al.*, 2003). These scalds are mainly from hot

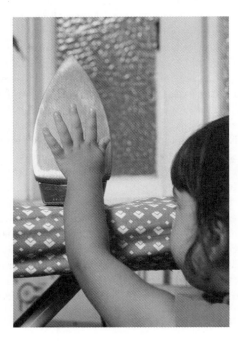

Fig. 10.1 Most burns in children occur in the under-5 age group and in the home.

water, but many other hot liquids being heated cause burns (Figure 10.2). Contact burns from household appliances such as oven doors, hot irons and wood stoves are also common (Brady *et al.*, 2002; Street *et al.*, 2002). Electrical burns occur in young children exposed to electrical cords, plugs, outlets, and poorly maintained electrical devices (Hemeda, 2003; Ramakrishnan *et al.*, 2005; Lui *et al.*, 2003). Flammable liquid burns are common from cooking accidents in developing countries and in adolescent boys experimenting with petrol and other accelerants (Henderson *et al.*, 2003).

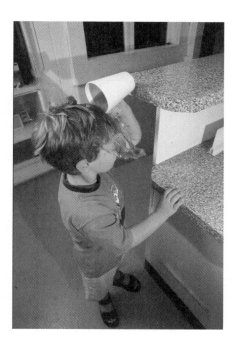

Fig. 10.2 Hot-beverage scalds account for up to a quarter of all burns in children.

A multidisciplinary service approach

Care of paediatric burns patients involves a great deal more than just treatment of the wound. A multidisciplinary team is required to ensure that every aspect of the child's physical, psychological and social needs is met during hospitalisation and following discharge. Complex social issues often impact the delivery of a child's care and therefore require skilled personnel to manage adjustment to hospitalisation. Even the smallest percentage area burn, if deep, requires long-term follow-up as the child continues to grow and develop. Early intervention is the key to ensuring that children receive optimal care during their hospitalisation.

From initial presentation, the multidisciplinary team becomes involved in assessing and planning the care for the child. The referral process plays a large part in capturing the needs of the child. The clinical nurse consultant for burns coordinates the referral process to the multidisciplinary team including: physiotherapy, occupational therapy, psychiatry, acute pain service, social work services, dietetics and play/music therapy. Each team member plays a vital role in determining the needs of the child and will consult separately with the patient and family upon admission. Dressings and operative procedures are planned in consultation with all the team members and the family. Twice weekly team meetings are vital in ensuring that communication is optimal between team members, and complex issues are discussed with the aim of care planning towards solutions and goals for the patient and family.

Clinical assessment of burn severity

History taking

The history from the child and their parents can give valuable information as to the nature and severity of the burn, and bring to light the possibility of other injuries. Flame and contact burns are commonly deeper than scalds. With scalds, it should be noted whether the child was wearing clothing, as burn depth is not only related to temperature but also contact time, and scalds under clothes often are deep as it takes time to remove clothing. Electrical injuries are important to ascertain by history as damage to underlying tissues can often be more extensive than clinical inspection would reveal. If a flame burn occurred in an enclosed space or an explosion from a gas or petrol fire, smoke inhalation should be suspected. If the child has a chemical burn, the responsible substance should be identified as the optimum treatments will vary. It should be ascertained whether adequate first aid was carried out at the scene or subsequently, as it is probably still beneficial up to 3 hr post-burn (see section on First Aid). It is also important to determine if any topical treatment has been given. Many traditional topical agents are used by people over the world, and some may make burn assessment difficult. A full past medical history should be taken from the caregivers including current and past medical problems, previous anaesthetics, medications, allergies and vaccinations (especially tetanus) (Hettiaratchy & Papini, 2004). Children with neurological disability such as spina bifida or diabetes may have reduced sensation predisposing to the burn. These same children are also at highest risk of a latex allergy. Previous psychiatric illness in children with burns is much less common than is seen in the adult burns population, but when present should be documented.

A carefully taken history may raise suspicion concerning a non-accidental injury. Factors that would make one suspicious include:

- conflicting histories from caregivers and the child;
- if the burn distribution and severity do not match the mechanism given by the caregivers;
- unreasonable delay in seeking medical attention;
- the presence of other injuries, including previous injuries;
- certain patterns of injury including cigarette and rope marks, or glove and stocking distribution of a forced immersion in hot water.

Any child who has a history or signs of a non-accidental burn needs to be referred to a Suspected Child Abuse & Neglect Team (SCAN) for assessment and appropriate action. This team should work independently from the burns team.

Clinical examination

The examination of the burned child should be the same as for any child with trauma. It should follow the guidelines for advanced trauma life support (British Burn Association, 1996).

A – Airway

Hot gases can cause a burn to the airway above the vocal cords and may swell up over time to be worst between 12 and 36 hr, compromising the airway. This is a particular problem in young children who have a relatively narrow airway and short necks with soft tissues, which are readily distorted by oedema (Hettiaratchy & Papini, 2004). A compromised airway requires prompt intubation.

Signs suggestive of significant airway injury are:

- singed nasal hairs;
- productive cough;
- croup-like breathing;
- respiratory difficulty;
- rib retraction;
- flaring of alar nasae.

A useful formula for the endotracheal tube size is $4 + \frac{1}{4}$ age in years, or the same width as the child's little finger. There will be instances where endotracheal intubation is not possible and tracheostomy or cricothyroidotomy will be required.

B – Breathing

Oxygen should be given by facemask to all cases of moderate to severe burns in children (12 litres/min). Nasal prongs are less effective, but can be used with oxygen at 2 litres/min (higher flows are not tolerated by children). Deep dermal or full thickness circumferential burns to the chest will compromise respiration and may necessitate escharotomies (see section on Escharotomies). If the child has been involved in a blast injury, lung contusions can have occurred and ventilation and gas exchange may be compromised. Blast injuries can also cause penetrating chest trauma with a resulting pneumothorax (often under tension). These children need to be treated with an intercostal catheter and underwater seal drainage. Eardrum perforation is a good sign of a significant blast injury.

Smoke inhalation can cause acute respiratory distress syndrome with multiorgan failure and will increase dramatically the morbidity and mortality of a burn. Changes in the voice or cry and burns or soot in the nose, mouth or pharynx should be looked for. Other features suggestive of smoke inhalation include: a productive cough, croup-like breathing, respiratory difficulty with rib retraction or flaring of the alar nasae. The products of combustion, though cooled by the time they reach the lungs, act as direct irritants to the lungs, leading to bronchiospasm, inflammation and increase in secretions. The ciliary action of respiratory epithelium is impaired, and if the inflammatory exudate is not cleared, then atelectasis and pneumonia result. The situation is particularly severe in children with pre-existing asthma (Hettiaratchy & Papini, 2004). Systemic toxicity follows absorption of the products of combustion producing systemic acid–base disturbances (carbon dioxide, ammonia and hydrochloric acid), while hydrofluoric acid may produce hypocalcaemia. Carbon monoxide poisoning classically gives a cherry red appearance to the skin. Carbon monoxide binds to deoxyhaemoglobin with 40 times the affinity of oxygen, and also binds to intracellular proteins, particularly those of the cytochrome oxidase pathway. These two effects lead to intracellular and extracellular hypoxia. Treatment should be with 100% oxygen, which displaces carbon monoxide from bound proteins six times faster than atmospheric oxygen (Hettiaratchy & Papini, 2004). Carbon monoxide bound to the cytochromes will be washed out of the cells in the next 24 hr, producing a secondary rise in serum carboxyhaemoglobin, and further symptoms of intoxication. Post-intoxication encephalopathy may be the serious sequelae of this phenomenon (Australia and New Zealand Burns Association, 2002).

C – Circulation

Burns greater than 10% TBSA in small children and greater than 15% in older children should be treated with intravenous resuscitation. Optimally, two intravenous canulas should be inserted and crystalloids given in the form of Hartmann's solution or Ringer's lactate (see section on Fluid Management). The ideal way to monitor whether a child is adequately hydrated is by monitoring hourly urine output with a urinary catheter (see below). The increased physiologic reserve of the child allows the maintenance of most vital signs in the normal range, even in the presence of severe shock. A 25% diminution in circulating blood volume in a child is required to manifest the minimal signs of shock. Tachycardia and poor skin perfusion often are the only keys to early recognition of hypovolaemia; however, tachycardia may be a sign of anxiety or inadequate analgesia. Blood pressure is very misleading in a child as they need to have lost 45% of their blood volume to become hypotensive. A child's systolic blood pressure should be 80 mm Hg plus twice the age in years, and the diastolic pressure should be two-thirds of the systolic blood pressure (American College of Surgeons, 1997).

D – Neurological disability

All children should be assessed for responsiveness, as they may later drop their conscious level due to hypoxia, hypovolaemia or sepsis in delayed cases. The Glasgow Coma Scale is the most widely used scale for this (Hettiaratchy & Papini, 2004).

E – Exposure with environment control

Examination of the whole of the child should now take place, with an estimation of body surface area burned. Other injuries should be looked for. It is also important that these children do not become hypothermic by prolonged exposure (Hettiaratchy & Papini, 2004). A space blanket should be used to prevent heat loss. Jewellery that could be constrictive should be removed.

Classification of burn depth

The accepted classification of the depth of a burn has changed over the past few years. Traditionally, burns were classified as 1st, 2nd or 3rd degree, depending on whether the burn to the skin was superficial, partial thickness or full thickness.

The term 4th degree has been often used to describe burns that also involved underlying tissues e.g. muscle and fascia. In 2001, Dr. Peter Shakespeare, the then Editor of the journal *Burns*, proposed a classification system that could be universally adopted. This system is now the main system used throughout the world:

- *Superficial burns* involve only epidermis
- *Superficial partial thickness burns* involve only papillary dermis and epidermis
- *Deep dermal partial thickness burns* involve epidermis and dermis to reticular dermis
- *Full thickness burns* evidently involve the whole thickness of the skin and possibly subcutaneous tissue.

This classification system is not that different from the classical description with superficial burns corresponding to 1st degree burns, superficial partial thickness burns and deep dermal partial thickness burns corresponding to shallow and deep 2nd degree burns respectively, and full thickness burns corresponding to 3rd degree. Instead of using 4th degree, a better term proposed was: 'full thickness burn injury with involvement of underlying tissues' (Shakespeare, 2001).

Determination of burn depth

Examination of the burn wound can usually reveal information as to the depth, but can be difficult if the burn is deep dermal partial thickness, infected or has had previous topical treatment with creams, herbal therapies and dyes.

Superficial burns: Superficial burns are erythematous, have intact epithelium and blanch when touched. Blistering is unusual.

Superficial partial thickness burns: These have blistering as a common feature. They are typically painful as they have intact sensation with exposed nerves. Here, the epidermis is raw where the blisters have broken and is erythematous and blanches to touch.

Deep dermal partial thickness burns: These are difficult to assess as the wound may change in characteristics over the first 48 hr. Here, blistering is uncommon and discomfort less. Originally, the raw wound surface may blanch but will not do so 24–48 hr later as these superficial vessels cease functioning, leaving a pale wound eschar of dead cells and exudate.

Full thickness burns: These are easier to identify with their thick leathery layer of eschar and total loss of sensation. Sometimes deep dermal partial thickness and full thickness burns have a red appearance that does not blanch to touch. The reason for this phenomenon is that red blood cells have extravasated and lie in the eshcar.

Laser Doppler scanning

Many burn centres are equipped with a Laser Doppler scanner that can determine the depth of injury within 3–5 days of the burn. It works by scanning the skin with a low-power laser penetrating 1 mm into the skin to determine blood flow. These instruments have been extensively studied in children, and when used by trained personnel are very accurate in predicting which children require skin grafting (Holland *et al.*, 2002; La Hei *et al.*, 2006). Analgesia and sedation are often required to keep the child still for the scan, which can take up to several minutes to complete. Eye protection for the child is mandatory.

Electrical burns

Electrical burns are most likely to be low-voltage injuries in the home environment where children are exposed to electrical cords, plugs, outlets and poorly maintained electrical devices (Lui *et al.*, 2003) (Figure 10.3). Older children, especially boys with

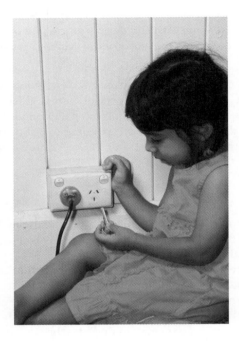

Fig.10.3 Electrical burns are most likely to be low-voltage injuries in the home environment.

risk-taking behaviour, present with high-voltage injuries from contact with high-tension cables. In all electrical injuries, entry and exit points should be looked for, and an expectation for the degree of injury to be more extensive in the deeper tissues than external inspection would reveal. An electrocardiogram should be obtained on admission of all children with an electrical injury. If the child has suffered a cardiac arrest at the scene, or the passage of current has been through the chest, then they are at risk of serious dysrhythmia. Such children should be monitored in a hospital after the injury for 24 hr as a dysrhythmia may occur even after an initial normal trace phenomenon (Australia and New Zealand Burns Association, 2002). Most low-voltage injuries will result in small full thickness defects. High-voltage injuries may result in deep muscle damage in the limbs. The damaged muscle and red blood cells release myoglobin and haemoglobin respectively into the blood stream, and are excreted in the urine, making it pink to red in colour. Both, however, can precipitate in the renal tubules, producing an acute tubular necrosis picture. Myoglobin precipitation is accentuated by acid urine and decreased by alkaline urine. The treatment consists of keeping the urine output greater than 1 ml/kg/hr with administration of intravenous Hartmann's or Ringers lactate solution until the pigment load has decreased. Sometimes mannitol is required to maintain this level of output. In addition, sodium bicarbonate is useful to maintain urine pH $\geqslant 7$ in order to minimise pigment precipitation. The extensive muscle damage seen in high-voltage injuries will often cause a compartment syndrome and require fasciotomies (Demling *et al.*, 2000–4).

Chemical burns

Children are burned less frequently with chemicals than adults. However, chemicals are commonly found in households and children do present with chemical burns. Drain cleaners and paint removers are usually strong alkalis and disinfectants are phenols or hypochlorites. Sulphuric acid is sometimes used to clean toilets, and phosphorus is found in fireworks, insecticides and fertilisers. Dry chemicals should be dusted off, and wet chemicals should be irrigated off with copious quantities of water. One guide to how much irrigation is required is the presence of pain, the supposition being that as long as there is pain, the chemical is still active and continuing to cause damage (Herndon, 2002). Since it is impossible to remember the systemic sequelae of all the chemicals to which a child might be exposed, the chemical should be identified and information sought from the regional or national poison centre. It is important to determine if there has been ingestion of the chemical and instigate the appropriate management (chemical ingestions are not dealt with in this chapter).

Calculation of burn surface area

The rule of nines for the calculation of burn surface area should not be used in small children and infants. The reason is that a child's head represents a significantly larger percent of total body surface area and their legs represent a smaller percent than that of an adult. However, the rule of nines can be modified for infants and small children by doubling the head from 9% to 18% and decreasing each lower limb to 14%. For each year of life above the first, the head decreases in relative size by approximately 1% and each leg gains 0.5% in comparison with total body surface area. The Lund and Browder method uses narrower age ranges and divides the body into smaller anatomic regions to account for age-related changes in surface area. It is more accurate than a modified rule of nines. For small areas, a good rule is that the child's palm including the fingers is 1% of body surface area (Jose *et al.*, 2004; Nagel & Schunk, 1997). It should be noted that erythema never becomes included in the calculation of total burn surface area.

Management

First aid

Cooling burns with water has been shown in both humans and animal models to lessen the eventual depth of a burn. Therefore, burn wounds should be cooled with running tap water or other non-contaminated water (8–25°C) for 20 min (McCormack *et al.*, 2003). If water is in short supply, then recycling the irrigation fluid with a basin would be appropriate. Irrigation also removes noxious agents and reduces pain, and may reduce oedema by stabilising mast cells and histamine release (Huspith & Rayatt, 2004). The use of ice has not been shown to be beneficial, and has the potential to cause hypothermia. Cooling is best done immediately after the burn, but can also be beneficial up to 3 hr after the injury has occurred (Australia and New Zealand Burns Association, 2002). It is important while cooling the burn to keep the child warm with a blanket. Small children cool down much faster than adults because they have a larger body surface to mass ratio than adults, and have less body fat and muscle bulk. It should be remembered that children under 1 do not have a shivering reflex.

Acute pain management on presentation

Cooling the burn with water as a first aid measure and covering with a dressing will alleviate much of the pain associated with burns. However, superficial burns can be extremely painful, and titrated intravenous morphine is the best analgesic in the acute situation. Intramuscular injections should be avoided as absorption cannot always be predicted. Splinting and elevation of limbs can also make the child more comfortable. It should be remembered that with the limbs unsplinted, the position of comfort is also the position of contracture, and although it can be painful applying splints, the child will quickly settle down (see also section on Pain Management via Acute Pain Service).

Fluid management

Burns greater than 10% TBSA in small children and greater than 15% in older children should be treated with intravenous resuscitation. It is important that superficial burns (erythema) should not be used in this calculation. Crystalloids in the form of Hartmann's solution or Ringer's lactate solution should be administered. Using the Parkland formula (4 mls × body weight (in kg) × % body surface area burned) will estimate the amount of fluid required in the first 24 hr. Half of the volume is given in the first 8 hr and half over the next 16 hr. The fluid replacement should be calculated from the time of the burn, and so there is always some catch up to be made. In children, maintenance fluids need to be given on top of these calculated losses. This should be given in the form of dextrose 4% saline 1/5 (or equivalent maintenance solution containing dextrose and saline). Daily maintenance fluids for small children can be calculated using:

- 100 mls/kg for the first 10 kg of body weight plus;
- 50 mls/kg for each kg over 10 kg and less than 20 kg body weight plus;
- 20 mls/kg for each kg over 20 kg of body weight.

The addition of glucose is necessary in small children because of their decreased glycogen stores and the speed with which hypoglycaemia can occur, particularly in association with hypothermia. Ideally, four hourly blood sugar levels should be measured in small children during initial stabilisation.

It must be made quite clear that these are only guidelines, and the best way to monitor how much fluid to give a child is on urine output measured with an indwelling urinary catheter. One would aim for 2 mls/kg/hr in the under 1-year-old children, 1 ml/kg/hr in 1–5-year-olds and 0.5 ml/kg/hr in older children. Additional fluids are commonly needed with inhalation injuries, electrical burns and associated trauma. However, cerebral oedema is more likely in small children with fluid overload, particularly with hyponatraemia. This risk can be reduced by using a 'head up' position for the first 24 hr (Australia and New Zealand Burns Association, 2002). If peripheral intravenous access cannot be achieved initially, then a choice between central access, surgical cut-down onto a vein and intra-osseous administration can be made.

Escharotomies

With circumferential deep burns to the limbs, distal pulses should be checked. If absent, then mid-axial escharotomies may be limb saving. Limbs should be elevated above the heart level to reduce swelling (no more than 45°). In circumferential chest burns, escharotomy may also be necessary to relieve chest wall restriction and improve ventilation. In small children whose breathing is principally diaphragmatic, the problem can be seen when only the anterior and sides of the chest and abdomen are burned. Here, incisions are made longitudinally along the anterior axillary lines to the costal margin or to the upper abdomen if this is burned, and are connected by two cross incisions, which may be convex upwards across the upper chest below the clavicles and across the upper part of the abdomen (Australia and New Zealand Burns Association, 2002). Escharotomies can be easily performed with a scalpel or diathermy, and division should only be through the firm eschar, not subcutaneous tissue. The child requiring escharotomies is usually ventilated, but if awake will still require analgesia and sedation (even though theoretically they should have little sensation).

Decompression of the stomach

After a moderate to severe burn, gastric ileus can be problematic. Small children can also swallow large quantities of air during crying. A nasogastric tube if available should be inserted early in these children prior to transfer, and left on free drainage. If the child has had morphine, this can also diminish peristalsis. In moderate to severe burns, gastrointestinal perfusion decreases and motility is slowed. Increased gastrointestinal permeability allows for the translocation of gram-negative bacteria and endotoxins into the circulation. However, there is good evidence that enteral nutrition given early may prevent enteral complications including reducing sepsis, and this should be commenced on arrival to the burns centre. Ideally, this should be protocol and be supervised by the centre's dietician.

Burn wound care

Cleaning the burn

The wound should be cleaned with water containing an antiseptic solution such as 0.1% chlorhexidine gluconate (made by diluting a 5% solution). Chlorhexidine gluconate is desirable because of its antimicrobial activity against common skin flora. Loose, devitalised tissue should be gently trimmed away (a practice known as epluchage), and should not cause any pain or bleeding.

Burn blisters

The case for debriding blisters and treating with topical antimicrobial agents is supported by studies that demonstrate that blister fluid depresses immune function by impairing the function of neutrophils and lymphocytes and also increases inflammation. The fluid and devitalised skin are also a medium for bacteria growth (Moss, 2004; Rockwell & Ehrlich, 1990). The alternative argument is that a blister is indicative of a superficial partial thickness burn, which should heal on its own. For the first few days, the fluid in the blisters will remain sterile as the underlying skin heals. Leaving blisters intact may also reduce the need for analgesia and dressings and therefore reduce costs (Moss, 2004). A compromise between these two arguments is probably the best policy. Large blisters should be completely removed, and moderate and small ones can be pricked to express fluid and left intact.

The burns dressing

The ideal burn dressing has the following attributes: broad-spectrum antimicrobial activity, requiring infrequent changing with minimal discomfort, and finally, promotion of re-epithelialisation. The practicalities are also that the dressing must be cost-effective. Antimicrobial activity in the dressing has been shown to decrease wound-related infections and morbidity when used appropriately. It does this by controlling microbial colonisation, thus preventing development of invasive infections (Palmieri & Greenhalgh, 2002). Infrequent dressing changes are desirable to decrease what is a distressing procedure, especially in children. Increasing the rate of re-epithelialisation is important because if a burn re-epithelialises within 2 weeks, it will generally do so without scarring. If it takes more than 3 weeks, it will inevitably scar. When it comes to what dressings should be recommended for the treatment of burns in children, no two centres can agree on appropriate dressings. Some centres use dressings that have no antimicrobial properties such as paraffin gauze. Their argument is that all antimicrobial dressings delay wound healing and they accept a higher rate of burn wound infection. Other centres try and decrease this increased infection rate by taking children to theatre for surgical debridement prior to the application of a non-antimicrobial dressing, which will then stay on until the wound is healed or grafted. There is merit in this latter approach, as removing debris and burn eshcar will decrease bacterial load prior to dressing application under aseptic conditions.

Dressing changes under general anaesthesia

Dressing procedures can cause pain and distress not only to the child, but also to the attending staff and family. The child's pain and anxiety are often difficult to safely manage with conscious sedation, and general anaesthetic is often the best option.

The following criteria are used for consideration for general anaesthetic:

- Anxious children who have failed conscious oral sedation.
- Children less than 1 year of age requiring painful dressing changes that may involve airway management due to excess sedation from narcotics.
- Difficult areas to dress such as circumferential hand burns requiring complex bandaging and splinting.
- Removal of dressings for children with large body surface area burns (>10% burn surface area).
- Removal of dressings 5–7 days after grafting procedure for large surface area burns and/or removing skin staples.

- Specialty dressings, such as application of negative pressure dressings to difficult areas.
- Painful procedures, such as ranging and splinting for severe contractures.

Preparation for theatre

Education for parents and guardians

Burns are associated with significant emotional overlay in the child and their parents or caregivers. Feelings of grief and loss are common and are normal accompaniments of burns. In addition, feelings of guilt, self-reproach, fear, depression and often anger in the parents need to be addressed (Australia and New Zealand Burns Association, 2002). Long-term emotional outcome after a paediatric burn is more dependant on the whole family's emotional care than in adult burns where the concentration is on the patient. Therefore, early and adequate care of the family is essential, and this starts from the moment of injury.

Prior to any procedure, it is important to recognise that the child and their family require education that meets their current needs; however, social and emotional issues will impact upon how much information is accepted and processed. Generally, when procedures are discussed with caregivers, careful attention is taken not to discuss plans of care in front of the younger child. Young children often misinterpret and become overly anxious by adult language and require specialised procedural education aimed at their developmental level. Complex families often involve more than two parents. The burns team social worker should assess these families and help with the education process. Often, each set of parents requires separate education sessions, and extended families also require education as they may play a large role in the rehabilitation of the child in the future. Mediation during education sessions is sometimes advised owing to parent guilt and blame of themselves or others.

Consent

The clinical nurse consultant or suitably trained burns nurse should give the preoperative education sessions utilising simple written information on debriding and grafting and the option of an accompanying photo presentation. These education sessions are planned preferably 2 days prior to the procedure to allow reclarification and questioning prior to the procedure. After the education sessions have occurred, medical staff should then obtain informed consent.

The child

Age-appropriate procedural preparation with the child is often the role of the occupational therapist. This is facilitated in young children with cartoon books that provide a simple story about theatre, operations, skin grafting, dressing changes and what to expect in a hospital (Broome, 1990; Hunsberger *et al.*, 1984). For older children and adolescents, a more formal education package is used, in order to engage participation in the planning of their own care. Caregivers are often encouraged to attend these sessions to support and help their child to understand and learn.

One day prior to theatre

Prior to theatre, medical preparation and results are obtained including preoperative bloods (full blood count, blood typing and crossmatching if necessary). Multiresistant organisms cultured must be notified to operating theatre as this may impact on the cleaning of theatres and order of the list. Informed consent should be obtained with the legal consenter and must be obtained in advance for children under social services orders. The surgical site should be marked and the sites being used as donors should be written on the consent form. Children should be given a sponge bath in soap and water, as their dressings usually remain intact until theatre. An allergy/reaction history to medications, skin preparations, tapes and other products (including latex) should already have been documented, but is reviewed again at this time. Religious limitations should be noted and counselling may be required (e.g. blood transfusion and Jehovah's Witness patients). A preoperative anaesthetic consultation is important as premedication is often helpful for the anxious child. Nutrition and nasogastric feeding fasting times are calculated and communicated to parents, child and staff.

Theatre procedures

There are a variety of reasons children will be taken to the operating theatre for a general anaesthetic including: debridement with or without split skin grafting, change of dressings, removal of graft dressings, staple removal, escharotomies and fasciotomies, scar injection with steroids and reconstructive surgery.

Dressing care in the operating theatre

Each burns centre will use different dressings depending on local experience and preferences. Ideally, burns medical staff, nursing staff, the occupational therapist and physiotherapist will be present in the theatre working together. Some basic principles do however apply.

(1) *Dressings for the acute burn:* See section on The Burns Dressing.
(2) *Non-meshed split skin grafts:* These wounds require a dressing that is easy to remove, that also allows exudate to flow through the dressing with some absorbency and protection against sheering and trauma. This can be achieved with a silicone mesh or paraffin gauze dressing covered with an absorbent layer and crepe bandage.
(3) *Meshed split thickness skin grafts:* These grafts tend to be used to cover larger surface areas. The nanocrystalline silver dressings are useful for this purpose when moistened with a simple water irrigation tube. The use of this dressing has beneficial outcomes in that it prevents overcolonisation, and studies have shown faster epithelialisation of the holes in the meshed skin (Demling & DeSanti, 2002). Alternatively, paraffin gauze can be used.
(4) *Donor sites:* These require an absorbent, dressing, that will allow new epithelium to grow with minimal trauma upon removal. Donor sites tend to be heavily exudative for the first 48 hr, which require extra reinforcement. Depending on the patient history of colonisation, donor sites tend to be dressed with non-antimicrobial dressings and left intact for 7–10 days in order to ensure that healing is not interrupted for traumatic removal of dressings. Satisfactory results

can be achieved with a polyurethane film dressings placed onto the donor site after haemostasis is achieved with topical adrenalin, then covered with an absorbent foam dressing and crepe bandage.

(5) *Full thickness grafts:* Usually used in reconstruction of burn scar contractures. Covering dressings should be non-stick and facilitate adherence to the wound bed. Dressings such as paraffin gauze under an absorbent layer or acriflavine-treated wool work well in this situation. Negative pressure dressings are also useful for wound bed adherence and removal of tissue fluid.

(6) *Splinting:* Splinting in the operating theatre is performed by the therapists at the end of the procedure whilst the child is still under general anaesthetic. The advent of thermoplastic splints has allowed for custom-built splints to be moulded for the individual's requirements (Figure 10.4).

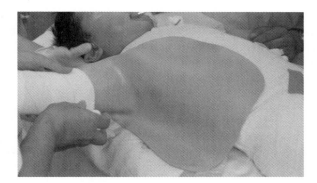

Fig. 10.4 A thermoplastic axilla splint being applied under general anaesthetic

Pain management via acute pain service

A skilled paediatric pain service is invaluable to any burn centre. The service should provide a 24-hr on-call service, and a twice-daily pain rounds. Pain scoring and ongoing assessment should be recorded hourly on observation charts by nursing staff using appropriate tools. For very young children, the FLACC (Faces, Legs, Activity, Cry and Consolability) pain assessment tool is appropriate (Manwaorren & Hynan, 2003). For verbalising 4–8-year-olds, a good tool is the FPS-R (Revised Faces Pain Scale) (Hicks *et al.*, 2001). Finally, for children older than 8, the self-reporting VAS (Visual Analogue Scale) is very useful (De Jong *et al.*, 2005). Pain scoring is then utilised to identify and communicate ongoing pain issues if modifications to medications are required.

Patient Controlled Analgesia (PCA) pumps are utilised with a background infusion of morphine for children who are developmentally capable (generally above 7 years of age) (Gaukroger *et al.*, 1991). As the patient progresses and pain is well controlled, oral medications such as slow-release morphine are instituted, with a view to ceasing intravenous medications as soon as possible. Fast-acting oral opioid medication is useful for breakthrough pain (such as oxycodone), when intravenous morphine is ceased and slow release has started. If breakthrough medications are needed, the slow-release morphine can then be titrated up until breakthrough medications are not necessary.

Pruritis is always problematic to the burned child in the recovery phase. Itch control is difficult, but can often be managed in the short term by oral medications such as antihistamines. Long-term oral medications are often considered for neuropathic pain and itch control, but owing to the excess cost and excessive reports of side effects, this is carefully considered on an individual-patient basis (Vitale *et al.*, 1991; Gordon, 1988; Bell *et al.*, 1988; Matheson *et al.*, 2001).

Procedural pain is treated on an individual basis in consultation with the pain service. General anaesthetic is considered for patients in early stages of admission. When the child has progressed past skin grafting and donor sites are fully healed, conscious sedation is considered. Often, anaesthetic personnel are booked to attend for the first two baths after general anaesthetic has ceased. Oral conscious sedation is often given via nasogastric tube, with anaesthetic staff present during the bath if any further medication or airway management is required (Humphries *et al.*, 1997; Sharar *et al.*, 2002; Day *et al.*, 2006).

Age-appropriate strategies for distraction during procedures to reduce pain and anxiety have been effective. These include traditional distracters such as music therapy (Presner *et al.*, 2001), play therapy and movies (Landolt, 2002) and also newer systems such as augmented reality and virtual reality (Das *et al.*, 2005).

Post-operative care

The child is returned to the ward with monitoring of vital signs including: temperature, pulse, respiration rate and oxygen saturation. The child should be nursed in a heated room at 28–31°C as hypothermia can become a significant problem after extensive and prolonged theatre procedures. Dressing checks should be made regularly, looking for excessive blood loss and dressing slippage. Splints are checked every 4 hrs as pressure ulcers can develop if the child is poorly positioned or the splint slips. Circulation observations of affected limbs are performed for the first 24 hrs post-operatively as tight dressings and poorly positioned splints may compromise blood flow.

Physiotherapy

Physiotherapy plays a vital role in post-operative recovery. Chest physiotherapy will be required for the ventilated or immobile child. After the initial post-grafting period, physiotherapy sessions ideally should be daily to twice daily to encourage active movement of all affected areas to prevent contracture. The physiotherapist will have to facilitate active assisted and passive ranging of movements depending on the child's ability to move the affected area independently. Muscle strengthening, mobilisation and gait training are commenced when appropriate. Hydrotherapy can be utilised when the skin has sufficiently re-epithelialised with minimal open areas as it enhances the rehabilitation process.

Infection control

The commonest cause of mortality in the burned child is sepsis. Burns render children markedly susceptible to a host of infectious complications of which most are bacterial, but viral and fungal infections can also occur (Sheridan, 2005). Early signs of infection include increased redness, warmth, pain and swelling of the wound. Early burn wound infections tend to result from gram-positive organisms such as *Staphylococcus* and *Streptococcus*, which are normal cutaneous flora (Palmieri & Greenhalgh, 2002). Red streaking, extending from the wound in a child is indicative of a streptococcal infection and mandates intravenous antibiotics in addition to a topical antimicrobial dressing. Gram-negative wound infections tend to predominate after 7–10 days in larger, deeper burns. Gram-negative infections are heralded by increased greenish exudate from the wound, high fevers and pain (Palmieri & Greenhalgh, 2002). Many burn wounds that are colonised rather than infected by gram-negative organisms will also have a green exudate. Clinical correlation is required in these cases prior to the institution of unnecessary systemic antibiotics. Colonised wounds in children are best treated with daily cleansing and topical antimicrobial dressings. If sepsis is suspected, cultures of both the wound and blood should be taken. Often, antibiotics can be withheld until positive cultures are returned with antibiotic sensitivity. However, it is sometimes necessary to administer antibiotics in an empirical manner to reduce the complication of multiorgan failure and death (Kreger *et al.*, 1980). Skin surveillance is conducted twice weekly, with dry swabs taken from the nose, groin and axilla. Children who grow multiresistant organisms are nursed in isolation in hepa-filtered rooms until they have three negative cultures.

Toxic shock syndrome

Toxic shock syndrome is a rare complication of a *Staphylococcus aureus* infection and was first described in children with burns in 1985 (Frame *et al.*, 1985). Twenty per cent of the strains of *S. aureus* are capable of producing toxic shock syndrome exotoxin, a superantigen, which causes the classic picture of toxic shock syndrome owing to overstimulation of T-cells (Trop *et al.*, 2004). Classically, it affects young children with small partial thickness burns, which would be expected to fully re-epithelialise.

Symptoms and signs of toxic shock syndrome consist of (Trop *et al.*, 2004):

- high fever;
- diffuse macular erythroderma rash;
- desquamation (1–2 weeks after onset of illness, particularly of palms and soles);
- hypotension.

and involvement of three or more of the following organ systems:

- gastrointestinal (vomiting or diarrhoea);
- muscular (myalgia);
- mucose membrane (vaginal, oropharyngeal or conjunctiva hyperaemia);
- renal (renal failure or leukouria);
- liver (raised bilirubin or transaminases);
- haematological (reduced platelets);
- central nervous system (disorientation or alteration in consciousness).

A survey looking at burn units in the UK revealed that toxic shock syndrome affected approximately 2.5% of all children admitted (Edwards-Jones, *et al.*, 2000). In this survey, the authors could not find a relationship between the dressings used and developing the condition. However, it is clear that in the UK, many children are treated with non-antimicrobial dressings and this is the highest rate reported in the world. In contrast, The Royal Children's Hospital in Brisbane, Australia, is a busy tertiary-level Paediatric Burns Centre, treating up to 500 new children per year. Here only antimicrobial dressings are used, with a resultant extremely low rate of sepsis, and no cases of toxic shock syndrome were seen in the past 35 years.

Pseudomonas aeruginosa

Pseudomonas aeruginosa is an opportunistic gram-negative pathogen. Its virulence depends on the production of many enzymes (including penicillinases) and toxins. *Pseudomonas* organisms are mobile, possessing a flagellum. Adherence of the bacterium to both biological cell membranes and inert surfaces is mediated through pili or fimbriae and by the production of large amounts of alginate or slime. Together, this makes the organism very difficult to treat or eradicate, and predisposes the burn wound and medical equipment in burn units to *Pseudomonas* infection and contamination (Tredget *et al.*, 2004).

Tetanus

Tetanus immunisation status should be checked, and if not up to date, toxoid should be given along with tetanus immunoglobulin if the burn wound is contaminated.

Human immunodeficiency virus (HIV)-positive children

Children who are HIV positive have an increased mortality with burns, which is usually sepsis related. However, HIV-positive children who do not develop infection or recover from an episode of infection have a similar hospital stay, need for skin grafting and graft take, as non-HIV children (James *et al.*, 2003; Kimble & Smith, 2004). It is clear, therefore, that these children should be treated just the same way as non-HIV children.

Scar management

Contact media and pressure garments have become the standard in scar management. Custom-made pressure garments are measured and fitted when the child's skin is able to withstand pressure (Figure 10.5). Garments will be required until the scar is mature, a process that can take anywhere from 6 to 18 months. New garments will be required as the child grows and develops or when garments are damaged or have lost sufficient tension for adequate pressure. For control of itch, patients are instructed to apply moisturiser four times a day under the garment, often combined with oral medication. Contact media with silicone under the garment will enhance scar maturation and reduce the degree of hypertrophic scarring. Sensitivity reactions to silicone are common and non-silicone contact media can be alternatively used.

Discharge planning

As the child and family progress, the discharge planning process begins. Preparation of parent and child in dressing care and garment application is required. Parents will begin to attend baths and take over dressing care 1–2 weeks prior to expected discharge. This is to allow the parent or guardian to feel comfortable with wound care and garment application and general problem solving within a safe and secure

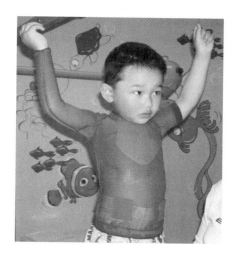

Fig. 10.5 Custom-made pressure garments are measured and fitted when the child's skin is able to withstand pressure.

environment. Assessment of home environment may be required for complex patients, and often modifications and assistive facilities must be sought to accommodate the needs of the child prior to discharge. Assessment of the parent or guardian to care and maintain the child in a safe environment is sometimes necessary for children who are under social services orders, or for children with high needs. In preparation for discharge and return to school, the occupational therapy service will often make a school visit to provide education sessions to teachers and students. For children living considerable distances from the burns centre, rural services are contacted for nursing, physiotherapy and occupational therapy needs. Telemedicine video-link follow-up consultations with the burns multidisciplinary team and local services are invaluable to avoid long trips back to the burns centre and ensure that the child receives the same service in their local community as offered in the metropolitan areas (Kimble & Smith, 2004; Smith *et al.*, 2004a, b; Johansen *et al.*, 2004) (Figure 10.6). For patients within the metropolitan area, dressing care, scar management and

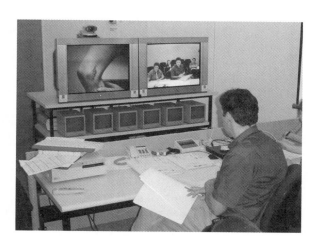

Fig. 10.6 Teleconferencing for follow-up for burns patients is effective and avoids long trips for the child and family.

ongoing follow-up are provided ideally by a multidisciplinary burns outpatient service. Appointments are made initially weekly then graduate to fortnightly and then monthly, depending on the progress of the child. All children with significant burns should be followed-up to adulthood to monitor for contractures and to recognise and treat psychological problems as they arise. Transition at an appropriate time to an adult burns centre will often be required.

References

Ahuja, R.B., Bhattacharya, S. (2004). Burns in the developing world and burn disasters. *British Medical Journal*, 329: 447–449.

Al-Shehri, M. (2004). The pattern of paediatric burn injuries in Southwestern Saudi Arabia. *West African Journal of Medicine*, 23: 294–299.

American College of Surgeons. (1997). *Advanced trauma life support for doctors. Instructor course manual, book 1*, 6th ed. American College of Surgeons, Chicago.

Ansari-Lari, M., Askarin, M. (2003). Epidemiology of burns presenting to an emergency department in Shiaz, South Iran. *Burns*, 29: 579–581.

Australia and New Zealand Burns Association. (2002). *Emergency management of severe burns manual*, 7th ed. Australia and New Zealand Burns Association, Kelvin Grove.

Bangdiwala, S.I., Anzola-Perez, E., Romer, C.C., *et al.* (1990). The incidence of injuries in young people: 1: Methodology and results of a collaborative study in Brazil, Chile, Cuba and Venezuela. *International Journal of Epidemiology*, 19: 115–124.

Belba, M.K., Belba, G.P. (2004). Review of statistical data about severe burn patients treated during 2001 and evidence of septic cases in Albania. *Burns*, 30: 813–819.

Bell, L., McAdams, T., Morgan, R., *et al.* (1988). Pruritis in burns: A descriptive study. *Journal of Burn Care and Rehabilitation*, 9: 305–311.

Brady, D., McGrady, M., Simons, M., Plaza, A., Kimble, R.M. (2002). Hot iron burns in children. *Burns*, 28: 587–590.

British Burn Association. (1996). *Emergency management of severe burns course manual, UK version*. Wythenshawe Hospital, Manchester.

Broome, M. (1990). Preparation of children for painful procedures. *Pediatric Nursing*, 16: 537–541.

Burd, A., Yuen, C. (2005). A global study of hospitalized paediatric patients. *Burns*, 31: 432–438.

Burke, J.F., Bondoc, C.C., Quinby, W.C. (1974). Primary burn excision and immediate grafting: A method of shortening illness. *Journal of Trauma*, 14: 389–395.

Cope, O., Laugohr, H., Moore, F.D., Webster, R. (1947). Expeditious care of full-thickness burn wounds by surgical excision and grafting. *Annals of Surgery*, 125: 1–22.

Cryer, H.G., Anigian, G.M., Miller, F.B., Malangoni, M.A., Weiner, L., Polk, H.C. Jr. (1991). Effects of early tangential excision and grafting on survival after burn injury. *Surgery, Gynecology and Obstetrics*, 173: 449–453.

Das, D.A., Grimmer, K.A., Sparnon, A.L., Thomas, S. (2005). The efficacy of playing a virtual reality game in modulating pain in children with acute burn injuries: A randomised control trial. *BMC Pediatrics*, 5: 1.

Davies, E.N., Mewton, J.F., Barlow, K., *et al.* (2003). Bathroom scalds in children. *Journal of Burns & Surgical Wound Care*, 2: 9.

Day, P.F., Power, A.M., Hibbert, S.A., Paterson, S.A. (2006). Effectiveness of oral midazolam for paediatric dental care: A retrospective study in two specialist centres. *European Archives of Paediatric Dentistry*, 7: 228–235.

De Jong, A., Bremer, M., Schouten, M., Tuinebreijer, W., Faber, A. (2005). Reliability and validity of the Pain Observation Scale for young children and the Visual Analogue Scale in children with burns. *Burns*, 31: 198–204.

Demling, R.H. (1983). Improved survival after massive burns. *Journal of Trauma*, 23: 179–184.

Demling, R.H., DeSanti, L. (2002). The rate of re-epithelialisation across meshed skin grafts is increased with exposure to silver. *Burns*, 28: 264–266.

Demling, R.H., DeSanti, L., Orgill, D.P. (2000–2004). High tension electrical burns. *burnsurgery.org section 7*. Available from http://www.burnsurgery.com/Modules/initial/part_two/sec7.htm (accessed 21 January 2008).

Dewar, D.J., Magson, C.L., Fraser, J.F., Crighton, L., Kimble, R.M. (2004). Hot beverage scalds in Australian children. *Journal of Burn Care and Rehabilitation*, 25: 224–227.

Edwards-Jones, V., Dawson, M.M., Childs, C. (2000). A survey into toxic shock syndrome in UK burn units. *Burns*, 26: 323–333.

Engrav, L.H., Heimbach, D.M., Reus, J.L., Harnar, T.J., Marvin, J.A. (1983). A randomized prospective study of early excision and grafting of indeterminant burns less than 20 percent TBSA. *Journal of Trauma*, 23: 1001–1004.

Frame, J., Eve, M.D., Hacket, M.E.J. (1985). The toxic shock syndrome in burned children. *Burns*, 11: 234–241.

Gaukroger, P.B., Chapman, M., Davey, R.B. (1991). Pain control in paediatric burns – the use of patient controlled analgesia. *Burns*, 17: 396–399.

Gordon, M. (1988). Pruritus in burns. *Journal of Burn Care and Rehabilitation*, 9: 305.

Hemeda, M., Maher, A., Mabrouk, A. (2003). Epidemiology of burns admitted to Ain Shams University Burns Unit, Cairo, Egypt. *Burns*, 29: 353–358.

Henderson, P., Hoehlriegel, N., Fraser, J.F., Kimble, R.M. (2003). Flammable liquid burns in children. *Burns*, 29: 349–352.

Herndon, D. (2002). *Total burn care*, 2nd ed. Elsevier, Edinburgh.

Herndon, D.N., Barrow, R.E., Rutan, R.L., Rutan, T.C., Desai, M.H., Abston, S. (1989). A comparison of conservative versus early excision: Therapies in severely burned patients. *Annals of Surgery*, 209: 547–553.

Hettiaratchy, S., Papini, R. (2004). Initial management of a major burn: I – overview. *British Medical Journal*, 328: 1555–1557.

Hicks, C., von Bayer, C., Safford, P., Korlaar, I., Goodenough, B. (2001). The Faces Pain Scale revised: Toward a common metric in pediatric pain measurement. *Pain*, 93: 173–183.

Holland, A.J., Martin, H.C., Cass, D.T. (2002). Laser Doppler imaging prediction of burn wound outcome in children. *Burns*, 28: 11–117.

Humphries, Y., Melson, M., Gore, D. (1997). Superiority of oral ketamine as an analgesic and sedative for wound care procedures in the paediatric burns patients. *Journal of Burn Care and Rehabilitation*, 18: 34–36.

Hunsberger, M., Love, B., Byrne, C. (1984). A review of current approaches used to help children and parents cope with health care procedures. *Maternal and Child Nursing Journal*, 13: 145–165.

Huspith, J., Rayatt, S. (2004). First aid and treatment of minor burns. *British Medical Journal*, 328: 1487–1489.

James, J., Hofland, H.W., Borgstein, E.S., Kumiponjera, D., Komolafe, O.O., Zijlstra, E.E. (2003). The prevalence of HIV infection among burn patients in a burns unit in Malawi and its influence on outcome. *Burns*, 29: 55–60.

Janzekovic, Z. (1970). A new concept in the early excision and immediate grafting of burns. *Journal of Trauma*, 10: 1103–1108.

Johansen, M., Wootton, R., Kimble, R.M., Mill, J., Smith, A.C., Hockey, A. (2004). A feasibility study of email communication between the patient's family and the specialist burns team. *Journal of Telemedicine and Telecare*, 10 (Suppl. 1): 53–55.

Jose, R.M., Roy, D.K., Vidyadharan, R., Erdmann, M. (2004). Burns area estimation – an error perpetuated. *Burns*, 30: 481–482.

Kimble, R., Smith, A.C. (2004). Post-acute burns care for children. In: Wootton, R. & Batch, J. *Telepediatrics: Telemedicine and Child Health*. Royal Society of Medicine Press, London.

Komolafe, O.O., James, J., Makoka, M., Kalongeolera, L. (2003). Epidemiology and mortality of burns at the Queen Elizabeth Central Hospital Blantyre, Malawi. *Central Africa Journal of Medicine*, 49: 130–134.

Kreger, B.E., Craven, D.E., McCabe, W.R. (1980). Gram-negative bacteremia. IV. Revaluation of clinical features and treatment in 612 patients. *American Journal of Medicine*, 68: 344–355.

La Hei, E.R., Holland, A.J., Martin, H. (2006). Laser Doppler imaging of paediatric burns: Burn wound outcome can be predicted independent of clinical examination. *Burns*, 32: 550–553.

Laloe, V. (2002). Epidemiology and mortality of burns in a general hospital of eastern Sri Lanka. *Burns*, 28: 778–781.

Landolt, M.A., Marti, D., Widmer, J., Meuli, M. (2002). Does cartoon movie distraction decrease burned children's pain behaviour? *Journal of Burn Care and Rehabilitation*, 23: 61–65.

Lui, P., Tildsley, J., Fritsche, M., Kimble, R.M. (2003). Electrical burns in children. *Journal of Burns & Surgical Wound Care*, 2: 8.

Manwaorren, R., Hynan, L. (2003). Clinical validation of FLACC: Preverbal patient pain scale. *Pediatric Nursing*, 29: 140–147.

Matheson, J.D., Clayton, J., Muller, M.J. (2001). Reduction of itch during burn wound healing. *Journal of Burn Care and Rehabilitation*, 22: 76–81.

McCormack, R.A., La Hei, E.R., Martin, H.C. (2003). First-aid management of minor burns in children: A prospective study of children presenting to the Children's Hospital at Westmead, Sydney. *Medical Journal of Australia*, 178: 31–33.

Moss, L.S. (2004). Outpatient management of the burn patient. *Critical Care Nursing Clinics of North America*, 109–117.

Nagel, T.R., Schunk, J.E. (1997). Using the hand to estimate the surface area of a burn in children. *Paediatric Emergency Care*, 13: 254–255.

Palmieri, T.L., Greenhalgh, D.G. (2002). Topical treatment of pediatric patients with burns. *American Journal of Clinical Dermatology*, 3: 529–534.

Presner, J., Yowler, C., Smith, L., Steel, A., Fratianne, R. (2001). Music therapy for assistance with pain and anxiety in burn treatment. *Journal of Burn Care and Rehabilitation*, 22: 83–88.

Pruit, B.A. Jr., O'Neill, J.A. Jr., Moncrief, J.A., Lindberg, R.B. (1968). Successful control of burn-wound sepsis. *Journal of the American Medical Association*, 203: 1054–1056.

Ramakrishnan, K.M., Sankar, J., Venkatraman, J. (2005). Profile of paediatric burns. Indian experience in a tertiary care burn unit. *Burns*, 31: 351–353.

Rockwell, W.B., Ehrlich, H.P. (1990). Should burn blister fluid be evacuated? *Journal of Burn Care and Rehabilitation*, 11: 93–95.

Shakespeare, P.G. (2001). Standards and quality in burn treatment. *Burns*, 27: 791–792.

Sharar, S., Carrougher, G., Selzer, K., O'Donnell, F., Vavilala, M.S., Lee, L.A. (2002). A comparison of oral transmucosal fentanyl citrate and oral oxycodone for pediatric outpatient wound care. *Journal of Burn Care and Rehabilitation*, 1: 27–31.

Sheridan, R.L. (2005). Sepsis in pediatric burn patients. *Pediatric Critical Care Medicine*, 6: S112–S119.

Smith, A.C., Kimble, R.M., Bailey, D., Mill, J., Wootton, R. (2004a). Diagnostic accuracy of and patient satisfaction with telemedicine for the follow-up of paediatric burns patients. *Journal of Telemedicine and Telecare*, 10: 193–198.

Smith, A.C., Youngberry, K., Mill, J., Kimble, R.M., Wootton, R. (2004b). A review of three years experience using email and videoconferencing for the delivery of post-acute burns care to children in Queensland. *Burns*, 30: 248–252.

Street, J., Wright, J., Choo, K., Fraser, J.F., Kimble, R.M. (2002). Woodstoves uncovered: A paediatric problem. *Burns*, 28: 472–474.

Tarim, A., Nursal, T.Z., Yildirim, S., Noyan, T., Moray, G., Haberal, M. (2005). Epidemiology of pediatric burn injuries in southern Turkey. *Journal of Burn Care and Rehabilitation*, 26: 327–330.

Tredget, E.E., Shankowsky, H.A., Rennie, R., Burrell, R.E., Logsetty, S. (2004). Pseudomonas infections in the thermally injured patient. *Burns*, 30: 3–26.

Trop, M., Zobel, G., Roedl, S., Grubbauer, H.M., Feierl, G. (2004). Toxic shock syndrome in a scald burn child treated with an occlusive wound dressing. *Burns*, 30: 176–180.

Van Niekerk, A., Rode, H., Laflamme, L. (2004). Incidence and patterns of childhood burn injuries in the Western Cape, South Africa. *Burns*, 30: 341–347.

Vitale, M., Fields-Blache, C., Luterman, A. (1991). Severe itching in the patient with burns. *Journal of Burn Care and Rehabilitation*, 12: 230–233.

11 Paediatric transplantation

Rebecca Smith and Susan Tame

Introduction

Techniques in organ donation are advancing rapidly, and the morbidity and mortality associated with this has reduced in the last three decades for both adult and paediatric recipients of organs. In the UK, approximately 50 children become organ donors each year. A donor is considered to be a paediatric donor if the patient is 15 years of age or under.

This chapter details the care of children and families who (a) undergo organ transplants and (b) are donors, in the UK. It would take too much space to give specific details for all countries, but the UK model is one that is similar to that used in many countries, and the surgical procedures and subsequent nursing care is similar internationally. Reference to international perspectives of organ donation and transplants is provided at the end of this chapter.

Donors are found in many hospitals, but the British Transplant Society (2003) recommends that recipients should be transplanted in specialist centres. Therefore, whilst many readers of this book will encounter organ donors, few will be present in the recipient side of the transplantation process. Whilst this is a book covering paediatric surgery, the literature indicates that the emotional upset and distress perioperative nurses experience, especially during the retrieval of organs for transplant, is related to a lack of understanding of the nature and diagnosis of brainstem death and the care provided to the patient pre-, intra- and post-operatively (Carter-Gentry & McCurren, 2004; Levvey, 2006; Regehr *et al.*, 2004; Bothamley, 1999; Duke *et al.*, 1998).

For these reasons, in this chapter we address these issues and provide the theatre nurse with a comprehensive overview of the paediatric transplantation processes from a donor and a recipient perspective, beginning with the process of becoming an organ donor. Having discussed the actual patient care provided to both the donor and recipient children, the chapter concludes by looking into the future and the developments that are currently ongoing, which will advance the described organ donation processes.

Becoming an organ donor

Traditionally, a person could carry an organ donor card to indicate their wish to become an organ donor. In 1995, UK Transplant introduced the National Organ Donor Register (ODR), a database on to which a person could put their details indicating that they wished to donate their organs in the event of their death.

Previously, although carrying a donor card and/or being on the ODR gave an indication of the person's wishes, these wishes could still be overridden by the person's relatives. The Human Tissue Act (2004) (Department of Health, 2004), which came into practice on the 1 September, 2006 now states that being on the ODR is consent and this cannot be overridden by relatives. A donor card, the known wishes of the deceased and a will also count as consent.

This opting-in model, which requires an action from the individual, is not without its critics, primarily because whilst approximately 80% of the public state that they support organ donation, only 27% have put themselves on the ODR (UK Transplant, 2009). Given the small number of people who died each year in a way in which they can donate their organs, this leads to many potential donors not becoming donors because the family did not know the patient's wishes.

Thus, there have been calls for an opting-out system in which the individual would have to indicate that they do *not* wish to become a donor. If they have not done this, then they are presumed to have consented, hence consent is an omission. However, there are worries that such an authoritarian system may produce a backlash against organ donation, whereas at the moment there is a feeling that the general public cherishes the 'gift' notion. Second, there are vulnerable groups who may not have the resources to opt out and may end up becoming organ donors against their wishes.

There are children on the ODR, and the position of a competent child who has consented is legally the same as that of an adult (for more information about children and consent, please see Chapter 3). A younger child can also be put on the ODR by his/her next of kin; the problem is that as an adult that person will remain on the ODR perhaps without their knowledge and contrary to their wishes. However, in reality, for children, the person with parental responsibility will always be approached for permission to proceed with donation. If there is a conflict because an older child has put him/herself on the ODR but their next of kin do not want donation, then the transplant co-ordinator must try to resolve those objections. If they prove to be irresolvable, there is a clause that allows the transplant coordinator to use their discretion to decide whether to proceed with the donation or not.

UK NB: In November 2007, the government appointed a task force to look at the opting-in model again; at the time of publication, it has not yet reported its recommendations.

Types of donation

There are four different ways of donating organ and tissues and it is useful to clarify the differences between them.

Solid organ donation following brainstem death

Also known as 'heart beating donation'. Here, the patient has been certified brainstem dead. However, they remain on the ventilator following certification of death. Whilst ventilated, their heart will continue to beat ensuring that all the internal organs are receiving an oxygen supply. This allows time for the donation process to be put into place. The organs that can be donated following brainstem death are heart, lungs, liver, kidneys, pancreas and small bowel.

Solid organ donation following cardiac death

This is known as 'non–heart beating donation' (NHBD), and since 2002 has been undergoing a revival in an attempt by UK Transplant to turn around falling donor numbers. There are five categories of NHBD. The British Transplant Society (BTS) has recently reviewed the categories and these are described below. Each category is further classified as either controlled or uncontrolled.

Box 11.1 Maastricht criteria (1995)

Category I: Dead on arrival at hospital (uncontrolled)
Category II: Unsuccessful resuscitation (uncontrolled)
Category III: Awaiting cardiac arrest (controlled)
Category IV: Cardiac arrest in a brainstem dead donor (controlled)
Source: Zaltzman (2007).

In the *controlled* situation, the patient's injury is deemed unsurvivable by the caring team and there is a plan to withdraw treatment (normally ventilation and/or inotropic support). There must be a distinct line between the decision to withdraw treatment and the decision to pursue organ donation. The donation team is called and treatment is withdrawn once they are set up in theatre. Once the patient's heart has stopped beating and death has been certified, the patient is taken to theatre. The retrieval operation has to commence within 10 minutes of asystole, hence a rapid retrieval technique is used. With this technique, the kidneys, liver, lungs and pancreas can be retrieved.

In *uncontrolled*, withdrawal of the patient's treatment is not planned, and the donation retrieval team must respond and attend the unit within several minutes after the patient has been certified dead. Abdominal cooling and perfusion are commenced immediately and then the donor is taken to theatre. In this situation, only kidneys may be retrieved.

Tissue donation following cardiac death

Tissue donation is not as well known as organ donation; however, it can bring about an increased quality of life for many people. Tissues can be retrieved up to 48 hr following death, and unlike organ donation the patient does not have to have died within a critical care area in order to be able to donate tissues. Consequently, many more people can donate tissues than can solid organs. Tissues that can be donated after death are corneas, skin, bone, heart valves, tendons, meniscus and costal cartilage. The age limits that apply for tissue donation are:

Corneas – 1 year upwards (no upper age limit)
Skin – 17 years upwards (no upper age limit)
Bone – 17 years upwards (no upper age limit)
Heart valves – 32 weeks gestation (or over 2.5 kg) – 60 years
Tendon – 17–60 years
Meniscus – 17–50 years

NB: Age limits occasionally change, so it is always advisable to check with the tissue services.

Live donation

The most common form of live donation is of course blood donation; however, other tissues can also be retrieved from a living donor, such as bone marrow, skin, bone, eggs, sperm and birth membranes. In terms of solid organs, the most well known is live renal donation, and there are several active programmes running in the UK. However, in recent times, there have also been innovations in live liver donation and lung donation. In liver donation, the left lateral section of the liver is removed and donated. The operations to date have been exclusively parent to child. For live lung donation, the lower lobe of the right lung is donated, and this can be performed between adult to adult. Both these forms of live donation are in their infancy, and the mortality risks for the donors are significantly higher than for live renal donors.

The British Transplantation Society (2003) recommend that all children with end-stage renal failure should be on the waiting list for transplantation. A living donor may be found who has the same tissue type as the recipient. This donor may or may not be related to the recipient, or a paired donation in line with new guidelines as outlined in the Human Tissue Act (2004). In a paired donation, a donor and recipient who are not compatible but willing to donate and need a kidney are paired with a donor and recipient who again are not compatible but willing to donate. In this situation, these pairs may be matched. The Act also makes legal altruistic donation where a stranger may donate their kidney into the national pool, following stringent assessment.

Box 11.2   Definition of brainstem death

Brain Stem Death

> 'The irreversible loss of the capacity for consciousness, combined with the irreversible loss of the capacity to breathe'.
>   (Department of Health, 1998)

Death is a complex subject, and there is a remarkable variation of beliefs surrounding it. It is at the centre of most religions and is accepted as an inevitable end to a human life. Finding the exact point at which we die has long been at the centre of medical and philosophical debates. The notion of death itself has changed, and continues to change, both with the development of technology and changing beliefs about the world we live in. One such major change took place in the 1970s and this was the introduction of the concept of Brainstem Death (BSD).

The 1950s and 1960s saw substantial growth in intensive care therapy, primary with the ability to effectively maintain a person on a ventilator. In 1959, two French physicians Mollaret and Goulon described a group of patients they had observed on ventilators, whose cardiac and respiratory functioning could be maintained whilst the patients appeared devoid of brain function (Mollaret & Goulon, 1959). They gave this phenomena the name 'coma dépasse', literally meaning a 'state beyond a coma'. In 1968, the Ad-Hoc Committee of Harvard Medical School was appointed to examine the definition of brain death; they clearly reported that the clinical state of brain death should be regarded as death as well as giving the tests required to diagnose the condition (Beecher, 1968). In 1971, a second major conceptual advance occurred when Mohandas and Chou, two Minneapolis neurosurgeons, made the 'suggestion that in patients with known irreparable intra-cranial lesions, irreversible damage to the *brain stem* was the "point of no return'" (Pallis & Harley, 1996), and this became the concept of BSD. The Minnesota Criteria gave guidelines for diagnosis, and this became the foundation for the codes developed by most countries. The UK adopted the BSD criteria as a legal definition of death in 1976.

The anatomy and physiology of the brain

The brain is divided into three areas: the cortex, or cerebrum, in which all cognation (thinking, knowing, memory, emotions etc.) occurs, the cerebellum and the brainstem, which controls vegetative functions (breathing, blood pressure, temperature, motor output and sensory input) (Figure 11.1). As well as the brain, the skull contains blood and central spinal fluid (CSF).

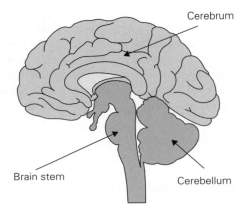

Fig. 11.1   Anatomy of the brain.

When damaged, the brain has certain compensatory mechanisms it will try to use to protect itself. These centre around the fact that the skull is a ridged box and therefore there is little room for swelling or bleeding to occur. It will decrease CSF production and increase CSF absorption; it will also reduce blood flow. All these strategies are trying to make room in the skull for the swelling and/or bleeding. However, if these continue despite the reduction in circulating fluids, then brain damage will start to occur. If it is severe enough, then this may progress to BSD. If left ventilated, the clinical course of a BSD patient is short, and they normally will become asystolic with 72 hr.

The most common causes of BSD are:

- intercranial haemorrhage;
- head injury;
- brain tumour;
- infection (e.g. meningitis);
- hypoxia.

Brainstem death tests

BSD testing in the UK is regulated by Department of Health guidelines (Department of Health, 1998). If a patient is thought to be BSD, then the doctors can carry out the

BSD tests to ensure that the patient fulfils the criteria. Two doctors who are registered with the GMC, of whom one must be a consultant, carry these out. This involves:

- ensuring that certain preconditions have been met before testing commences (such as excluding hypothermia or sedatives);
- ensuring that there is a known cause of the coma;
- a clinical examination of the patient, looking for any evidence of brainstem functioning.

The tests are done twice to exclude the possibility of human error. The time of death is timed at the completion of the first set of tests; it is not the time when ventilatory support is withdrawn.

The Code of Practice applies to adult and children; however, in 1991, the British Paediatric Society and the Royal College of Physicians produced additional guidance for the testing of children. These stipulate that below the age of 37 weeks gestation, BSD cannot be applied because of the developmental state of the brain. Between the ages of 37 weeks gestation and 2 months, it is rarely possible to confidentially diagnose BSD; however, it is up to the clinician to decide whether to test or not. The standard criteria apply for over 2 months of age, although the precise techniques used may need to be adapted slightly depending upon the size of the child.

Role of the transplant co-ordinator

Transplant co-ordinator is a term that actually covers several distinct roles. Broadly speaking, there are recipient transplant co-ordinators and donor transplant co-ordinators, although there can be further subdivisions within these two branches. Furthermore, some transplant co-ordinators play dual role, meaning that they undertake both donor and recipient work. Such diversity means that the outlines below are very broad and intended to give a general idea of the transplant coordinator's role.

Recipient transplant co-ordinators

Recipient co-ordinators cover specific organs, thus there are renal recipient co-ordinators, liver recipient co-ordinators and cardiac recipient co-ordinators (covering both heart and lungs). Some recipient co-ordinators work on-call. The main responsibilities of the role include the following:

1. Assessment and workup of the patient prior to go on the transplant waiting list.
2. Management of the waiting list – this includes registering patients for transplant, providing them with transplant information and being a contact point for patients on the waiting list.
3. Calling patients in for transplant and organising the actual operation.
4. Providing post-transplant follow-up care.

Live recipient transplant co-ordinators

Some centres run live related transplant programmes for renal transplants (although as advances in live liver and lung donation continue, there maybe future expansion of the live co-ordinator role). These co-ordinators focus on assessing the suitability of the potential live donors (physically and psychologically). The workup period can take several months and they work closely with the families during this time. They are then responsible for organising the operation and providing follow-up care and advice.

Donor transplant co-ordinators

Donor transplant co-ordinators are traditionally based in a transplant hospital and from there cover all the hospitals within a defined region. They work on-call and their role involves the following:

1. Assessing the suitability of a potential multiorgan donor by reviewing notes, interviewing the family, physical examination and speaking to the patient's GP.
2. Predonation information and counselling for potential donor relatives.
3. Obtaining written consent from the relatives.
4. Co-ordinating the retrieval teams and operation.
5. Organising the allocation of the organs (with UK Transplant).
6. Assisting in theatre.
7. Providing follow-up support for the donor family.
8. Providing education sessions and support for the regional hospitals.

In-house donor transplant co-ordinators

In recent times, UK Transplant has moved towards employing donor transplant co-ordinators to work in hospitals that have a large donor potential (as opposed to working from the transplant centres), and this is based on a successful Spanish model for transplant co-ordination. These co-ordinators have responsibility for project managing and promoting the donation services within that one hospital, although they may also undertake regional on-call work.

Dual role co-ordinators

Some donor transplant co-ordinators also cover the recipient co-ordinator role; this is normally either renal or liver recipient work. However, as the recipient workload has increased and in response to concerns over potential conflict of interests, there has been a trend to separate the two roles and employ more recipient-only co-ordinators.

Tissue co-ordinators

Tissue co-ordinators work on a national on-call rota as opposed to a regional one. They co-ordinate the whole tissue donation process over the phone. After taking the initial referral, they ring the families of the potential tissue donor at home at a pre-arranged time. They get a past medical and behavioural history of the patient and obtain consent (recorded with the permission of the family member); they also contact the patient's GP. After this, if the patient is suitable, they liaise with the coroner, mortuary and tissue retrieval services to organise the retrieval. They will also provide family follow-up care as required.

NB: A recent report from the government Organ Donation Taskforce (January 2008) has recommended a complete separation between donor and recipient co-ordinators. It also recommends a doubling of co-ordinator numbers and a further move towards donor transplant co-ordinators working in donor hospitals.

Donor care and management

This section will look at the care and management of a paediatric donor and their family throughout the donation process. The approach of the family, donor assessment and management, the interoperative period and what happens post-op will be discussed.

Making the donation request

At such an emotionally distressing time, it can be daunting for the staff to raise the issue of organ donation. However, there is evidence to demonstrate that if done in a planned and sensitive manner, the request will not increase the distress of the family, and for some families it can give them comfort. Thus, it is important that all families are informed that they have the option of donation.

There have been attempts to be prescriptive in the way in which families are approached about organ donation, and each method has research to support it. However, it can be argued that ridged prescriptions do not always work when dealing with human nature and emotions. Thus, outlined below is a range of 'best-practice' methods that a practitioner can draw from in order to best suit the situation and family that they find themselves with.

Understanding of death

The family needs to understand that the patient is dead, because if they still believe that they are alive, and that there is a chance of recovery, they are not going to agree to donation. BSD should be explained carefully to them, and their understanding checked. They should be given the option of observing the BSD testing; for some, this may help their comprehension, as might the use of visual aids (Sque *et al.*, 2003). The requestor should begin the interview by checking their understanding of BSD and going over it again if required.

Mini-conversations

Before BSD testing, some families may start to ask questions about what will happen after the tests. The doctors and nurses looking after the patient are in a good position to explain to them that they will be asked about organ donation. This is not a request to which they are expected to give a reply, but a warning that they will be approached. This can provide useful thinking time for the family without the pressure of having to give an instant (and often instinctive) answer. These bedside conversations are often a useful format for providing information about donation whilst not being in the setting of a formal discussion with a consultant. An experienced and confident nurse may gently direct these conversations to prompt the family to ask questions and re-enforce the patient's diagnosis (Verbel & Worth, 2002).

A quiet and private place

It may seem obvious to say but it does make a difference if the request is made in a private room that has been set out beforehand. Gortmaker *et al.* (1998) found that the consent rate increased by 24% if the request is done in a quiet and private place.

Information giving

Many families say no to donation on the basis of misconceptions about what becoming an organ donor entails. Therefore, it is vital they are given that information before they make a decision. This is not always easy to achieve. Verbel and Worth (2002) suggest a technique in which the requestor tells the family that they are going to give them some information about donation, tell them that they will be able to ask them some questions and then they will be given time to make their decision. This allows the requestor control of the conversation and chance to give the family the appropriate information before a decision is made.

Planned and collaborative requesting

Transplant co-ordinators are trained to make requests, they are also the experts in their field, and thus they are in the best position to give information about donation and answer questions. Gortmaker *et al.* (1998) found an increase of 19% in the consent rate when a transplant co-ordinator and the hospital staff made the request together. In its strictest sense, collaborative requesting means that the co-ordinator and the doctor go to the family together to make the request. However, it can also mean that the patient is discussed with the transplant co-ordinator first, and they give the doctor guidance on how best to conduct the request (if needed). This form of planned requesting is particularly useful if geographical distance is an issue.

Decoupling

Gortmaker *et al.* (1998) found that if the conversation in which the family is informed about the results of the BSD tests is separated from the conversation about donation, then consent rates went from 53% to 71%. The recommended practice is for the doctor to go to the family and confirm that BSD has occurred. They will then inform the family that they will give them a few minutes and then come back and have a further discussion with them. For the second conversation, the transplant co-ordinator, if present, can accompany the doctor to discuss about donation.

Preoperative care of a potential paediatric donor

Donor assessment

Every effort has to be made to ensure that potential recipients are protected from the risk of infection or disease when receiving an organ. To this end, a comprehensive donor assessment is required. Because it is obviously impossible to interview the patient, the transplant co-ordinator has to draw from a variety of sources available to them. These include:

1. reviewing the patient's medical notes;
2. contacting the patient's GP – if the donation is occurring out of hours, this has to be done retrospectively;
3. physically examining the patient, particularly looking for any suspicious moles or lumps, evidence of IV drug abuse and old operation scars;
4. interviewing the family to ascertain their knowledge of the patient's past medical history and behavioural history (particularly alcohol intake, smoking history, drug abuse and sexual history).

None of these methods are perfect; obviously, the family and/or GP might not know what lifestyle activities the patient has been engaging in. Even for paediatrics, the family may not know e.g. if their 15-year-old child is sexually active or not. However, by drawing on all fours, a good picture of the patient should emerge. On top of these, the transplant co-ordinator will examine, or initiate, further investigations to assess the patient and individual organs. Most commonly, these are:

1. measuring height and weight;
2. chest X-ray;
3. ECG;
4. echocardiogram;
5. sputum and urine culture and sensitivities;
6. blood group;
7. full blood count;
8. urea and electrolytes;
9. liver function tests;
10. amylase;
11. blood glucose;
12. virology screen (standard screening includes HIV, hepatitis B and C, CMV, toxoplasmosis, syphilis);
13. arterial blood gases for oxygenation levels.

There are only two absolute contraindications to solid organ donation: HIV and CJD. However, there are also relative exclusions such as malignancy, undertaking high-risk behaviour (e.g. IV drug abuse), hepatitis B and C. In the instances where the patient falls into one of these categories, they should be discussed with the transplant team.

Donor management

The principle of donor management for any potential donor is to maintain organ integrity in order to maximise the likelihood of a successful transplant. Following BSD, the body undergoes many physiological changes that make successful donor management challenging. Various therapies may be put into place in order to protect/improve the quality of the organs prior to theatre. However, whilst national guidelines for the management of an adult organ donor exist (Intensive Care Society, 2005), to date there are no such guidelines for paediatric management. Nonetheless, many of the principles of management for adult organ donors are directly transferable to paediatrics, e.g. good chest physiotherapy and temperature regulation. However, a great deal of donor management involves the administration of fluids and medications. This can pose a problem; some of the recommended adult therapies, such as the use of tridothyronine, have not been proven in children. This perhaps can be attributed to the low number of paediatric donors each year, making conclusive studies difficult. Given this, it is important to manage a paediatric donor in collaboration with the attending paediatrician.

Potential donors need to be managed holistically; the instigation of some treatments can have wide-ranging and potentially negative systemic effects. For example, diabetes insipidus if left untreated, or incorrectly managed, can lead to profound electrolyte imbalance, affecting all organ systems. However, if such problems can be anticipated, monitored for and treated promptly, such major complications can be avoided. Donor management is often seen as a primarily ICU role, however, many donors can be in theatre for up to 6hr (or even longer if there are any delays). Hence, it is vitally important that assessment and good donor management continue during the interoperative period.

Endocrine changes

Endocrine changes underpin many of the problems that occur in the body following BSD. Therefore, it is worth looking at those changes before discussing individual organ management.

The anterior pituitary gland stimulates the thyroid gland to produce tridothyronine (T3) and thyroxine (T4). Amongst other roles, these hormones in turn stimulate the adrenal glands to produce adrenaline and noradrenaline, which regulate the body's cardiac output and blood pressure. The body titrates the release of these hormones to meet its own requirements. However, during the process of becoming BSD, the pituitary gland ceases to function, and in its final moments it floods the body with hormones, resulting in a massive surge of adrenaline and noradrenaline, often called a catecholamine storm. The patient is difficult to manage during this stage, as they can be extremely hypertensive and tachycardic then bradycardic; occasionally, patients will even suffer a cardiac arrest at this point. This is known as 'Cushing's response' and is a classic sign of brainstem herniation (Figure 11.2). However, very shortly after this, there is no further release of T3 and T4 (and consequently adrenaline and noradrenaline), and thus the patient will become markedly hypotensive.

Antidiuretic hormone, which regulates the body's fluid balance, is produced in the posterior pituitary gland. Following BSD, this production stops and most of these patients develop diabetes insipidus, the main symptom of which is an excessive urine output. One consequence of this is that the patients become hypernatraemic and they tend to be treated with large volumes of dextrose fluids. Coupled with the increased levels of catecholamines and reduced insulin production, these patients will often also become hyperglycaemic.

Cardiac management

The cardiac muscles in a BSD patient are under stress. They have undergone an intense period of autonomic activity followed by profound hypotension, often then

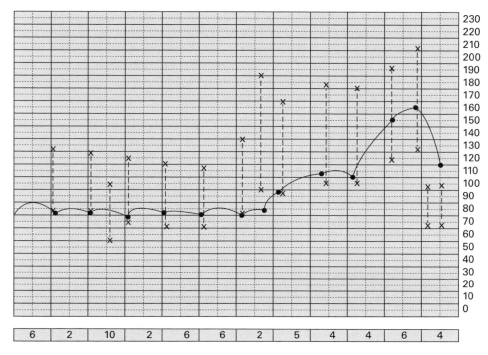

Fig. 11.2 An example of 'Cushing's response' during brain herniation.

controlled by infusions of adrenaline and noradrenaline. They are further stressed by blood gas and electrolyte abnormalities. These multifactorial changes lead to ischaemic damage and ECG abnormalities. In order to protect the heart for transplantation, it is desirable to discontinue these as soon as possible. Hence, after BSD testing, these patients may be started on an infusion of T3 and/or vasopressin. The rationale is that by giving the patient the hormones that stimulate the body to produce its own adrenaline and noradrenaline, a satisfactory blood pressure is maintained at minimal cost to the heart. This HRT has been proved to be effective in adults, but there is no evidence that it is of value in paediatrics, hence it is prudent to liaise with the caring paediatrician.

If a patient develops diabetes insipidus, they can quickly lose potassium and become hypokalaemic. If this is left untreated, then the patient will have cardiac ectopics and eventually, should the potassium drop far enough, a cardiac arrest. In the first instance, the diabetes insipidus should be treated. However, blood potassium levels should be monitored closely and if they do drop, they should be treated with a potassium chloride infusion.

Lung management

The lung is the organ that is most easily damaged by the event that led to the death and the subsequent ventilation. This is because following a severe head injury (no matter what the cause) these patients often vomit, and because of the nature of head injury, they can no longer protect their own airway, and hence aspiration is a common problem. Furthermore, Intermittent Positive Pressure Ventilation (IPPV) and oxygen therapy, whilst both necessary, can damage the delicate lung membranes coupled with the fact these ventilated patients are susceptible to chest infections. They can also develop neurogenic pulmonary oedema owing to increased permeability of capillary, and alveolar endothelium allows protein-rich fluid to shift into the extravascular spaces.

Therefore, there is intense focus on good lung management, and lung recruitment strategies can be implemented to 'turn around' borderline lungs. The aim of lung management is to keep the lungs clear of sputum and infection and to maximise oxygen exchange with the lowest possible oxygen requirement. These patients need regular chest physiotherapy to remove secretions. If they have a chest infection, it is important that they continue on their prescribed antibiotic regime. If they do not have a chest infection, they should be commenced on a broad-spectrum antibiotic as a prophylaxis along with steroidal medication.

Renal management

The kidneys are very susceptible to hypoxic damage, and if the patient has had a hypoxic event during their initial injury or afterwards, it may be that renal function deteriorates, and thus it needs to be closely monitored. However, if there is no sign of renal failure, then the principles of renal management are quite simple i.e. to keep the kidneys well-hydrated and oxygenated. Hence, their management is dependent upon good cardiovascular management. It is important that the patient has standard maintenance fluids running; they are monitored for diabetes insipidus and this is treated quickly if it develops. For a child, diabetes insipidus is defined as 5 mls/kg/hr combined with a urine specific gravity of less than 1.005 (Saborio *et al.*, 2000). It maybe that they are already on a vasopressin infusion for cardiovascular management. However, a bolus dose maybe required to keep excessive dieresis under control.

Liver management

The liver does not require specific management as such. However, if the patient develops diabetes insipidus, then they may become hypernatraemic, which, if high enough, can make the liver unsuitable for transplant. Thus, the focus of treatment is, as before, to treat the diabetes insipidus, ensuring that the maintenance fluid is one with low sodium content. If the sodium does not improve with this, then sterile water down the nasogastric tube can be given.

Temperature management

BSD patients have no ability to regulate their temperature, as the hypothalamus is no longer functioning. Hence, preventative measures should be taken before the patient becomes hypothermic. Generally, close monitoring and a warming blanket will be sufficient, but in some cases, fluid warming, warm humidified air and ambient temperature control may be required.

Haematological management

The ischaemic brain tissue can release thromboplastin, causing a significant disruption to the coagulation pathway. Hence, although uncommon, BSD patients can develop Disseminated Intravascular Coagulation (DIC). This should be monitored for and if it develops treated with fresh frozen plasma and/or platelets.

Organ allocation

The UK Transplant is responsible for the allocation of organs. It classes a paediatric donor as a child under the age of 15. Their organs will go into a paediatric allocation system with different sequencing orders for each organ, and these are outlined below. However, it should be noted that the allocation systems are regularly reviewed and amended if needed; hence, this information is provided to give an idea of how the allocation systems work.

Heart

1. Urgents – a national pool of adult and paediatric patients who are deemed to be so sick that they only have a few days left to live
2. Offered on a rotation basis to the paediatric cardiac centres (including adults registered as paediatrics)
3. Offered on a rotation basis to adult centres.

Lungs

1. Offered on a rotation basis to the paediatric cardiac centres (including adults registered as paediatrics)
2. Offered on a rotation basis to adult centres.

Liver

1. Local Super Urgents – patients who are deemed to be so sick that they only have a few days left to live (adult and paediatric)
2. National Super Urgents of a compatible blood group
3. Paediatric small bowel and liver combined
4. Local paediatric patients (including adults registered as paediatrics)
5. National patients – paediatric and adult.

NB: An adult under 45 kg can be registered as a paediatric and has equal entitlement to paediatric organs.

Kidney

For kidneys, the donor's tissue type (HLA) is sent to UK Transplant and they undertake a national matching run to identify the most suitable recipients. The matching run goes first on tissue type and second on age, and it will try to match the recipient closely with the donor's age. Hence, a paediatric kidney is more likely to go to a paediatric, but this is not guaranteed.

Small bowel

If the donor is under the age of 16, then the small bowel is offered to the one centre in the country that undertakes paediatric small bowel transplantation.

Perioperative care

Once it has been agreed that a child will donate their organs, the tests explained above have been conducted and a recipient(s) for the donated organ(s) is located through UK Transplant, then it is the role of the transplant co-ordinator to liaise with the theatre staff and negotiate a suitable time when the child can go to theatre for organ removal. It is necessary to locate recipients for the heart and lungs, as this reduces the cold ischaemic time; i.e. the period of time between the cessation of the blood supply from the donor to the blood supply being re-established in the recipient.

Surgical teams

Each organ requires specialist care during its removal to preserve it in a condition that will promote optimal function when grafted to the recipient, and each organ requires a separate surgical team who will operate. Thus, the teams that are present at a retrieval process are dependent upon the organs to be removed, and this can mean that there are many more people in theatre than for other types of surgery.

The teams consist of a number of people all of whom perform vital roles within the retrieval process. They are usually provided from the hospital where the transplant is to occur, and as such may not be known to the permanent staff in the theatre where the retrieval will take place. The constituent members of each team who attend an organ retrieval are provided in Table 11.1. This table assumes that each organ is being removed in isolation from the others, whereas in reality, with paediatric donors, it is usual for more than one organ to be removed from a donor, and as such some of these roles may be shared depending on the organs to be taken. There may also be variations to the staff travelling as a part of a retrieval team due to other factors.

Table 11.1   Personnel involved in organ transplants

Team	Surgeon	Surgeon's assistant	Perfusionist	Scrub nurse	Donor physiologist
Heart and lung	✓	✓	✓	✓	In some teams
Liver, kidneys and small bowel	✓	✓	✓*	✓	
Pancreas	✓			✓	

*In some cases, the role of the perfusionist is undertaken by the transplant co-ordinator.

Depending on the hospital in which the retrieval takes place, the visiting teams may provide their own scrub and circulating practitioners as a part of the teams, or the hospital itself may provide these staff. The transplant co-ordinator will be present, and there will be an anaesthetist and operating department practitioner or anaesthetic nurse present to support the patient. In addition, there may also be student members of the professions listed, adding to the number of personnel present in theatre.

In some teams, there will be a donor physiologist present during the retrieval, and this is a role that is likely to become more prominent in the future.

Each organ has a time where it is in the optimal condition for transplantation into the recipient, after which the condition of the organ begins to deteriorate, meaning that the chances of graft survival are reduced. This is known as the cold ischaemic time. If the cold ischaemic time of the organ is exceeded, then the organ is unable to be transplanted into the recipient.

To ensure the best use of the donor organs, in any retrieval, adult or paediatric, the organs are always removed in the following order: heart, lungs, pancreas, liver and then the kidneys. Children do not require pancreas transplants because the indications are for end-stage diabetes. However, a pancreas, especially from a larger child, may be donated to an adult.

The patient will come to theatre and will continue to be monitored and with any infusions running, and ventilated if appropriate. In theatre, the child will be given muscle relaxants, prophylactic antibiotics and a bolus dose of steroid to aid lung function. The anaesthetist remains in theatre with the child to maintain the donor's cardiovascular and ventilatory systems.

NB: This may change in the future because the Organ Donation Taskforce (January 2008) has recommended the establishment of dedicated retrieval teams complete with their own anaesthetist and theatre staff.

Intraoperative care

Patient preparation

The patient is placed in a supine position, with both arms close by their sides, and their abdomen is prepared with an antimicrobial solution from neck to mid-thigh and to the operating table laterally. Sterile drapes are then applied as for a laparotomy; i.e. large drapes to cover the patient's legs and head, and also smaller drapes are used as side drapes to cover the lateral aspects of the prepared area.

All organ retrievals are conducted under strict aseptic conditions, ensuring that the integrity of the sterile field is not breeched. Using a size-10 blade, a vertical midline incision is made through the patient's skin to the fascia from the xiphoid to the pubis. Langenbeck retractors are then used to retract this tissue whilst the fascia is incised using another size-10 blade and the external oblique muscle is split and retracted, followed by the internal oblique muscle and transverse muscles.

The peritoneum in then grasped with non-toothed forceps, and an incision made with a scalpel. This incision is then extended to the length of the wound using a pair of scissors to reveal the abdominal contents, and ice is placed into the abdominal cavity to rapidly cool the organs. At this stage, the organs for which parents have given consent to be removed are examined visually for any defects, which may not have been identified during the preoperative investigations. A self-retaining retractor is inserted to maintain the opening in the abdomen to allow good vision of the internal organs and allow the removal of the organs for which consent has been obtained.

If the heart, lungs and liver are to be retrieved, the wound extends up to the patient's neck. In this case, following the laparotomy, the sternum is divided into two using an air-powered saw, allowing vision into the cardiopulmonary cavity.

Retractors are then inserted to ensure that the ribs remain separated, enabling good vision of the heart and lungs. The patient is placed onto cardiopulmonary bypass prior to the commencement of surgery.

The surgical team must work quickly to remove the donor organs to ensure that the cold ischaemic time is minimised. Each organ must be removed carefully in order to preserve its main arteries and veins, to maximise the chances of its function in the recipient. It is usual to follow the order set out below to the removal of organs, if all are to be removed, as this respects the maximum cold ischaemic times for each organ, helping it to remain in a condition suitable for reimplantation in the recipient, and also allows planning to be performed in a routine way, maximising the efficiency of the teams involved.

Heart

Minimum age for donation: can be donated from birth
Patient criteria: lack of underlying cardiac pathology
The heart that is to be donated must be of a similar size to that the recipient requires. Following sternotomy, the pericardium is opened. A PA catheter may be inserted at this stage or the surgeon may take direct pressure measurements from each chamber of the heart. The surgeon will then inspect the heart visually and identify the aorta, pulmonary artery, vena cavae. The aorta is cross-clamped, and the heart vented through an incision in the inferior vena cava and cold saline is used to cool the heart internally; along with ice slush, this reduces the temperature of the heart to bring about a rapid cardiac arrest. Working quickly, the donor heart is removed, starting by excision of the inferior and superior vena cavae, followed by the aorta, pulmonary artery and the left atrium and lastly the pulmonary veins. The length of the vein removed is dependent upon the intended recipient's condition and the reason for which they require cardiac transplant. Once excised and removed from the chest, the heart is again inspected for any defects on the back table by the scrub nurse, prior to placing this into ice-cold, sterile saline. The blood vessels are flushed with saline until the solution runs clear. The heart is then transferred to clean saline, ready for transportation to the hospital in which the recipient child is being prepared to receive the heart.

Lungs

Minimum age for donation: can be donated from birth
Patient criteria: good O_2/CO_2 gas exchange (PO_2 above 40 mmHg on 100% FiO_2), lack of respiratory disease
Retrieval of the lungs is through *en bloc* removal via a sternotomy. Both pleura are opened, and the lungs inspected visually prior to their removal. If there are no obvious defects, then the trachea, superior and inferior vena cavae, pulmonary artery and pulmonary vein are identified. The aorta is cross-clamped and the ascending aorta is dissected away from the pulmonary artery, and the posterior pericardium incised between the ascending aorta and the superior vena cava to allow exposure of the trachea. The right side of the heart is decompressed by ligating the superior vena cava and incising the inferior vena cava with a scalpel blade. The heart is vented by

removing the tip of the left atrial appendage. UW solution is then used as a flush. It is essential throughout to continue to ventilate the donor's lungs to avoid alveolar collapse, however, overinflation should be avoided, as this is associated with increased allograft dysfunction in the post-operative stages (Mendeloff, 1998). Immediately prior to their removal, the surgeon asks the anaesthetist to hyperinflate the lungs using 100% oxygen. The trachea is then clamped and dissected. Once the lungs have been removed, they are placed on the back table and visually inspected by the surgeon, prior to being bagged in the perfusion fluid and quickly taken to the recipient hospital.

Liver

Minimum age for donation: can be donated from birth
Patient criteria: adequate liver function
Following the laparotomy incision, the patient's vena cava and aorta superior and inferior to the kidneys and liver are dissected. The portal vein, hepatic artery, superior mesenteric artery and coeliac trunk and the common bile duct are identified and dissected, prior to the patient being heparinised, and systematically cooled. If the patient's heart is also to be retrieved, then it is at this point that this procedure would be carried out. The liver and pancreas may be removed *en bloc*; however, in children this is rare, and pancreatic transplants in children have not yet been performed.

Clamps are placed on the suprahepatic and infrahepatic vena cava and the hepatic artery and vein and the common bile duct prior to these structures being dissected. Once dissected, the liver is placed on a back trolley, inspected visually by the scrub nurse and a surgeon performs further dissection prior to flushing the vascular structures with UW solution until the solution runs clear. The organ is then placed into sterile bags and into a container of ice ready for transportation.

At this stage, if the kidneys are also to be donated, work commences on identifying and removing these as described below.

Kidneys

Minimum age for donation: 6 months
Patient criteria: not diabetic, HLA matching required, adequate renal function
In a live donation, it is usual to have two surgical teams working simultaneously, one removing the donor kidney and one to implant the removed kidney into the recipient. In the case of the cadaveric donor, the kidney is removed in the same way as in an open nephrectomy, with care being paid to not damage the renal vein, artery and ureter. Following the laparotomy described above, the colon is moved to one side, and the fascia and kidney are exposed by blunt and sharp dissection. The ureter is identified and ligated between double ligatures. Any adherences to other structures, including the vena cava and aorta, are dissected. The renal artery and vein are identified, dissected, clamped and ligated with a double ligature.

Once a kidney is removed, it is transferred to the back table where the scrub nurse visually inspects the organ, the renal artery and vein and also the ureters for any possible damage, which would render it unsuitable for transplantation. The removed kidney is then perfused with cold perfusion solution until the solution runs clear and the kidneys appear uniformly perfused. The same procedure is followed if the other kidney is also to be removed.

Anomalies in the donor and recipient anatomy can lead to complications in grafting the donor kidney. For this reason, a record of the vascular anatomy of the kidney and any damage is made and this accompanies the kidney to the transplant centre.

Small bowel

Minimum age for donation: can be donated from birth
Patient criteria: adequate bowel function, lack of bowel diseases

The consultant who will be carrying out the recipient's surgery will come to remove the small bowel from the donor. This ensures that a sufficient portion of the small bowel is taken. Following laparotomy, the surgeon inspects the bowel visually for defects. The vascular supply is maintained by the portal vein and the mesenteric artery, and these structures are also identified and the surrounding tissues dissected. The length of bowel required for the recipient is identified and two rows of staples applied transversely at the distal and the proximal end of this section. The bowel between the two staple lines is cut using diathermy. The blood vessels are ligated with two ties and dissected between using scissors, leaving as long a portion of vein and artery as possible connected to the small bowel to allow for reshaping of these prior to the recipient anastomosis.

Following its removal, the section of small bowel is removed to the back table where it is perfused with cold perfusion solution until the solution runs clear. The bowel and vascular structures are also inspected for any defects, which may impede successful transplantation into the recipient. The organ is then placed into sterile bags and ice ready for transportation.

What happens post-retrieval

Post-retrieval, nursing care must be offered to the donor child, and also the organs that are to be used for the recipient.

The laparotomy wound is closed by approximating the peritoneum and suturing this with a continuous suture. The skin edges are then sutured, again using a continuous non-absorbable suture. This suturing does not have any function in wound healing, but does prevent leakage of body fluids. It is also important that the final result is aesthetically pleasing as the parents may see the child's wound post-operatively. Having sutured the wound, this is covered with a sterile dressing. The drapes are then removed and any tubes and infusion lines are clamped.

The donor child has last offices performed by the theatre staff and the transplant co-ordinator in accordance with local hospital policy and the parents' wishes. This may include taking impressions of the child's hands and footprints in paint or plaster and also a lock of the child's hair as keepsakes for the parents. Theatre staff must pay careful attention to ensure that the child appears restful and relaxed prior to being viewed by the parents. Different centres where organ retrieval occurs have different policies regarding whether the parents will be allowed into the theatre or another area within the perioperative department to visit their child post-donation. Alternatively, in some centres, parents will be able to spend time with their child post-retrieval in the intensive care unit, or in the mortuary. The actual procedure for this will be included in the local hospital policy. Wherever this visit occurs, the parents, and family, will be supported by the organ transplant co-ordinator who has liaised with them throughout the process, as described above.

The organ transplant co-ordinator plays a pivotal role again post-donation, not only in supporting the parents at this time, but also in contacting the family of the donor child once organs have been grafted into the recipient child. The actual support that is provided in each centre will vary according to the local policy. Good practice guidelines set out in The National Donor Family Care policy outlines that the organ transplant co-ordinator should offer to contact the child's family the following day, and that a follow-up visit may be undertaken 1 month following organ retrieval to offer further support. The organ transplant co-ordinator will also send a letter to the family, thanking them for the decision to donate their child's organs, and if the family requests, brief details of the outcomes of the transplant for the recipient(s) of the child's organs. This letter is a great source of comfort to parents, as they are able to see those who have benefited from their act of kindness in allowing their child's organs to be donated. All information is kept confidential and anonymity is maintained in this letter.

In order to ensure that all the organs that are removed remain able to be transplanted into the recipient, the organs must be preserved in optimum conditions during their transit to other centres (if this is required) and that the cold ischaemic time for these organs is not surpassed. To preserve the organs, the arteries are flushed with UW solution as described above, and they are packed into crushed ice prior to their transportation to other centres. UW solution contains a mix of glucose and additives to support the deoxygenated tissues. The British Transplant Society (2003) provides current guidelines for the acceptable cold ischaemic times before which organs may be used, which are provided in Table 11.2. These guidelines are continually changing as new research is conducted and as new techniques are used, so they should be used only as a rough estimate of the cold ischaemic times of each organ.

Table 11.2 Cold ischaemic times

Organ	Time organ can be used after retrieval	Notes
Heart	2–4 hr	Donor and recipient must be operated on simultaneously Must be stored cold
Lungs	6 hr	Donor and recipient must be operated on simultaneously Must be stored cold
Heart–Lungs	Immediately or 4–6 hr	Donor and recipient must be operated on simultaneously Must be stored cold
Liver	12 hr	Must be stored cold
Kidneys	<24 hr	Must be stored cold
Small bowel	6 hr	Must be stored cold
Pancreas	6 hr	Must be stored cold

In the case of all organs, the longer they are out of the body and are not perfused, the lower the longer-term graft survival rate. Therefore, co-ordination of the donor and the recipient children is essential, to ensure maximum chances of survival of the donor organ.

Difficulties for theatre nurses

Appreciation is often given to the concerns and thoughts parents have when their child dies and they are approached to consider donation of their child's organs. It is less often thought that the nurses within theatre also have issues, which is relevant to explore.

The experience of the individual nurses relating to organ donation is dependent on their belief systems and their previous experiences, and as such is unique to the individuals. However, commonly, theatre nurses are not comfortable with the concept of organ donation, and these feelings are exacerbated when the donor is a child. This may be due to the fact that ward-based colleagues and departments such as intensive care liaise with relatives on the decision whether or not to enable patients to become organ donors, whereas this decision has already been made by the time the patient reaches the operating room doors, and the theatre nurse is often not educated in the diagnosis of BSD or the process by which patients are selected to become organ donors.

This means that the practitioners who are involved in the care of the child who is having their organs removed for transplantation may have many concerns, which relate to the difficulty theatre nurses have in accepting the diagnosis of BSD (Bothamley, 1999b). This is further emphasised by the fact that although perioperative nurses are intimately involved with the retrieval of organs for transplantation, they describe the process of organ donation as mutilating (Carter-Gentry & McCurren, 2004; Regehr *et al.*, 2004), and very few carry a donor card themselves (Regehr *et al.*, 2004).

These concerns are not initially apparent, but relate to the difficulties theatre nurses have distinguishing life from death; the child who presents in theatre for organ retrieval appears the same as any other anaesthetised patient presenting for surgery. In addition, this image is reinforced by the monitoring of vital signs and maintenance of ventilation as would be the case for any patient coming through the perioperative department. However, this image is shattered as the retrieval begins, with the many staff present working quickly to retrieve the organs and to preserve these for transplantation, which in the case of the heart may mean that this remains beating on the back table during its perfusion with UW solution, and culminates with the child's empty body cavity.

Bothamley (1999a) acknowledges that this appearance of the patient on the operating table and the routine monitoring of that person can cause conflict for the theatre practitioner. The practitioner knows that there will be a recipient patient or patients who will usually have a positive outcome from the donation; however, at the end of the surgery, there will be a dead patient, on whom they will have to perform last offices. One of the participants in Regehr *et al.*'s (2004) study described this as a 'sinking feeling' and depending on the organs that had been removed as though the person was empty inside. Similar findings were found by Carter-Gentry and McCurren (2004).

Coupled with the difficulty staff have in accepting the diagnosis of BSD, this is exacerbated by the presence of a larger-than-normal number of perioperative staff, some or all of whom may not be known to the theatre staff. In certain situations, this can lead to increased stress and anxiety for perioperative staff. This stress may be increased when that patient is a child or teenager, and some studies have reported that the nursing staff involved began to question whether they have been involved in the death of the donor patient (Bothamley, 1999b).

The staff within the theatre department can appreciate that their patient has been pronounced as dead, but through their treatment find this hard to comprehend as to all intents and appearances they receive the same treatment as a living patient. This extends to their rights as a human being under the Human Rights Act (1998) and also to provide informed consent for the removal of their organs, and nursing issues relate to codes of conducts for perioperative practitioner (NMC, 2004; HPC, 2003), which guide the practitioner to ensure that their actions or inactions do not cause harm to the patient. Every intervention that patients undergo must be performed only with their informed consent – i.e. they have been told exactly what the procedure will involve and the risks and benefits that may result from that procedure (Department of Health, 2001). Given that theatre nurses have issues regarding the diagnosis of brain-stem death, how can a layperson with little or no medical knowledge truly consent to organ removal following their death? This situation is further complicated when that issue of consent involves a child, the issue of which is discussed in Chapter 3.

Both the code by which nurses are guided in their conduct (NMC, 2004) and that by whose guidance ODPs work (HPC, 2003) describe how practitioners should do nothing that harms their patient, either through their action or inaction, and that they should remain their patient's advocate and only act in their best interests.

It is easy to see that the theatre practitioner faces an obvious ethical dilemma in retrieving their patient's organs for transplantation into another individual. Whilst the donor patient will not recover, this is balanced by the recipient whose quality of life will be improved by the receipt of a new organ. This is an interesting ethical dilemma that could be considered against the code of professional conduct for the professionals working within theatre.

The transplant co-ordinator writes a letter to the theatre staff present at the time of the organ retrieval. This letter thanks staff for their support in caring for the donor child and family during the retrieval and providing brief details of the outcomes of the retrieval in terms of the recipients of the donor's organs. As in the case of the letter sent to the child's parents, this letter is a source of comfort to the theatre staff, as they can see the positive aspects of what some regard as a traumatic procedure and how others have benefited by this act of generosity.

Recipient management and care

Introduction

It is usual for the donor child to be operated on in the hospital in which the child has been receiving treatment, whilst the recipient receives their transplant in a specialist centre, which are located nationally throughout the UK (Table 11.3). There are a number of centres that specialise in caring for paediatric patients, which are summarised in Table 11.3.

Table 11.3 National paediatric transplant centres, UK

Specialist centre	National locations
Heart	Great Ormond Street, Newcastle (Freeman)
Lungs	Great Ormond Street, Newcastle (Freeman)
Kidney	Belfast, Birmingham, Bristol, Glasgow, London (Great Ormond Street and Guys), Leeds, Manchester, Newcastle and Nottingham
Liver	Birmingham (Queens Elizabeth Hospital), Leeds (St James'), London (Kings College)
Small bowel	Birmingham

The recipient child is brought to theatre, and undergoes a general anaesthetic, consisting of an anaesthetic agent, administered either through inhalation or intravenous routes, analgesics, and muscle relaxants. The child will also be given a prophylactic dose of antibiotics intraoperatively; these will be continued post-operatively. They will be intubated using an endotracheal tube, and have routine monitoring attached. They will be positioned according to the operative procedure to be carried out, and care must be taken to ensure that correct anatomical positions are attained to reduce the risk of nerves, blood vessels or skin damage, using appropriate positioning aides. In the case of children, all fluids used for therapeutic purposes or for washing and cleaning must be warmed to reduce the risks of surgical hypothermia and the possibility of vasoconstriction hindering anastomoses of blood vessels.

The actual surgical techniques involved in the operation are dependent upon the organ to be implanted.

Cardiothoracic organs

Heart transplants

Indications for transplant: end-stage heart failure (life expectancy without transplant is 6–12 months); congenital heart disease is the main indication in children under 5 years; cardiomyopathy is the main indication in older children.

Contraindications: renal impairment, hepatic dysfunction, chronic infection

In the UK, there is on average 10–15 children waiting for a heart transplant at any one time.

The donor heart must be of a similar size to that which it will replace, therefore, these children are at a disadvantage because of the small number of paediatric donors a year. Consequently, the average mortality of children on the waiting list for heart transplants is higher than for other types of transplant, and may be as high as 15–20% (British Transplant Society, 2003). Recent innovations that try to address this problem include the use of ABO mismatch hearts (discussed in section on The Future) and the use of artificial assist devices to prolong the life of the child.

Lung transplants

Main indications in paediatrics: cystic fibrosis
Contraindications: hypertension, renal dysfunction, diabetes

In the UK, on average there are 10–15 children waiting for a lung transplant at any one time.

As with the heart, the donor must be the same size as the child. Coupled with the fact that viable lungs are difficult to maintain and retrieve from a donor, children waiting for lungs will wait on average three times as long as an adult waiting for a lung transplant. In the UK, lung transplants are performed on children aged 3 and above. This is partly because been prepared for lung transplant involves regular bronchoscopes for which small children need an anaesthetic. This is obviously problematic in children with poor lung function, and also because lung function is one of the first tests of rejection. Single-lung transplants (splitting the donor's lungs and transplanting them into two people) are possible in children, but rarely performed.

Heart/lung block transplants

Indications for transplant: end-stage diseases affecting cardiopulmonary systems, and congenital defect

Contraindications: hypertension, renal dysfunction, diabetes

In the UK, on average there are 5–8 children waiting for a heart/lung transplant at any one time.

These children have the same problems as children waiting for either a heart or a lung transplant in that the donor organs have to be a size match and that there are low numbers of potential donors for them. Domino heart transplants, where the patient receives a heart and lung transplant and then their heart is transplanted into a second recipient, are still occasionally performed. The rationale was that these patients had improved outcomes receiving a heart/lung block as opposed to lungs alone. However, the current line of thinking is that it is unnecessary to remove a healthy heart.

Preoperative care

When a child is called in for transplant, they undergo an assessment to ensure that they are well enough for transplant, which include taking bloods and a chest X-ray. Primarily, the team will want to make sure that they are infection free. Immunosuppressant therapy is then commenced before they go to theatre. The timing for transplanting cardiothoracic organs is extremely tight. Ideally, when a heart is removed from the donor's body, it needs to be transplanted within 2 hr, and the maximum time is 4 hr. Lungs can go for up to 9 hr, but again ideally they should be transplanted within 6 hr of been removed from the donor. Therefore, the child's own organs need to be removed before the donor organ arrives at the transplanting hospital. This poses problems in terms of organisation and ensuring that the donor organs are suitable for transplant before the child's organ/s are removed.

Intraoperative care

A heart transplant operation takes approximately 3–4 hr and a lung transplant takes approximately 5–6 hr. The principles of care are the same as for any child undergoing cardiothoracic surgery. The patient has skin preparation using an antimicrobial solution and drapes applied.

There are different methods used for implanting the donated heart into the recipient; the orthoptic transplant (replacing the recipient heart with the donated heart) and the heterotopic or 'piggy back' transplant (where the recipient heart remains in place and the donated heart is grafted onto this). Orthoptic transplants can be used as a treatment option for a range of congenital heart defects, whilst heterotopic transplants are used in the case of an undersized donor heart when immediate transplantation is required. The preferred technique for transplants is orthoptic, as the heterotopic has disadvantages including greater technical difficulty, increased risk of post-operative complications including thromboembolus.

The patient is laid supine and prepared with an antimicrobial solution from neck to foot and to the operating table laterally, prior to being draped with a sterile drape in the groin, under the legs and over the head. A sternotomy is performed using an air-powered saw. In an orthoptic transplant, many different methods may be used to implant the donor heart, depending on the condition for which the transplant is required. This is often more complicated in the paediatric patient than for cardiomyopathies in adults, due to the varied nature of the congenital defects with which the child presents. One example of a cardiac transplant implantation method is the biatrial technique.

In this instance, the patient is placed on bypass, by cannulating the inferior and superior vena cavae prior to cooling the patient to around 25°C. The pulmonary trunk and the aorta are identified and the aorta clamped using a Fogarty clamp. The pulmonary artery and aorta are dissected above their valves. The right side of the heart is incised, with care to preserve the left atrial wall and atrial septum to allow grafting of the donor heart. This incision is extended to the left side of the heart and to the left atrium. At this stage, the recipient's heart is removed.

The new heart is again inspected, and is placed inside the pericardium and orientated. The left atrium is the first to be anastomosed, using a double-ended, non-absorbable suture, followed by right atrium. End-to-end aortic anastomosis then occurs, aortic cross-clamp removed and checks are made for signs of haemorrhage. In the absence of haemorrhage, the cross-clamp is removed, allowing the heart to perfuse with the recipient's blood. Whilst reperfusion is occurring, the pulmonary artery anastomosis is made. Air is removed from the left side of the heart using a saline flush prior to the anastomosis of the pulmonary artery.

Once the new heart has been grafted into the recipient, it is necessary to make it start beating. This may be done by using a defibrillator and internal paddles, and a single direct current (DC) shock; however, spontaneous function should return with the correction of calcium and electrolytes, although inotropes are often also given at this point. A needle is inserted into the ascending aorta to allow any residual air to escape. Once the child has been weaned off the bypass, the cannulae in the aorta and vena cavae are removed, and the sternotomy closed using wire sutures, followed by suturing of the wound.

In the case of the lung transplant, the patient is laid supine and prepared with an antimicrobial solution from neck to thigh and to the operating table laterally prior to draping with towels, which leave the chest area exposed. A bilateral thoracosternotomy is made, and the child is placed on cardiopulmonary bypass. The pulmonary artery and veins are identified, and double ligatures placed around each of these; it is essential that there is sufficient vessel length to allow the formation of anastomoses of the donor and recipient vessels. These vessels are then divided. Each bronchus is then mobilised close to the carina and stapled before being divided, allowing removal of the lungs from the thoracic cavity.

The donor lungs are prepared by separating these and trimming the bronchi. The lungs are placed into the recipient, and the staple line removed from their bronchi. An end-to-end anastomosis is performed using a double-ended, absorbable suture for the membrane and the cartilage. The recipient and donor pulmonary artery and vein are anastomosed, also end to end, using a double-ended, absorbable suture. The patient is then weaned off of cardiopulmonary bypass, and reperfusion of the lungs is observed. Any signs of haemorrhage will also be observed and repaired using the same suture material.

The wound is closed by approximation of the sternum and closure with wire sutures. The skin and underlying tissues are closed using absorbable sutures, and a dressing applied.

If the patient is to undergo a combined heart–lung transplant, the decision is made by the surgeons to either remove the recipient's organs separately or *en bloc*. This involves the similar processes to those described above, and the same level of care must be taken not to damage any vascular structures. In the case of removing the organs separately, the cardiac transplant will be performed after the pneumonectomies have been performed.

Immediate post-operative care

Post-operatively, the child needs close monitoring and observations so that any problems can be detected without delay. For this reason, immediately following their transplant, patients are transferred to an intensive care unit. Here, they are monitored for complications arising from the surgery itself and also from the implantation of the donated organ. They will be ventilated on nitric oxygen and have inatropic infusions. However, these are rapidly weaned and if there are no complications, then the children will normally be extubated within a day. Lung recipients normally have four drains and heart recipients have two, and these are removed within a few days. Because they are immunosuppressed, these patients have to barrier-nursed in a cubicle for 1 week. If there is no sign of infection at this stage, they can come out but it will be a further 1–2 weeks before they can be discharged. Because of the immunosuppressants, they are monitored very closely for signs of rejection.

Surgical complications are not often encountered following the transplant, but when these occur, they are mainly related to bleeding. Haemorrhage may result from inadequate anastomoses of arteries and veins or from damage to other vascular structures near to the implanted organ. This requires the theatre staff, whilst the child is in theatre, and the intensive care nurse, once transfer to ICU has been completed, to monitor for the signs of post-operative haemorrhage. If this haemorrhage is not detected or managed, then this can lead to hypotension, tachycardia, reduced haemoglobin and coagulopathy. All potential indications that haemorrhage is occurring should be investigated as delay in this increases the effects on the child and also increases the risks that the organ may not remain viable. The longer the delay in reacting to the signs of haemorrhage, the greater the risk of coagulation-related problems, including thrombosis of vessels, embolus formation and the risk of anastomosis breakdown.

Complications that can occur when the patient is admitted to the ICU include:

- respiratory problems;
- cardiac problems – arrhythmias, hypertension, hypotension;
- fluid and/or electrolyte imbalance;
- renal dysfunction.

It is the role of the nurse to monitor the patient and to liaise with the surgical and anaesthetic and medical staff to ensure that the patient's problems are addressed and that the child reaches a state of physiological stability prior to their discharge from the ICU to a ward. It is common for the child to stay in ICU for 2–4 days following a transplant, although the child may stay for a longer time if there have been complications intraoperatively or immediately post-operatively. Discharge criteria from the ICU include that the child can breathe spontaneously on air or with low levels of oxygen and that their observations indicate they are physiologically stable. That is, they have a stable heart rate and blood pressure, and that their renal output is acceptable in terms of fluid and electrolyte balance. The child must have begun to eat and drink, either orally or via a nasogastric feed. If these criteria are met, then the child is discharged to a specialist paediatric ward, and is taken care of by paediatric nurses.

Liver

Indications: end-stage liver dysfunction, Wilson's disease, extra hepatic biliary atresia, malignancy
Contraindications: acceptable alternative treatment, connected secondary organ failure, including Alper's disease, Alagille syndrome, systemic infection
In the UK, on average there are 15–20 children waiting for a liver transplant at any one time.
Paediatric liver transplantation used to suffer from the same size–match problem that cardiothoracic transplantation does. However, in the 1980s, techniques were developed that enabled an adult liver to be reduced in size to fit the paediatric. This soon progressed into split liver grafts, where a single liver is split and divided between two recipients; normally, a child receives the left lateral segment and an adult receives the right lobe. The liver is sent to the centre where it will be transplanted, it is then split in theatre under normal operation conditions; this takes between 2–3 hr. This additional warm ischaemic time can damage the liver, thus only good livers from young healthy donors are normally considered for splitting.

Preoperative care

As well as normal preoperative preparation, on admission for transplantation, the child has to be screened to ensure that they are free from acute infections. They are then commenced on preoperative antibiotics.

Intraoperative care

A vertical midline incision is made using a size-10 blade and exterior and interior oblique and transverse muscles dissected and retracted. A sternotomy is performed.

A small cut is made in the peritoneum and extended using a pair of scissors. A self-retaining retractor is then inserted to allow the surgical team good vision of the abdominal connects. Following the laparotomy, the surgeon identifies the vena cava, hepatic artery and portal vein and the common bile duct and dissects these. At this stage, the child may be placed on cardiopulmonary bypass. The hepatic artery, portal vein and the superior and inferior vena cava are clamped, and the child's liver removed. The donor liver and the child's vascular system are connected through the anastomoses of the suprahepatic vena cava, infrahepatic vena cava and portal vein using a double-ended, non-absorbable suture. The clamps are released very slowly, to allow perfusion of the implanted liver, observing the anastomosis sites for signs of haemorrhage. If any signs of leakage are detected, the clamp is reapplied and sutures used over the site of the haemorrhage. The clamp is then again slowly released. This process occurs with each of all the clamps, and is repeated until no signs of leakage can be observed. If the child has been placed on bypass, this is removed. Focus is then turned to the anastomosis of the hepatic artery, which again is through the use of a double-ended, non-absorbable suture, with the clamp only being fully released when no sign of haemorrhage can be observed. The surgical team observes the new organ to determine its level of perfusion, and in some cases may perform an intraoperative Doppler to determine the perfusion of the organ.

Biliary reconstruction is performed usually by end-to-end anastomosis of the bile ducts. Drains are placed to drain any excess fluid and brought out through the skin. Having ensured that there are no signs of haemorrhage, the wound is then closed beginning with the peritoneum, followed by the different layers of tissue until finally the subcutaneous tissue and then the skin is sutured, usually using a continuous, absorbable suture prior to a dressing being applied.

Post-operative care

Similar to paediatric cardiac recipients as described above, these children are barrier-nursed initially on ICU where they are closely monitored for signs of infection, rejection and haemorrhage. If they continue to make good progress, they will be transferred to the ward within 2–3 days, and discharged home within 2–3 weeks.

Kidneys

Indication for the transplant: end-stage renal failure
Contraindications: malignancy, acute infection
Relative contraindication: HIV

In the UK, on average there are 120 children waiting for a kidney transplant at any one time. The smallest child who can receive a transplant would be between 10 and 15 kg, with children smaller than 15 kg being transplanted only if absolutely necessary.

Children should be transplanted, if possible, prior to their commencement on dialysis, as this results in improved growth and psychosocial development, and conserves peritoneal and haemodialysis for future use, should the graft fail. Most centres refer children for pre-dialysis transplant once the glomerular filtration rate falls below $10–15/min/1.73 m^2$, and it is likely that dialysis would be needed in 18–24 months, or the child's growth has begun to be affected. The smaller and younger the child, the increased risk of the graft failing, due to the size of their anatomy, and the risk of transplantation and the benefits of this must be determined on an individual basis.

Preoperative care

On admission for transplantation, the child has to be screened to ensure that they are free from acute infections. They are then commenced on preoperative antibiotics.

Intraoperative care

The patient is positioned supine and their skin prepared with antimicrobial solution from nipple to mid-thigh and also laterally to the operating table on the side where the transplant is to occur and to the opposite iliac crest. Drapes are applied to perineum, head and foot and to the sides to create a sterile field. The child is catheterised and their bladder filled with an antibiotic solution. The catheter is then clamped.

Following the laparotomy, as described for the liver, the aorta and inferior vena cava are identified and mobilised and dissected; loops placed around the vessels are used to aid this dissection, and also visualisation during the implantation of the donor kidney. The recipient aorta and vena cava are cross-clamped with a Fogarty vascular clamp across both vessels. It is not usually necessary to remove the recipient's kidney, and often this is left *in situ*, and the donor kidney placed in the iliac fossa.

Attention is then turned to the donor kidney, and the vessels trimmed to facilitate anastomosis of the vessels. The renal vein will be anastomosed to the vena cava and the renal artery to the aorta. The vena cava is incised and flushed with heparinised saline before the incision is extended using endarterectomy scissors to accommodate the size of the donor renal vein. An anastomosis of these vessels is then made using a double-ended, non-absorbable suture. The same process is used to anastomose the renal artery to the aorta. In the case of two donor arteries, the second is anastomosed to the proximal, anastomosis is to the aorta, and the distal to the common iliac artery. Once the suturing is completed, the Fogarty clamp is slowly released and the vascular anastomoses checked for signs of leakage; if present, the clamps are reapplied and the leakages sutured using the same non-absorbable suture material. The implanted kidney is also double-checked at this point for signs of damage or bleeding, and also its perfusion is checked.

The anterior wall of the bladder is grabbed with tissue forceps and a small incision made using a scalpel. The bladder wall is tunnelled and the donor ureter passed through the passage created, with any excess ureter removed. The ureter is then sutured into the bladder to allow the free drainage of urine from the kidney into the bladder. To facilitate this during the initial stages following the transplant, a ureteric stent may be inserted to overcome the effects of oedema whilst retaining the patency of the donor ureter. The bladder is then sutured with absorbable sutures. A closed suction drain may be inserted and brought out laterally through the skin. The muscle and fascia are then closed with non-absorbable sutures, and the subcutaneous layer with absorbable sutures. The skin is closed using absorbable subcuticular sutures.

As well as the length of ischaemic time, the time of release of the clamps to the production of the patient's first urine should be entered into the patient notes. All renal recipients are registered with the paediatric section of the National Renal Registry.

Throughout surgery, the most important thing to observe is the child's fluid balance. Once the transplanted kidney is reperfused, there will be a substantial drop in cardiac output due to the high cardiac output to the kidneys in paediatric patients (20–25%). Therefore, the CVP must be kept at 10 or above. These observations are important not only intraoperatively, but also extend into the post-operative phase.

Post-operative care

Post-operatively, the patient will be transferred to ICU if they weigh between 10–20 kg. If they are above this weight, they will be transferred to a paediatric ward and barrier-nursed for 1 week. They will be discharged after 2–3 weeks.

In addition to the general principles of post-operative patient care, as described elsewhere, it is particularly important in the renal transplant recipient to ensure that their fluid balance continues to be monitored, along with U&Es.

Small bowel, liver and multivisceral

Multivisceral is the transplantation of the liver and small bowel together with other abdominal organs (kidney/pancreas/stomach).

Indications: irreversible intestinal malfunction: intestinal atresia, Gastroschisis Crohn's disease

Contraindications: acute infection, stable on TPN

Small bowel transplantation is still relatively new. The intestine is highly immunogenic, and transplantation only became feasible with the development of new immunosuppressant agents. Hence, the first truly successful transplant occurred in 1988 (Woodward & Mayer, 1996). Despite its restrictions on lifestyle, Total Parental Nutrition (TPN) is a relatively safe treatment and is the preferred therapy for patients with intestinal failure. However, if the patient develops life-threatening complications related to TPN, then transplantation may be the only viable option for them. Children are more prone to such complications; consequently, they represent two-thirds of the UK waiting list for small bowel transplants, and on average there are 1–2 children waiting for a transplant at any one time. Because the small bowel is not sterile, the donor has to be treated with selective bowel decontamination via the NG Tube to flush the bowel before retrieval. Ideally, these grafts need to be transplanted as soon as possible with an upper limit of 6 hr.

Preoperative care

On admission for transplantation, the child has to be screened to ensure that they are free from acute infections. They are then commenced on preoperative antibiotics.

Intraoperative care

The patient will undergo a laparotomy and have the defective portion of their small bowel removed. The surgical team will identify the portion of the bowel to be removed, and clamp this using bowel clamps. The section of the bowel will be dissected, and the donor bowel orientated and placed into the child's abdomen.

The exact surgical procedure to implant the donor bowel will vary from patient to patient, depending upon the segment of bowel being transplanted and previous abdominal operations performed. However, as a general rule for small bowel, only the donor portal vein is anastomosed to the recipient's inferior vena cava and the superior mesenteric artery to the abdominal aorta (although the portal vein may be used if necessary). If transplanted with the liver or as a multivisceral, then donor aorta is required to form a conduit. For the intestine themselves, the proximal stapling is removed and the bowel trimmed to facilitate the proximal anastomosis to be carried out between the recipient's most distal small intestine and the proximal jejunum of the donor graft. The proximal stapling is removed and the bowel trimmed to facilitate the anastomosis at the proximal end, which can be done through suturing or using stapling. Attention is then turned to the distal portion of the bowel, and the same process is repeated. A stoma is then formed at the distal end and brought through to the child's skin. The recipient will also have a feeding jejunostomy placed in the proximal jejunum.

Post-operative care

The patients are initially nursed on an ICU, observing for routine post-operative complications. In addition, they are treated with 48 hr of prophylactic antibiotics and antifungal agents, and the functioning of the stoma is monitored. Because the intestine is non-sterile, there is a high risk of bacterial translocation, leading to sepsis and rejection in the immunosuppressed recipient (compounded by the highly immunogenic nature of the intestines). These patients need powerful immunosupressant therapy and careful management. Children under the age of 1 year require less immunosupressant therapy, perhaps due the immature development of the enteric immune system and the tendency to tolerate their grafts well.

The patient will remain on parental feeding, whilst enteral feeding is introduced gradually after transplant. Initially, this will be via the jejunostomy tube and then orally. There is evidence to suggest that early feeding improved graft function and reduces the risk of infection (Woodward & Mayer, 1996).

Reducing the risk of rejection of the new organ

Post-operatively, there is a risk that the new organ will be rejected by the recipient's body. If no actions were taken, the recipient's body would recognise this new organ as foreign material, initiating the child's immune responses. Rejection of an organ can take three forms:

(1) Hyperacute rejection – very rare due to meticulous compatibility testing between the donor and recipient child. This occurs when the antibodies in the recipient's body attack the antigens detected through sensitisation to the implanted organ, or ABO incompatibility.
(2) Acute rejection – occurs during the days following the transplant or early, following discharge of the child from hospital.
(3) Chronic rejection – a process that takes months or more, usually years, to occur. It is caused by infection, acute rejection that has not been controlled through the use of immunosuppressants and corticosteroid treatment, the effects of overuse

of immunosuppressants and their side effects, hypertension and lack of adherence to nutritional advice, leading to obesity.

To maximise the chances of the survival of the new organ, the chances of the recipient's body rejecting the donated organ as foreign tissue has to be minimised. A number of actions are taken prior to the transplant to ensure that the donor organ has the best chances of survival in the recipient's body.

The minimisation of risks relating to rejection of the organ begins preoperatively by ensuring the compatibility of the donor and recipient, as described above, and continues in the post-operative phase when the child is provided with drugs to suppress their immune system. These actions are taken to reduce the risk of the body's immune system attacking the new organ post-operatively and reduce the chances of rejection of the new organ.

These immunosuppressants are usually some form of corticosteroid. In some patients, immunosuppressive treatment has been shown to predispose a patient to a number of side effects including infection, inflammation of the pancreas, stomach duodenal ulcer, diabetes, damage to the liver or kidneys, osteoporosis and tumours of the lymphoid system (lymphomas). Whilst these side effects are not insignificant, and the possible occurrence of these should be explained to the child and their parents, the benefits of immunosuppression compared to organ rejection outweigh the risks.

As well as the length of ischaemic time, the time of release of the clamps to the production of the patient's first urine should be entered into the patient notes. All renal recipients are registered with the paediatric section of the National Renal Registry.

Longer-term post-operative care

Continuous monitoring of the child during their hospitalisation and on discharge from hospital will indicate whether they are at risk of acute or chronic rejection. This includes routine observations of physiological measurements, ultrasound, X-ray or CT scanning of the organ, blood monitoring, histological examination of tissue samples from the organ and psychological assessment of the child – including their adherence to post-operative regimes to reduce the risk of rejection of the organ.

In addition, depending on the organ that has been transplanted, other members of the multidisciplinary team may be involved in the child's immediate and ongoing treatment. In the immediate post-operative period, this includes 24-hr access to paediatric intensivists, paediatric anaesthetists, the operating surgeons, consultants with a knowledge of the systems and organs that have been transplanted, and in the longer term, other team members involved in continuing care are dieticians, social workers, teachers, play therapists and psychologists.

Psychological issues affecting children receiving transplanted organs

Much is reported in the literature relating to the effects of having someone else's organ within the recipient's body. These effects vary depending on the organ that has been implanted, but most include the recipient reporting that they take on some characteristics of the donor, despite anonymity and confidentiality being retained.

In some cases, depending on their age and maturity, the child may not have reached a developmental stage where they consider the donor. However, if the child is at an age where they are beginning to conceptualise the notion of death, then it may prey on their mind that their organ has been removed from a person who has lost their life. Realisation of this may have a profound psychological impact on the child, which can change their feelings regarding the organ they have received.

An additional consideration with children is their level of emotional and psychological maturity towards their health, and related to this their compliance with immunosuppressant regimes to minimise the risks of rejection. In order to appear 'normal' within their friendship circles, children may not adhere to these regimes or may ignore dietary and nutritional advice, which puts the viability of the organ into question.

Perceptions of sexuality can also influence a child's attitude towards their organ, even though these have no sexual function (Sanner, 2003). In some cases, this can lead to a dislike of having an organ from a donor of the opposite sex. An additional consideration, especially for young girls, is their altered appearance due to the effects of the immunosuppressants leading to the growth of facial hair.

For this reason, ongoing psychological assessment of the child, and their adherence to follow-up advice and guidelines, must be incorporated into the physiological assessments made on the organ itself. Some paediatric transplant units have psychologists attached, who monitor the psychological aspects of the child's health as a part of their ongoing care.

The future

The advances made in the field of organ donation and transplantation are considerable and growing all the time. The overriding aim of all of these developments is to increase the amount and quality of organs available, by either expanding the donor pool or improving the methods of preserving organs prior to transplant. To this end, the government established an Organ Donation Taskforce, which reported in January 2008. Its recommendations include the establishment of a central employing organisation, doubling donor transplant co-ordinator numbers, the establishment of dedicated organ retrieval teams and an emphasis on making donation an usual rather than unusual event in hospitals through the establishing of local donation committees and champions (Department of Health, 2008).

In term of expanding the donor pool, a significant change has been the reintroduction of non–heart beating donation (see section on Types of Donation). As heart beating donor numbers continue to decline, NHBD has provided a valuable source of donors (approximately 130 a year and increasing all the time as hospitals become more familiar with it). Furthermore, the possibility of NHB heart donation is being explored. NHB donation was initially restricted to adults, but as confidence and experience has grown, some centres have lowered their minimum age to 5 years. In reality, very few paediatric NHB donors occur each year (approximately 3–4 a year).

Live donation is also on the increase, and whilst kidneys are still the most common organ to donate, there have been internationally successful live liver and live lung transplants, and these are primarily parent to child. It can be expected that these numbers will grow as UK Transplant is considering funding live recipient co-ordinators for these organs. Other initiatives to increase the donor pool include the introduction of In-House Transplant Co-ordinators and concepts such as collaborative requesting in an attempt to increase the consent rates. For much further in the future research continues into areas such as stem cells and xenotransplantation, if these are ever successful, the desperate need for cadaveric organs may be alleviated. Finally, worldwide, the first face transplant and larynx transplant have been performed and will no doubt become more widespread in the future.

All the above serve to expand the donor pool, but sometimes an organ becomes available that cannot be matched to a recipient. This is especially true of paediatric cardiothoracic organs because of the need for a size match and the relatively small numbers waiting. One recent advance that addresses this problem is the use of an ABO mismatched hearts for transplant. This means that a child can receive a donor heart that is the right size but not the same blood group as them. It has been found that a child under the age of 18 months is less likely to reject a donor organ; this has been linked with them having an underdeveloped immune system (the oldest child to have had a mismatched heart is 2.5 years). Thus, even though the organ is from a different blood group, the child will be successfully transplanted with it and will still require less immunosupressant therapy post-op than other patients. This is also in its early stages, with approximately 50 transplants been performed worldwide.

Another way of maximising the organs that are available is to work on preservation techniques. The traditional method of placing removed organs into ice-filled containers for transportation carries with it the risk that the organ will be irreversibly

Box 11.3   Useful websites

UK:
  www.uktransplant.co.uk
  www.blood.co.uk

AUSTRALIA:
  http://www.transplant.org.au/
  http://www.medicareaustralia.gov.au/public/services/aodr/index.shtml
  http://www.healthinsite.gov.au/topics/Organ_donation

CANADA:
  http://www.transplant.ca/
  http://www.hc-sc.gc.ca/ahc-asc/media/nr-cp/2001/2001_36bk1_e.html

USA:
  http://www.organdonor.gov/
  http://www.unos.org/

NEW ZEALAND:
  http://www.donor.co.nz/donor/
  http://www.anzdata.org.au/

EUROPEAN UNION:
  http://www.etco.org/
  http://europa.eu/rapid/pressReleasesAction.do?reference=IP/07/718&format=HTML&aged=
  1&language=EN&guiLanguage=en

---

damaged should it come into contact with the ice as well as the problem of melting ice. The time until the organ can be transplanted is also quite limited. Advances have been made in how to better preserve the organs for transporting. Renal transporter machines are becoming commonplace; these continuously pump perfusion fluid through the kidney and maintain a constant cold storage temperate. There is also a machine for preserving heart perfusion for transport, and research continues into preservation machine for the other organs.

The field of organ donation is young and fast moving, with new innovations regularly occurring. But as yet, they are not matching the demand for donor organs. Paediatrics organs are a particularly precious commodity and every effort has to be made to ensure that they are maximised to the full, the key to which is good family communication, information and care at such a difficult time. Early involvement of the transplant co-ordinator and carefully considered donor management will help ensure that the potential for donation is maximised. This care continues into the theatre setting, and thus as advocates for their patients, perioperative nurses need to be aware of BSD and the intraoperative procedures. Perioperative nurses are key to ensure that the organ-donation processes in theatre run smoothly to ensure the maximum benefits for the recipients of the donated organs.

References

Beecher, H.K. (1968). A definition of irreversible coma. Report of the *ad hoc* committee of the Harvard Medical School to examine the definition of brain death. *Journal of the American Medical Association*, 205: 337–340.

Bothamley, J. (1999a). Education focus – organ donation 2: Consent and patients' rights. *British Journal of Theatre Nursing*, 9: 573–578.

Bothamley, J. (1999b). Education focus – organ donation 1: A review of the literature. *British Journal of Theatre Nursing*, 9: 521–529.

Bothamley, J. (1999a). Education focus – organ donation 2: Consent and patients' rights. *British Journal of Theatre Nursing*, 9(12): 573–578.

British Transplantation Society. (2003). *Standards for solid organ transplantation in the United Kingdom*. British Transplantation Society, London.

Carter-Gentry, D., McCurren, C. (2004). Organ procurement from the perspective of perioperative nurses. *AORN Journal*, 80: 417–431.

Department of Health. (2004). *Human tissue act*. The Stationary Office Limited, London. Available from www.opsi.gov.uk/acts/acts2004/20040030.htm (accessed 8 February 2008).

Department of Health. (2001). *Good practice in consent implementation guide: Consent to examination or treatment*. Department of Health, London. Available from http://www.Department of Health.gov.uk/prod_consum_Department of Health/idcplg?IdcService=SS_GET_PAGE&siteId=en&ssTargetNodeId=566&ssDocName=DEPARTMENT OF HEALTH_4005762 (accessed 8 February 2008).

Department of Health. (1998). *A code of practice for the diagnosis of brain stem death*. Department of Health, London. Available from http://www.Department of Health .gov.uk/prod_consum_Department of Health /idcplg?IdcService=GET_FILE&dID=25131&Rendition=Web (accessed 8 February 2008).

Department of Health. (2008). *Organs for transplant: A report from the organ donation taskforce*. Department of Health, London.

Duke, J., Murphy, B., Bell, A. (1998). Nurses' attitudes toward organ donation: An Australian perspective. *Dimensions of Critical Care Nursing*, 17: 264–270.

Gortmaker, S.L., Beasley, C.L., Sheehy, E., *et al.* (1998). Improving the request process to increase family consent for organ donation. *Journal of Transplant Coordination*, 8: 210–217.

Health Professions Council (HPC). (2003). *Standards of conduct performance and ethics.* Health Professions Council, London.

Intensive Care Society. (2005). *Guidelines for adult organ and tissue donation.* Available from http://www.ics.ac.uk/icmprof/downloads/Organ%20&%20Tissue%20Donation.pdf (accessed 8 February 2008).

Levvey, B.J. (2006). Nursing challenges associated with non heart beating organ donation. *Australian Nursing Journal*, 13: 43.

Mendeloff, E.N. (1998). Lung transplantation for cystic fibrosis. *Seminars in Thoracic & Cardiovascular Surgery*, 10: 202–212.

Mollaret, P., Goulon, M. (1959). *Le coma depasse (memoire preliminaire). Review of Neurology*, 101: 3.

Nursing and Midwifery Council. (2004). *The NMC code of professional conduct: Standards for conduct performance and ethics.* Nursing and Midwifery Council, London.

Pallis, C., Harley, D. (1996). *ABC of brainstem death*, 2nd ed. BMJ Publishing, London.

Regehr, C., Kjerulf, M., Popova, S.R., Baker, A.J. (2004). Trauma and tribulation: The experiences and attitudes of operating room nurses working with organ donors. *Journal of Clinical Nursing*, 13: 430–437.

Saborio, P., Tipton, G., Chan, J. (2000). Diabetes insipidus. *Pediatrics in Review*, 21: 122–129.

Sanner, M.A. (2003). Transplant recipients' conceptions of three key phenomena in transplantation and organ donation: The organ donation, the organ donor and the organ transplant. *Clinical Transplant*, 17: 391–400.

Sque, M., Long, T., Payne, S. (2003). *Organ and tissue donation: Exploring the needs of families.* Available from the British Organ Donor Society.

UK Transplant. (2009). *Transplants save lives.* Available from http://www.organdonation.nhs.uk/ukt (accessed 27.7.09).

Verbel, M., Worth, J. (2002). Fears and concerns expressed by families in the donation discussion. *Progress in Transplantation*, 10: 48–55.

Woodward, J., Mayer, D. (1996). The unique challenge of small intestinal transplantation. *British Journal of Hospital Medicine*, 56: 285–290.

Further reading

Bell, M.D.D. (2006). The UK Human Tissue Act and consent: Surrendering a fundamental principle to transplantation needs? *Journal of Medical Ethics*, 32: 283–286.

British Transplant Society. (2004). *Guidelines relating to solid organ transplants from non-heart beating donors.* British Transplant Society, London.

Department of Health. (2003). *Human bodies human choices.* Department of Health, London. Available from http://www.bts.org.uk/Forms/summaryofresponsestotheconsultation-report.pdf (accessed 8 February 2008).

Department of Health. (2007). *Saving lives, valuing donors – a transplant framework for England.* Department of Health, London. Available from http://www.dh.gov.uk/en/Policyandguidance/Organisationpolicy/Secondarycare/Transplantation/Transplantationframework/DH_4090069 (accessed 8 February 2008).

Department of Health. (2001). Seeking consent: Working with children. Department of Health, London. Available from http://www.Department of Health.gov.uk/prod_ consum_Department of Health /idcplg?IdcService=SS_GET_PAGE&siteId=en&ssTarget NodeId=566&ssDocName=DEPARTMENT OF HEALTH _4007005 (accessed 8 February 2008).

Ehrle, R., Shafer, T., Nelson, K. (1999). Referral, request and consent for organ donation: Best practice – a blueprint for success. *Critical Care Nurse*, 19: 21–33.

Koogler, T., Costarino, A.T. (1998). The potential benefits of the pediatric non-heartbeating organ donor. *Pediatrics*, 101: 1049–1052.

Mamode, N., Sutherland, D.E.R. (2003). Transplantation for diabetes mellitus. *British Journal of Surgery*, 90: 1031–1032.

Molzahn, A.E., Starzomski, R., McCormick, J. (2003). The supply of organs for transplantation: Issues and challenges. *Nephrology Nursing Journal*, 30: 17–28.

NICE. (2004). *Laparoscopic live donor simple nephrectomy.* Issue date May 2004. NICE, London.

NICE. (2006). *Living donor lung transplantation for end stage lung disease.* Issue date May 2006. NICE, London.

Neuberger, J. (2004). Developments in liver transplantation. *Gut*, 53: 759–768.

Silber, T. (2004). Ethical dilemmas in the treatment of children with disabilities. *Paediatric Annals*, 33: 752–761.

Stirling, J. (2005). Non-heart beating organ donation: A case study. *British Journal of Perioperative Nursing*, 15: 467–475.

Tejani, A. (2000). Pediatrics: Experts share data to improve future of transplantation. *Blood Weekly*, 7 September: 8–9.

Young, P.J., Matta, B.F. (2000). Anaesthesia for organ donation in the brainstem dead – why bother [editorial]. *Anaesthesia*, 55: 105–106.

Zaltzman, J.S. (2007). Organ donation after cardiocirculatory death: Allograft outcomes. Canadian Blood Services, CCDT. Available from http://www.ccdt.ca/english/publications/background-pdfs/Allograft-Outcomes.pdf (accessed 12 May 2009).

12 The care of children having endoscopic procedures

Janet Roper and Linda Shields

Introduction

Minimally invasive surgery (MIS) is 'surgical procedures that use small incisions and fibreoptic lighting to employ cameras and long specialized instruments during tissue manipulation and invasive intervention' (Phillips, 2007, p. 177). Endoscopy is defined as 'surgical procedures that use natural body orifices or percutaneous techniques, fibreoptic lighting to employ cameras and long specialized instruments during tissue manipulation and invasive intervention' (Phillips, 2007, p. 177). Examples of MIS include laparoscopy and mediastinoscopy, while colonoscopy, bronchoscopy and hysteroscopy are examples of endoscopic surgery.

The known history of such procedures dates back over a millennium, when an Arabian doctor, Abul Kasim (936–1013 AD), used reflected light to view the cervix (Ball, 2007) (see Box 12.1). The invention of the camera, and eventually fibre optics, allowed the development of MIS as we know it today, and no doubt it will not finish there, as new inventions are made all the time, and computer technology and artificial intelligence is being applied in surgery for the development of robotics for use in, e.g. cardiac (Simonite, 2007), or abdominal surgery where a robotic camera crawls around guiding the surgeon to the area to be excised (Graham-Rowe, 2006) (see Box 12.2). Endoscopy and MIS are widely used today, in most surgical specialities, including

Box 12.1 Websites and publications about the history of endoscopy

http://www.t-med.co.uk/files/History%20of%20laparoscopy%20May%202004.ppt
http://www.imaginis.com/endoscopy/
http://www.ncbi.nlm.nih.gov/pubmed/11801888

Accessed 10 September 2008.

Box 12.2 Websites about robotic surgery

Some information on robotic surgery:
http://library.thinkquest.org/03oct/00760/
http://electronics.howstuffworks.com/robotic-surgery1.htm

Accessed 10 September 2008.

abdominal surgery, especially for common procedures such as appendicectomy (Patrick, 2006), and also in gynaecology (Anastasakis *et al.*, 2007), urology (Kagadis *et al.*, 2006), neurosurgery (Gore *et al.*, 2006), orthopaedics (Lui, 2007), otorhinolaryngology (Stamm, 2006; Tichenor *et al.*, 2008), oral and dental surgery (Michaud *et al.*, 2007) and even veterinary surgical procedures (Geishauser, 2005).

MIS and endoscopy are now common procedures in surgery on children, used for many of the common paediatric surgical procedures, such as inguinal hernia repair (Handa, 2006), gastrostomy, appendicectomy (Aziz *et al.*, 2006), and others, including trauma (Feliz, 2006), and are often used for surgery on neonates (Becmeur, 2007).

Developments are regularly being superseded with new innovations; as with all care provided to children, the procedure and outcome must be safe and evidence based, and from an ethical perspective, the expected results for any endoscopic procedure must be at least comparable to those from an open-wound procedure. Along with the development of the design and function of surgical equipment techniques, knowledge and skills also advance. The child whose health status once may have excluded them from an endoscopic procedure may now find that, as a direct result of these advances, an endoscopic procedure can be applied. With the development of this technology and its ever-widening use for more and more procedures, children with complex co-morbidities coming for MIS and endoscopy present another dimension to the surgical team, anaesthetist, perioperative practitioner, facility and the child and family.

The perioperative nurse's role

There are many books that describe, in detail, MIS and endoscopy and the necessary techniques and care, such as *Alexander's Care of the Patient in Surgery* (Rothrock, 2007), and while this chapter includes summaries of equipment and its use, further detailed information can be found there. However, there are particular considerations for children that should be taken into account. Endoscopy provides the ability to view cavities and organs with a tube that can be rigid, semi-rigid or flexible that is inserted into an orifice or surgical incision, with a light source to illuminate the cavity. The scope is passed through one small incision, while further incisions may be made to accommodate the instruments used by the surgeon. Naturally, these incisions and the scopes, tubes and instruments passed through them for surgery in children are often very small, particularly in babies, neonates and preterm infants. The operating field provided with such techniques is essentially limited even in adults, but in children and babies it can be tiny.

Anatomically, children differ from adults, and some special considerations need to be made in preparation for the procedure (Phillips, 2007). It is important that the child has an empty bladder, and a general anaesthetic is usually used. For laparoscopy, decompression of internal structures may be required using a Foley's catheter or nasogastric tube. Sometimes, a radial dilating trochar is inserted into a tiny incision and the incision sequentially enlarged until the necessary size of incision is attained. Insufflation with carbon dioxide (CO_2), which is done to provide an open space in which the surgeon can work, should not exceed 8 cm H_2O in infants and 12 cm H_2O in children up to 8 years (Phillips, 2007). Laparoscopes with a 0–30° viewing angle are often used, and secondary trochars inserted under the laparoscope (Phillips, 2007).

Surgeons require a great deal of skill and training to undertake this surgery, as do the nurses who work in the team. It is not just the instrument nurse in the theatre who requires special skills and knowledge about MIS and endoscopy, all paediatric perioperative nurses need specialised education about it. The nurse who welcomes the child and family to the operating suite needs to know what the procedures involve in order to successfully undertake the preoperative checks and answer any questions the child and parents might have. The anaesthetic nurse needs knowledge of any specific anaesthetic requirements for MIS, while the nurse in the paediatric post-operative recovery unit (PPACU) must know about specific surgical outcomes and possible complications, such as pain and ooze from insertion sites, in the recovery period. All must be aware of the parents' and child's level of understanding of the procedure, and their expectations from it.

Box 12.3 shows types of endoscopes used for specialist surgery on children and an example of the endoscope used for each. Figure 12.1 shows some scopes.

Box 12.3   Some examples of endoscopes used for specialist surgery on children

- Respiratory, e.g. flexible bronchoscope
- Lower gastrointestinal, e.g. colonoscope, sigmoidoscope, proctoscope
- General surgery, e.g. laparoscope
- Cardiothoracic, e.g. rigid bronchoscope
- Neurosurgery, e.g. neuroscope
- Urology, e.g. cystoscope
- Gynaecological surgery, e.g. hysteroscope
- Ear nose throat, e.g. oesphagoscope
- Orthopaedics, e.g. arthroscope

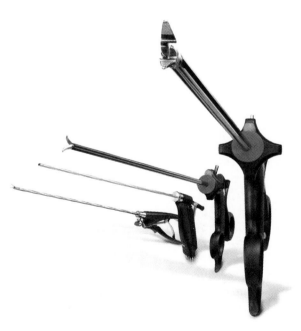

Fig. 12.1   Rigid scopes. Image courtesy of Olympus.

Preparing children for endoscopic procedures

An appropriate and relevant preparation before hospitalisation is known to be important for the emotional benefit of children (see Chapter 2). A study of children undergoing endoscopy found them to be afraid, beforehand, of smells associated with the anaesthetic, possible awakeness during the endoscopy, the potential for pain and lack of knowledge about the procedure. Parents were concerned about the anaesthetic, the procedure itself, diet after the endoscopy and were anxious about the results (Linden & Muller, 2004). Health professionals who care for children who are having endoscopic procedures and their families need to consider the same factors as they would for any family having surgery, but with the recognition that this technology can be even more frightening, as often it is not as well known to children and their parents as ordinary surgery, which, at least, is often represented in television shows.

Children may be chosen for MIS or diagnostic endoscopic procedures for a range of reasons. Laparoscopy is chosen as it gives good visual access of the surgical area for the surgeon, it reduces the formation of adhesions, post-operative pain is minimised, as is length of hospitalisation, and the tiny scars are aesthetically acceptable. There are several disadvantages, including the risk of intra-abdominal injuries, gas embolism, haemorrhage, longer procedure times and higher costs than open surgery. If the surgeon finds that he or she cannot perform the procedure, the child will then be subjected to an open technique (Harrington *et al.*, 2008).

Preparing children for an endoscopic procedure, similarly to other operations, requires significant preparation and education (see Chapter 3). However, the technology used needs some emphasis. Family members, e.g. grandparents and siblings, may have little knowledge of MIS, and so extensive education of the child, the parents and any other members of the family, e.g. siblings who may be concerned, should be included. Effective and supportive education requires a plan that can be standard for the OR or endoscopy unit, and could include an education package given to the family when the child is booked for the procedure, a pre-admission visit where the child and parents can see the equipment and ask questions about the procedure, a telephone call a few days before admission to provide support, make sure the child is physically well, and to answer further questions, and on the day of admission, further education about the process, and importantly, planning for discharge. Innovative techniques for education can be used, e.g. computer games, RSS feeds and other download technology with which children are familiar. A paper that gives comprehensive advice for nurses about preparation of children specifically for endoscopic procedures is Heard (2008).

Perioperative care

While MIS and endoscopic procedures are thought to reduce the length of hospital stay (Ravish *et al.*, 2007; Goers *et al.*, 2008), and to have reduced complications such as pain (Reismann *et al.*, 2007), this may not always be the case, as in a study of children in Australia, 60% suffered throat pain, 31% nausea and vomiting, over half did not attend school, nursery or day care the following day and half the parents had unplanned absences from work as a result (Melville *et al.*, 2007).

Endoscopy in adults is usually done with sedation, and many children, too, are given drugs such as midazolam to keep them still, calm and not anxious during the procedure. However, small children and infants may require general anaesthesia, and for procedures of MIS, this is usually the case. Parents are vital in this process, and should be allowed to stay with the child, at least until the anaesthesia or conscious sedation is working effectively. Preparation of the parents for this is of the utmost importance (see Chapter 3), as the sudden effects of anaesthetic induction can be frightening for parents who are not well prepared.

After a procedure in which the scope is passed through the mouth and throat, such as gastroscopy or bronchoscopy, children can have oedema in the area (Jin *et al.*, 2008), and this can be relieved with ice packs. The child must be carefully observed in PPACU for post-operative complications such as compromised respiration from swelling. Laryngospasm can occur when secretions collect over the anaesthetised vocal cords (McEwan, 2007) and if a local anaesthetic has been applied to the larynx, suction must be kept turned on and readily to hand. A drink before leaving PPACU will determine if the gag reflex has returned. Nonetheless, bronchoscopy has been shown to be a safe procedure in children, with relatively few complications (Bodart & de Bilderling, 1994).

Colonoscopy, where the scope is passed through the anus, is used to examine the large intestine. Children who have this done often have conscious sedation, and are usually required to ingest large volumes of fluid to eliminate faecal matter from their bowel before they arrive. If this has not been possible, an enema may have to be done after the child is sedated, and before the scope is passed. Children in the post-operative phase may pass a great deal of flatus (Pillitteri, 2007).

Bronchoscopies are done on children for diagnostic purposes (Brennan *et al.*, 2008), to introduce drugs, e.g. in children with cystic fibrosis (though there is some debate around this) (Bush & Davies, 2005), for surgical procedures (Abdel-Rahman *et al.*, 2002) and for the removal of foreign bodies (Martinot *et al.*, 1997). These are often done under general anaesthetic, though deep sedation is sometimes used in older children. Spraying of the vocal cords with a local anaesthetic, to immobilise and relax them to allow the scope to be passed, can result in ineffective respiration in the post-operative period. Oedema of the throat can occur, and children will often have a sore throat afterwards. Close observation of the child is necessary for at least 4 hr post-operatively (Pillitteri, 2007). Again, assessment of their gag reflex is important once they are able to drink.

Service perspectives

The National Institutes for Health and Clinical Excellence (NICE) provides evaluation of, and guidelines for, procedures, treatments and products used in health care in the UK, including advice on the use of endoscopy in children. Factors that may influence the surgeon's choice to provide endoscopic surgery are her/his experience, research, evidence-based practice, guidelines set by audit and policy organisations, studies and publications. All such decisions depend on the importance of having appropriately trained staff, in endoscopy and a range of related specialty practices. The facility/hospital must be able to provide a service of multidisciplinary teams so that the child's and family's needs are met throughout the hospital experience. This includes education of staff about the equipment. Some medical device companies provide specialist training for nurses and other health professionals, usually dependent on the hospital or centre purchasing their equipment.

There are benefits to both children and their families and to facilities in providing an endoscopic service. These include:

- offers the latest advances and options for surgery, impacting on reputation and ratings;
- promotes centres of excellence with regard to recruitment and retention of staff;
- decrease in procedure time, allowing more patients on to the list, thus influencing waiting times;
- earlier discharge leads to cost savings to the health authority as patients spend less time in hospital;
- reduction in the incidence of hospital-acquired infections;
- shortened hospital stay means early return to home, school, family and friends.

A district hospital or facility that wished to provide an endoscopic service for paediatric patients would need to weigh up the costs of setting up and maintaining an endoscopic facility against the option of referring a patient to a specialist paediatric facility. Examples of some challenges involved in setting up such a facility include:

- availability of funding for developing and maintaining the project;
- the ability to employ, and/or educate perioperative nurses, surgeons, anaesthetists with specialised training, competencies and qualifications, and experienced staff and facilities for the continuing care of the child and family;
- purchase of equipment;
- purchase of accessories comparing the costs and benefits of reusable items to single-use products;
- advancement in equipment and technique can lead to equipment and accessories becoming obsolete, resulting in further costs;
- process of decontamination and sterilisation of specialised equipment including staff training, facilities, environment to process this equipment;
- facilities/environment that have an appropriate procedural area, space for the storage of equipment and storage of reusable and single-use items;
- regular audit and validation of the facilities and staff providing the service;
- audit and review of the quality of care provided to the patient;
- maintenance of service to the required standards.

Box 12.4 contains some resources for information on the requirements for paediatric endoscopic services.

Box 12.4   Information on requirements for paediatric endoscopy service

Purchasing endoscopic equipment: http://bspghan.org.uk/information/guides.shtml (British Society of Paediatric Gastroenterology, Hepathology and Nutrition 2008).

   An example of a quality analysis undertaken by a children's hospital, which demonstrates the multifactorial and multidisciplinary aspects of managing services in an acute paediatric facility offering endoscopic services can be found at http://www.health.qld.gov.au/wwwprofiles/rch_hsd_rch_mq.asp

Accessed 10 September 2008.

Equipment for MIS and endoscopy

Equipment and checks will be different according to the endoscopic procedure being performed. It is essential that staff are trained and deemed competent prior to using equipment.

Safety

When one accepts the responsibility to care for a patient, the fundamental principal of perioperative practice and indeed a requirement from registration bodies is to meet the standard of duty of care, and under first principles, is do no harm. Endoscopy and MIS care, as with all perioperative care, includes management and risk assessment of the environment and equipment, so before undertaking any task, it is wise to undertake a risk assessment of one's own practice. A specialist competency framework allows progression of training and knowledge according to standards, procedures and protocols within the perioperative environment, thus ensuring patient safety.

Training

All staff must receive training and show competence before using MIS and endoscopy equipment. A database system should be developed to record all staff's competence on equipment and procedures.

Legal issues

By keeping an accurate record of training, health care institutions would have the reassurance that all safety issues are controlled. This sends out a strong safety message to patients that staff have achieved competence on equipment and procedure. Staff can use this as a developmental tool, and it can be an integral part of the staff appraisal system.

Manufacturers set guidelines and protocols on the use of equipment. Importantly, if changes, however small, are made to a product in any way, or if it is used for some other reason than its stated purpose, insurance and indemnity cover is compromised. A good example of such a practice is if a single-use item is reused on another patient (Waller, 2004).

Access to the manufacturer of all products is most important. One should not be using this equipment without sufficient training. Most companies who sell equipment such as endoscopy items and their sterilising systems will provide highly trained representatives who will stay in the facility for several days to weeks to ensure that the staff in a facility are trained in the proper and safe use of a product. Training is often part of the business and purchasing agreement, and material such as a training manual is usually left in the unit for reference. It is imperative that all staff who use such equipment have access to both the training and to up to date reference materials.

The most important point to raise in this section is that equipment must be used only according to manufacturer's instructions. Never change the design, e.g. never bend or shape a piece of equipment such as a scope to fit something for which it was not designed. Not only will it not be safe, but the person who has made the adaptation will not be covered legally. If there are concerns regarding the safety of equipment, always state and obtain expert/senior assistance. Extensive manuals are provided with all equipment and these must be easily and readily available to all staff using the equipment.

Preparation of equipment and accessories

All equipment should be checked to ensure it is safe and functioning prior to the patient's arrival in theatre. Use a general environment check including such items as operating and room lights, suction, diathermy, table and positioning accessories. Box 12.5 shows an example of an equipment check for laparoscopic and endoscopic equipment.

Integrated theatres is one of the latest developments offered to surgery. This is a computerised system where information gathered via the stack system is observed, stored or delivered to computers or teleconferencing networks within the department, hospital or even internationally. This new system requires the same respect that

Box 12.5   An example of laparoscopic endoscopic equipment check

- *Stack*: Laparoscopic stack is complete and functioning. Position according to the surgery being performed. The stack may be moved away from table while the child is being transferred and positioned onto the operating table. Ensure that all stack movement is monitored so that equipment and leads are not damaged or cause harm.
- *Light source*: Check if the light source turns on and intensity can be increased or decreased. Observe whether lamp life is within the accepted limits. This routine check ensures that the lamp has enough life to run throughout the case. Some hospitals have a policy that lamps are to be changed by the hospital medical engineer. Ensure that correct attachments are available to accept the sterile light cable. Once the light source is checked, place it on standby.
- *Monitor*: Switch on and set to the correct function and mode. Check if accessory monitor (slave) is on and then visually observe the monitor functions via camera.
- *Video camera*: Attach camera to the correct outlet, taking care not to burr pins on insertion. Check the camera view via the monitor to ensure that it is focused and correctly orientated. If required, ensure that correct coupling is attached to accept the sterile scope. Following function check, place the camera head within the specific bracket to hold the camera. Be aware that movement of stack may cause damage to the hanging lead of camera if not placed in correct bracket.
- *Gas insufflator*: Check if the cylinder is marked 'CO_2' (carbon dioxide). CO_2 is the gas of choice as it does not support combustion. Turn on gas cylinder, then switch on the insufflator to check volume of gas within cylinder. By ensuring that you physically turn on the cylinder, you will also ensure that the device mechanism (wrench) to turn cylinder on is available for use during the case. Check the function of the insufflator by manually going through its settings and functions, and set delivery volume according to surgeon's preference, zero volume.
- *Data collection device*: This may be a DVD or a video. Ensure that these function and accessories available.
- *Diathermy*: It may be positioned on the stack or as a stand-alone unit. It is essential that all staff members are aware of the function and the risks associated with the diathermy, especially relating to paediatric endoscopic surgery. Some risks include direct coupling, capacity coupling and insulation failure. All of these will lead to accidental burns to the patient. Access local standards and diathermy manuals to read how these risks can be minimised and prevented.

is given to any new equipment purchased. Thorough training and monitoring of the staff to ensure quality and safe use of the equipment is necessary. The perioperative nurse must embrace new technology; however, when using more advanced equipment, they must maintain the focus on the task at hand. For the paediatric perioperative nurse, situational awareness and the ability to clearly communicate any potential problems are necessary skills.

The Alliance for the Safety of Patients, supported by the Royal College of Surgeons England (2008), recognised the importance of the need for improvement in patient safety in theatres, and developed, planned and implemented the Safer Surgical Teams Pilot Project funded by the Health Foundation. Several hospitals are participating in the Safer Surgical Teams Pilot Project; an example is The Hospital for Sick Children, Great Ormond Street, London. This will be a valuable development for the perioperative practitioner as this project addresses the true 'team' with training and development to include all members of our everyday practice team. Paediatric perioperative nurses who work in MIS or endoscopy theatres require skills that enable them to facilitate a multidisciplinary team where short procedures, with sometimes extreme degrees of complexity and close work, and concerned parents and children with emotional needs related to what is happening to them, are part of the equation.

Instruments

The perioperative paediatric nurse requires specific knowledge when choosing the equipment required for an endoscopy list. It is essential to know the child's age and weight when choosing the length and diameters of scopes and instruments. Instruments are made specifically for the varying size of the paediatric patient. As instruments may be packaged so that size cannot be viewed, it is important that the perioperative team is familiar with the written information on the outside packaging so that only the instruments required are opened. Cost implications for opening unnecessary equipment include reduction in lifespan of the instrument from unnecessary reprocessing, the cost of the process to render the item sterile and time lost as a direct result of inadequate knowledge of correct equipment required.

Cannulated instruments need to be checked for any sign of break in the integrity of the insulated outer sheath. The child could sustain a burn through arcing when the diathermy is used. The perioperative nurse must be vigilant to assess the safety function of the instruments offered.

The perioperative nurse should also possess knowledge about the correct use of any instruments for which they are responsible. Some instruments require assembling by the nurse prior to the case. It is essential that new staff are provided time for training, and time to become familiar and efficient at assembly and function of an instrument prior to patient contact. The same respect should be given to disposable instruments as to reusable instruments. Companies will provide trainers to come into the department to give teaching sessions on the safe use and function of their product.

Rigid scopes

Rigid and flexible scopes have bundles of glass fibres within them, so naturally, this makes a scope susceptible to breakage. As rigid scopes may be finer and smaller than other scopes, great care must be taken when attaching the light lead and camera to ensure that the weight of the camera and light lead does not bend or damage it. Never rest heavy objects on instruments and scopes. Monitor the surgical staff to ensure that the scope is protected from damage. By understanding the design of a product, one is more likely to handle it properly. A check should be done immediately after the rigid scope and light source are removed from their sterile packaging to see that the fibre optics are clear and functioning. Hold the scope towards a room light, look into the eyepiece (taking care not to render the item non-sterile) to check that the view is clear. If dark spots are present, first clean both ends with a soft instrument wipe, and view again. If dark spots persist, replace with another scope. If the lens is blurred or has black spots, the surgeon will not have a clear view of the child's anatomy. The light lead is checked in a similar manner by holding one end to light and looking into the other end. Never leave a light lead switched on in an unattended area or resting on drapes, as there are documented cases of patients suffering burns (Hensman *et al.*, 1998).

Laser surgery requires extreme vigilance and safety measures. All staff who use lasers should undergo an accredited course on safe use of lasers. In some countries such as Australia, it is a legal requirement for surgeons to be licensed to use the laser, and nurses who work in areas where lasers are used should always be educated in their use and safety. Fire is a threat in surgery where lasers are used, and every facility will have safety procedures in place to protect patients, staff and the facility itself (Werder, 2003).

Decontamination and sterilisation of scopes

One of the best fundamental principles on which to base any writing on sterilisation is 'if it is not clean it cannot be sterile'. Thorough, correct and quality-controlled cleaning procedures must be in place in any facility that provides endoscopy services.

It is important to always check to what process equipment can be subjected. Flexible scopes are not able to be autoclaved, nor are some rigid scopes, but some endoscopic cameras are. The most important message here is always to check the manufacturer's directions before beginning the sterilisation process. However, as with any instrument that is being placed in the body, the item must be rendered sterile. Scopes can be automatically washed and sterilised, though some facilities may not have an automatic washer and steriliser, so it is necessary to manually decontaminate and sterilise the scope. The perioperative nurse should follow local policies and guidelines (that should reflect national and international guidelines) to ensure that safe and correct process is followed. Good practice when processing flexible scopes includes the following:

- Follow the manufacturer's recommendations on decontamination and sterilisation process and review policy and guidelines on decontamination and sterilisation of scopes.
- Always remove bio-burden (any tissue, blood, body fluids etc.) and rinse scope through to prevent body fluid and debris drying within the channel of the scope. This is necessary for any cannulated instrument. Remember always to submerge the open ends of the item being flushed under the solution to prevent aerosol spraying of droplets of contaminated fluid.

- An endozymatic solution should be used to break down bio-burden.
- Follow manufacturer's advice and instruction for cleaning and sterilising product.
- Undertake the process in a 'non-clean' area.
- Staff members must wear protective clothing for the process. Read the local health and safety act, and check the local policy on infection control. If an injury is sustained, and the staff member is not wearing protective attire, he/she may not be able to claim compensation benefits.
- A leak test is carried out before the decontamination process takes place. A leak test failure identifies that there is a fault or break to the outer covering of the scope, which will affect the integrity of the scope. Microorganisms and debris from the previous case may remain within the scope, preventing it from being rendered sterile. As well, if the process of decontamination continues, further damage will be caused to the scope as a direct result of fluid entering through the damaged surface to the inner workings. The item must be dried, packaged and identified as a contaminated scope, and the department or manufacturer that repairs scopes must be alerted to the scope's contaminated state before they accept the scope for repair.
- The same principle applies to all instruments and accessories. It is imperative to thoroughly examine each item to ensure that it is safe for use.
- It is important to use a new single-use brush following an individual patient event. Where a contaminated brush is used, bacteria and bio-burden could contaminate the following scopes and infect following patients. Second, it is unlawful to use an item deemed as single-use more than once unless a written agreement exists between the health service and manufacturer. This agreement would be put in place following a risk assessment and acceptance that no harm would be caused from reusing the item.

Specific guidelines exist for Creutzfeldt–Jakob Disease (CJD). All hospitals and centres must ensure that national guidelines are followed for the management of instruments, scopes and equipment for patients with CJD or any suspected case of CJD (British Society of Gastroenterology Decontamination Working Group and the ACDP TSE Working Group Endoscopy and vCJD Sub-Group (2005)). The British Department of Health (1999) published specific documentation relating to endo-scopes, such as the health service circular *HSC1999/178: Variant Creutzfeldt-Jakob disease (vCJD): Minimising the risk of transmission.*

Many professional and specialist associations have standards and guidelines that are an excellent source for updating any information about the decontamination and sterilising of scopes, and these have a real effect on practice. In 2004, in Northern Ireland, an enquiry into cleaning scopes found that processes were insufficient, thereby putting patients at risk (Health Protection Agency, 2005). The report from this incident resulted in national guidelines being developed and implemented by users of endoscopic fibre-optic scopes within the UK, with a flow-on effect internationally.

Peracetic acid is often used to sterilise endoscopic equipment. The Steris™ System uses peracetic acid (vinegar) to kill bacteria at 50°C. The system has a sealed chamber in which peracetic acid is diluted to a 0.2% solution and heated to between 50 and 55°C. The cycle runs for 12 mins and automatically drains off all the fluid once the solution has been neutralised by the automatic injection of a buffering agent into the chamber. Items are then rinsed in sterile water. Steris sterilises immersible surgical and diagnostic items. As with all sterilising techniques, it is effective only if cleaning has been adequate before immersion. Instruments with a lumen and other possible contamination traps must be cleaned with bacteriostatic or protein neutraliser product. Steris™ has been found to be of particular use in the sterilisation of scopes, and research has indicated that while it is more expensive than other methods, it is less toxic than gluteraldehyde, and it is usually more effective (Cronmiller *et al.*, 1999; Society of Gastroenterology Nurses and Associates Inc., 1999; Vesley *et al.*, 1999; Tandon & Ahuja, 2000; Herron & Shields, 2003).

Potential anaesthetic and surgical problems

Laparoscopic surgery: carbon dioxide gas (CO_2) is used for insufflation and extension of the abdomen. CO_2 does not support combustion, thereby reducing the risk of explosion. It must be noted that the gas is being delivered under pressure and there is a risk that gas emboli may enter the circulation. CO_2 usually dissolves quickly in the blood, however, as this risk factor exists, careful monitoring of the patient for signs of hypercarbia is required. Even though the insufflation pressure is selected by the surgeon for the age and weight of the child, the increased abdominal pressures along with positioning of the patient (such as reverse Trendelenberg or Trendelenberg) to allow access to the surgical site may result in changes in the patient's respiratory, cardiac and other body systems. It is essential that the perioperative nurse is aware of the flows and pressures set on the insufflator, takes heed of any alarms and ensures that the surgical team responds (Harrington *et al.*, 2008).

Prior to skin closure, the surgeon will use the scope to view organs and tissues beyond the surgical incision to check for any signs of perforation, burns or bleeding. Extra care is taken when insufflation is stopped so that there is no further bleeding (Ball, 2007).

Positioning

Prior to the child arriving in the department, it is essential that the teams are aware of the child's needs to ensure safety when positioning. Some children present with limited physical movement and as a direct result will need extra care and attention to position the body and limbs. No child should sustain any tissue or nerve damage or discomfort following surgery from improper positioning. Surgical access is essential; however, the patient's safety is paramount. Some examples of good practice are as follows (Harrington *et al.*, 2008):

- Prevent falls, ensure that the child is secured with appropriate supports and restraints. Always have a member of the team at the child's side so that if there is any movement, they are able to take immediate action and summon help.
- Limb, nerve, tissue damage is averted by care when positioning the patient. Check for misalignment of the body, or any pressure or undue stress or stretch placed on tissue or limbs. Use gel, padding and supports to prevent nerve damage. Aim to reduce post-operative discomfort.
- Reduce shear forces during patient positioning by practicing good manual-handling techniques.

- Ensure airway, vascular and other medical devices are secured, supported and checked during positioning so that any disconnections, trauma or tissue damage is averted. Monitors must be checked when the child is placed in the new position, for functioning and correct readouts.
- Ensure that the child's bladder is emptied before surgery, or a catheter may have to be passed if the child is anaesthetised with a full bladder. Because children have a shallow pelvis, the chance of bladder damage when the trochar is inserted is real.
- Repositioning of the patient may be required throughout surgery. Staff must engage with the anaesthetist in this process and be competent in the function of the table and accessories. All positions and devices used to move and support the patient should be documented on the patient care plan.
- Endoscopy involving the child's airway: It is imperative that all staff stay alert to the likelihood of any physical trauma occurring to the patient's airway. As these procedures require a shared airway, i.e. the anaesthetist and surgeon require access to the airway, it is imperative that good communication and procedure is followed. Fires have occurred within airways during surgery. Extra care must be taken by the team to ensure that the patient's airway is not compromised whilst surgery is performed.
- All children undergoing surgery should have their body's thermoregulation closely monitored, and this is particularly important with infants and small children whose temperature-regulating systems are not well developed. There are many actions that can be taken to ensure that the child's temperature is maintained within acceptable limits, such as warming insufflation gas, IV fluids, wrapping limbs in cotton wool, using warming blankets etc. The perioperative nurse must document all such care provided on the care plan. The perioperative nurse and surgical team will evaluate and take appropriate action on the patient's response to warming methods.
- For genitourinary endoscopic surgery, where sterile irrigating fluids are administered to distend the bladder to allow visualisation of the anatomy, irrigate and remove resected tissue, the solution is warmed to prevent hypothermia. However, it is important that fluids are not overheated. Ensure that the solution is safe to use with diathermy. The solution chosen by the surgeon will be the one that will cause the least risk to the patient if absorbed into the blood stream, and so a clear non-electrolytic and isosmotic solution should be used (Ball, 2007).

In PPACU

Some adult patients complain of shoulder pain following laparoscopic procedures (Ball, 2007), and this has been recorded in children (De Lagausie, 2006). This occurs when CO_2 delivered under pressure irritates the phrenic nerve, and thus pain is referred to the shoulder. Children may not be able to verbalise or describe their pain. Careful observation and administration of pain relief is required for all children post-surgery.

Following airway surgery, some children may require humidified oxygen and medication to alleviate oedema within the airway. The child should be positioned to enhance breathing and comfort.

Conclusion

Parents entrust their children to nurses for care, so it is important to remember that no matter what position within the theatre a nurse holds, the nurse is the child's and parents' advocate and it is part of the role to ensure that the family receives the best care. This is as relevant for MIS and endoscopy as it is in any other surgical specialty. Endoscopy is engulfed with modern technology that is forever developing and bringing benefits and some risks to the patient and health facilities. Paediatric perioperative nurses working in such a highly specialised role and environment need specialist education at the highest level, and part of the advocacy for children and parents includes political lobbying to ensure that recognition and funding are provided for such education. The care of children and their families having MIS and endoscopy will benefit.

References

Abdel-Rahman, U., Ahrens, P., Fieguth, H.G., Kitz, R., Heller, K., Moritz, A. (2002). Surgical treatment of tracheomalacia by bronchoscopic monitored aortopexy in infants and children. *Annals of Thoracic Surgery*, 74: 315–319.

Anastasakis, E., Protopapas, A., Daskalakis, G., Papadakis, M., Milingos, S., Antsakilis, A. (2007). Transforming a conventional theatre into a gynaecological endoscopy unit. *Clinical and Experimental Obstetrics and Gynaecology*, 34(2): 99–101.

Aziz, O, Athanasiou, T, Tekkis, P.P., *et al.* (2006). Laparoscopic versus open appendectomy in children: A meta-analysis. *Annals of Surgery*, 243(1): 17–27.

Becmeur, F., Reinberg, O., Dimitru, C., Moog, R., Philippe, P. (2007). Thoracoscopic repair of congenital diaphragmatic hernia in children. *Seminars in Pediatric Surgery*, 16(4): 238–244.

Ball, K.A. (2007). Surgical modalities. In: Rothrock, J.C., McEwan, D.R. (eds). (2007). *Alexander's care of the patient in surgery*. Mosby Elsevier, St. Louis, MO.

Bodart, E., de Bilderling, G. (1994). Fibreoptic bronchoscopy under local anaesthetic in infants is a safe and a useful technique with numerous indications. *European Journal of Pediatrics*, 153(3): 209.

Brennan, S., Gangell, C., Wainwright, C., Sly, P.D. (2008). Disease surveillance using bronchoalveolar lavage. *Paediatric Respiratory Review*, 9(3): 151–159.

British Society of Gastroenterology Decontamination Working Group and the ACDP TSE Working Group Endoscopy and vCJD Sub-Group (2005). *Endoscopy and individuals at risk of v CJD for public health purposes*. Available from http://www.advisorybodies.doh.gov.uk/acdp/tseguidance/endoscopy-consensus.pdf (accessed 8 September 2008).

Bush, A., Davies, J. (2005). Early detection of lung disease in preschool children with cystic fibrosis. *Current Opinions in Pulmonary Medicine* 11(6): 534–538.

Cronmiller, J.R., Nelson, D.K., Salman, G., *et al.* (1999). Antimicrobial efficacy of endoscopic disinfection procedures: A controlled, multifactorial investigation. *Gastrointestinal Endoscopy*, 50(2): 152–158.

De Lagausie, P., Ramella, B., Roquelaure, B. (2006). Left shoulder pain during meals: A rare complication after laparoscopic Toupet procedure in children. *Surgical Laparoscopy, Endoscopy and Percutaneous Technology*, 16(5): 368–369.

Department of Health (1999). *HSC 1999/178: Variant Creutzfeldt–Jakob disease (vCJD): Minimising the risk of transmission*. Available from http://www.dh.gov.uk/en/PublicationsAndStatistics/LettersAndCirculars/HealthServiceCirculars/DH_4004969 (accessed 8 September 2008).

Feliz, A., Shultz, B., McKenna, C., Gaines, B.A. (2006). Diagnostic and therapeutic laparoscopy in pediatric abdominal trauma. *Journal of Pediatric Surgery*, 41(1): 72–77.

Geishauser, T., Querengasser, K., Querengasser, J. (2005). Teat endoscopy (theloscopy) for diagnosis and therapy of milk flow disorders in dairy cows. *Veterinary Clinics of North America – Food and Animal Practice*, 21(1): 205–225.

Goers, T., Panepinto, J., Debaun, M., *et al.* (2008). Laparoscopic versus open abdominal surgery in children with sickle cell disease is associated with a shorter hospital stay. *Pediatric Blood Cancer*, 50(3): 603–606.

Gore, P.A., Nakaji, P., Deshmukh, V., Rekate, H.L. (2006). Synchronous endoscopy and microsurgery: A novel strategy to approach complex ventricular lesions. Reports of three cases. *Journal of Neurosurgery*, 105(Suppl. 6): 485–489.

Graham-Rowe, D. (2006). Robot set loose to film your insides. *New Scientist*, 189(2536): 26.

Handa, R., Kale, R., Harjai, M. (2006). Incidental inguinal hernias on laparoscopy. *Asian Journal of Surgery*, 29(1): 28–30.

Harrington, S., Simmons, K., Thomas, C., Scully, S. (2008). Pediatric laparoscopy. *AORN Journal*, 88(2): 211–236.

Health Protection Agency. (2005). Independent review of endoscope decontamination in Northern Ireland. *CDR Weekly*, 15: 3. Available from http://www.hpa.org.uk/cdr/archives/archive05/News/news1305.htm#endoscope (accessed 8 September 2008).

Heard, L. (2008). Taking care of the little things: Preparation of the pediatric endoscopy patient. *Gastroenterology Nursing*, 31(2): 108–112.

Hensman, C., Hanna, G.B., Drew, T., Moseley, H., Cuschieri, A. (1998). Total radiated power, infrared output, and heat generation by cold light sources at the distal end of endoscopes and fiber optic bundle of light cables. *Surgical Endoscopy*, 12(4): 335–337.

Herron, A., Shields, L. (2003). Infection control: Sterilizing. In: Shields, L., Werder, H. (eds). *Perioperative Nursing*. Greenwich Medical Media, London.

Jin, F., Mu, D., Chu, D., Fu, E, Xie, Y., Liu, T. (2008). Severe complications of bronchoscopy. *Respiration* (DOI: 10.1159/000151656).

Kagadis, G.C., Siablis, D., Liatsikos, E.N., Petsas, Nikiforidis, G.C. (2006). Virtual endoscopy of the urinary tract. *Asian Journal of Andrology*, 8(1): 31–38.

Linden, A.I., Muller, S. (2004). Endoscopy and children: Dealing with fears. *Gastrointestinal Gastroscopy*, 59(5): 142.

Lui, T.H. (2007). Arthroscopy and endoscopy of the foot and ankle: Indications of new techniques. *Arthroscopy*, 23(8): 889–902.

Martinot, A., Closset, M., Marquette, C.H., *et al.* (1997). Indications for flexible versus rigid bronchoscopy in children with suspected foreign-body aspiration. *American Journal of Respiratory and Critical Care Medicine*, 155(5): 1676–1679.

McEwan, D.R. (2007). Laryngolic and head and neck surgery. In: Rothrock, J.C., McEwan, D.R. (eds). *Alexander's care of the patient in surgery*. Mosby Elsevier, St. Louis, MO, pp. 674–703.

Melville, D., da Silva, M.S., Young, J., McCann, D., Cleghorn, G. (2007). Postprocedural effects of gastrointestinal endoscopy performed as a day case procedure in children: Implications for patient and family education. *Gastroenterology Nursing*, 30(6): 426–434.

Michaud, R.M., Schoolfield, J., Mellonig, J.T., Mealey, B.L. (2007). The efficacy of subgingival calculus removal with endoscopy-aided scaling and root planing: A study on multirooted teeth. *Journal of Periodontology*, 78(12): 2238–2245.

Patrick, D.A. (2006). Prospective evaluation of a primary laparoscopic approach for children presenting with simple or complicated appendicitis. *American Journal of Surgery*, 192(6): 750–755.

Phillips, N. (2007). *Berry & Kohn's operating room technique*, 11th ed. Mosby Inc., St. Louis, MO.

Ravish, R., Nerli, R.B., Reddy, M.N., Amarkhed, S.S. (2007). Laparoscopic pyeloplasty compared with open pyeloplasty in children. *Journal of Endourology*, 21(8): 897–902.

Reismann, M., von Kampen, M., Laupichler, B., Suempelmann, R., Schmidt, A.I., Ure, B.M. (2007). Fast-track surgery in infants and children. *Journal of Pediatric Surgery*, 42(1): 234–238.

Rothrock, J.C. (2007). Alexander's care of the patient in surgery. 13th ed. Mosby Elsevier, St. Louis, MO.

Simonite, T. (2007). Creepy-crawly robot to mend a broken heart, *New Scientist*, 194(2600): 26.

Society of Gastroenterology Nurses and Associates, Inc. (1999). Guideline for the use of high-level disinfectants and sterilants for reprocessing of flexible gastrointestinal endoscopes. *Gastroenterology Nursing*, 22(3): 127–134.

Stamm, A.M. (2006). Transnasal endoscopy-assisted skull base surgery. *Annals of Otology, Rhinology & Laryngology*, 196(Suppl): 45–53.

Tandon, R.K., Ahuja, V. (2000). Non-United States guidelines for endoscope reprocessing. *Gastrointestinal Endoscopy Clinics North America*, 10(2): 295–318.

The Royal College of Surgeons England. (2008). *Safety and Leadership for Interventional Procedures and Surgery (SLIPS)*. Available from http://www.rcseng.ac.uk/education/courses/safety_and_leadership_intervention.html (accessed 8 September 2008).

Tichenor, W.S., Adinoff, A., Smart, B., Hamilos, D.L. (2008). Nasal and sinus endoscopy for medical management of resistant rhinosinusitis. *Journal of Allergy and Clinical Immunology*, 121(4): 917–927.

Vesley, D., Melson, J., Stanely, P. (1999). Microbial bioburden in endoscope reprocessing and an in-use evaluation of the high-level disinfection capabilities of Cidex PA. *Gastroenterology Nursing*, 22(2): 63–68.

Waller, F. (2004). Singled out? *British Journal of Perioperative Nurses*, 14(3): 122–125.

Werder, H. (2003). Safety measures. In: Shields, L., Werder, H. (eds). *Perioperative nursing*. Greenwich Medical Media, London.

13 Ethical and legal issues in paediatric perioperative care

Linda Shields

Patients' rights

The United Nations Convention on the Rights of the Child (UNICEF, 2007) ascribes to every child the right to the best health care possible, and this affects every aspect of a child's experience in a health service. Every child and her or his family, regardless of sex, race, religion or class, has the right to expect to be cared for with dignity and respect in the perioperative area. Extraordinary procedures, an alien environment, odd smells and sounds, people in bizarre clothes and strange surroundings make up the *milieu* of the operating room suite. Many think they know what an operating theatre is like from watching television, but the reality is nothing like their expectations. Some children and their families are terrified at the thought of entering such a place, as it appears totally foreign to them. Any child and parent who comes to the operating theatres needs support, and nurses are the best people to give that support. Nurses have the communication skills to make children less frightened; nurses know the value of touch, of reassurance, of being beside the child, talking and explaining what is happening, and the best way to communicate with their worried parents.

Children and parents have the right to know that their safety is assured while in the care of perioperative nurses. This includes emotional and spiritual safety as well as physical. Often, children have operations for life-threatening illnesses and are frightened about what will be found; often, they are having palliative care operations to improve their quality of life and know that their lifespan will be shortened. Children and their parents often accept the risks of a new procedure in the hope that the child's life will be improved. Often, parents accept these responsibilities for their children. These are frightening situations, and nurses are most often the ones who recognise this and support the family most effectively.

People from a culture different to the prevailing culture of the hospital have a right to have their particular needs met, including religious and spiritual needs. As an example, Muslim families will feel much more comfortable having an operation for removal of a body part if they know they have the choice to decide if that body part will be given to them to dispose of according to their religious laws. Nurses are best situated to find out the wishes of people and to afford them the opportunity of having their wishes respected.

Ethical dilemmas surround contentious issues. While advocating for the child and family, the nurse must be aware of the laws of the country and act accordingly. However, it is important that the nurse knows the wishes of a child and his or her parents and ensures that they are respected.

Self-determination

Children and their families always have choices and it is an important part of operating room procedure to ensure that those choices are considered. If, at the last minute, a family decides that their child cannot go through with a procedure, then those wishes are respected. However, if a child decides at the last minute, then a dilemma occurs. Who has the final say? How much autonomy should a child be granted in this situation? Is the maxim of 'best interests of the child' relevant? Conclusive answers to such dilemmas do not exist, and they require skilful handling by nurses and doctors with effective communication skills who are well versed in the ethics and legalities of the situation.

Good counselling skills are vital for perioperative nurses who care for children and their families. A nurse can talk with the child and parents, help address any queries and issues and allow them to discuss the issues with the appropriate person, be it the surgeon, the anaesthetist or both. Often, these problems are complicated if the child has had premedication of some sort and may not be thinking clearly. The nurse assumes the role of patient advocate and co-ordinates communication for the child and family so their best interests are assured.

Privacy

A child's privacy can be greatly compromised within the operating theatre. The child is unconscious and has no control over what is happening. At the same time, his or her body is exposed for the operation and there are a number of people within the operating theatre at any one time. Theatre suites often have little provision for private conversations, and procedure boards with patients' names and details are often on view to anyone who enters the suite. It is incumbent on all perioperative nurses to ensure that children's privacy is respected at all times. Keep the child covered as much as possible, restrict visitors to the operating theatres and conduct conversations about private information away from heavy-traffic areas. Surgeons often brief parents on completion of a procedure; this is best done in a separate room away from other people.

Children need a great deal of privacy. Even the smallest children do not appreciate their bodies being exposed; in fact, some children are extremely 'body-aware'. To expose them unnecessarily is to affront their personal dignity, more so if they are anaesthetised and do not know what is happening to them. A special word about infants is needed here. While we have no knowledge of an infant's concept of body and nakedness, we cannot assume that it is not important. The tiniest baby requires the same degree of respect and privacy as any other patient.

Confidentiality

As in all health care, children undergoing operative and anaesthetic procedures have the right to expect that their personal details will be handled in a confidential manner. Operating departments, while closed areas, require a large staff of many different professions and trades, many of whom have no need to have access to patients' charts or details. Charts should not be left in places where they can be seen by any persons whose roles do not involve direct patient care. When interviewing the child's family to inform them of the progress of the operation, the surgeon needs a private room or area where he can explain confidential information in privacy.

Consent

Hospitals these days have strict, mandatory policies to be followed when obtaining consent for an operation from a patient. Scenario 13.1 demonstrates how informed consent can be utilised with a child. The principle of 'Gillick competence' covers consent by and for minors, and this is true in many countries. For an excellent, simple explanation of Gillick competence in medical treatment, see the Oxford Radcliffe Hospital's (2007) website: http://confidential.oxfordradcliffe.net/Gillick. While it is widely recognised in the UK, Australia (Queensland Commission for Children and Young People and Child Guardian, 2007) and New Zealand (McLean, 2000), it is also part of the legal framework for children in other countries. In short, it says that a child who is intellectually able to understand and make a decision can and should consent for his or her own treatment. Most places, though, also ask parents to sign consent forms, and there is a deal of legal discussion about merits in law of Gillick competence (Potter, 2006; Cavell, 2007). Scenario 13.2 shows how Gillick competence can guide decisions.

Scenario 13.1 Informed consent

In the preadmission clinic, Tom, aged 11, faces the surgeon, Uyen, who is going to remove a haemangioma from Tom's chest wall, and she has gone to great pains to explain to Tom's parents the procedure, its sequelae and probable results. However, Tom could not understand what Uyen has said, and has told them he does not want to have the operation done. Uyen calls on the nurse, David, and explains the problem. David and Uyen take Tom and his parents to the playroom in the clinic, where there are dolls, medical equipment, a miniature operating theatre and anaesthetic machines and equipment. Using the dolls for illustration, David explains to Tom what the procedure is and why it has to be done. He shows Tom the machines that will be used, shows him how the IV will be inserted and allows Tom to handle and examine all the equipment. Tom asks both David and Uyen questions about what will happen to him if he does not have the operation and what could potentially go wrong during it. They answer truthfully, but in ways that Tom can understand and that are not frightening. They then tell Tom that while his parents legally have to sign the consent form before Tom goes into theatre, Tom also can sign it. Tom is very pleased with this – he feels he is very much in control of what is going to happen to him, and is confident that Uyen will do a good job. He agrees to have the operation.

Scenario 13.2 Legal consent

Annabel is 14 years old, and has cystic fibrosis. She has had a series of chest infections, the last three resulting in prolonged ventilation in ICU. Annabel is on the list for a lung transplant, and one day the call comes. Her parents are overjoyed and take Annabel to the hospital, but Annabel is not so sure. Some of her friends have had transplants, and all but one have died after going through even more severe treatment than for their cystic fibrosis. In the OR reception, while she is being checked in, Annabel decides she does not want to go through with it and refuses to sign the consent form. Her parents have signed, but under the precepts of Gillick competence, Annabel is legally able to sign her own consent form. As a consequence of her refusal to sign the consent form, Annabel's operation cannot proceed.

Usually in the case of children, the parents and/or accompanying family can give consent (Kerridge *et al.*, 1998). In some hospitals, the right of children to sign consent forms is being recognised, and providing the parent countersigns it, older children are signing their own consent forms. The same principles stand – the child must understand what he or she is signing, must understand what the operative procedure is and what it is for and must be informed of the risks involved. Any communication with a child has to be age-appropriate, and tools such as puppets and calico dolls are good ways to help explain the procedure to a child.

It is important that any child and parent giving consent for any operative procedure should be fully informed as to the reason for the operation, what is going to happen to him or her and the risks involved. In many countries, it is the duty, in law, of the surgeon to explain the procedure and accompanying risks (Breen *et al.*, 1997), while the anaesthetist has the responsibility of explaining the anaesthetic and its implications to the child and parent before the operation (Australia New Zealand College of Anaesthetists, 2006). It is the nurses' responsibility to ensure that they have been told and that they understand what has been said (Murphy, 2000). Nurses in the ward confirm that the child and parents know and fully understand, as do the nurses who receive them in the operating suite. In some hospitals, it is the admitting nurse in the operating suite who must check that the consent form has been signed, in other words, the patient cannot leave the ward to be transported to the OR until the consent form is signed. In extreme emergencies, an operation can begin without a signed consent form; however, this occurrence is very rare (see Chapter 3).

If a child or parent does not seem to understand what is happening to the child, or if the consent form has not been signed, it is the nurse's responsibility to contact the surgeon and/or the anaesthetist. The doctor will see the child and ensure that the child and parent are adequately informed and the consent form signed. It is important that, in the case of a child who can consent themselves, this be done prior to administration of premedication.

Checking that the child and parents understand what is going to happen requires good, and age-appropriate communication skills. The best way is to ask the child and parents outright, however, some may say that they understand because they do not want to look foolish, or are frightened to say they do not understand. Asking the child and parents to explain in their own words what is going to happen will show the nurse how much they understand.

Nurses are ideally placed to tell patients about what the operation will be like and what will happen to them, not just in the operating theatre, but in the lead up to, and following, the operation. Children and their parents need to know what to expect. Even for the most informed, intelligent and knowledgeable person of any age, operating theatres and procedures are frightening, anxiety-causing events. The role of the perioperative nurse is to alleviate as much anxiety as possible.

Legal perspectives

Litigation is a real risk for perioperative nurses (Cox, 2000; Shinn, 2001; Singapore Nurses Association, 2005). Although many hospitals take vicarious liability for the nurse, it is imperative that perioperative nurses hold indemnity insurance to cover them for any potential legal action that may be taken against them. New technologies such as endoscopy and laser, and the increase in responsibility taken by nurses in situations where they become the surgeon's assistants have changed the boundaries of what could reasonably be expected of a nurse in the OR. Under the duty of care owed to patients undergoing surgical procedures, adherence to standards and guidelines for safe practice and detailed, objective documentation ensures that nurses' actions will be considered reasonable in a legal action.

Nurses may find themselves involved in lawsuits even though they may not have participated in an adverse incident. Nurses must be able to access legal counsel to protect their interests. In many countries, professional and industrial bodies provide such coverage, usually, though, only to their members. It is incumbent on nurses to join their organisations and ensure that their membership remains current.

In a survey of claims against perioperative nurses, the cases for which legal action was taken included retained foreign objects, pressure injuries, medication errors, equipment faults and operations at the wrong site (Murphy, 1997). If nurses document everything carefully, as well as ensure that their own standards of education and competence are kept up to date, that they keep abreast of rising technologies and act in accordance with policies, guidelines and principles in place in their hospital, then they will be sure of being able to attest to the reasonableness of their actions should the need to do so ever arise in a court of law.

Medical futility

A value conflict with which the perioperative nurse has to deal is medical futility, in other words, is it right to do an operation just because it can be done? While strict codes of ethics govern medical practice, as they do nursing practice, surgeons sometimes fail to see that an operation might be futile to the patient. While it is easy to dictate that nurses must become patient advocates in these situations, in reality, it becomes a difficult dilemma when a colleague's work is to be questioned, and nurses may often have to accept what they see as inappropriate activities. In these situations, the nurse can do several things (Schroeter, 1997). First, the nurse can assess if the child and parents have consented freely to the operation, and fully understand what is involved. The rest of the surgical team needs to be consulted, and this is usually done in an open meeting. While it may be difficult to stand back and watch what they see as a procedure of little benefit performed, nurses must accept the child's and parents' decision to have the operation. If perioperative nurses are aware of their own values systems and can identify and understand fully their own feelings and principles, then they will be better able to deal with problems such as these.

Some health care organisations have a qualified ethicist on staff, and/or staff counsellors. For any perceived conflict of ethical values, the nurse in charge of the unit can refer nurses in his or her charge to these people.

Conclusion

Because of the unique culture of the operating theatre, legal and ethical issues there can be confusing, and create dilemmas not seen elsewhere in health and nursing practice. A good knowledge of the ways to resolve such dilemmas and the rights and responsibilities of nurses, staff and parents and children will ensure that ethical practice, which is at the same time legal, will be paramount.

References

Australia New Zealand College of Anaesthetists. (2006). *PS7 Recommendations on the pre-anaesthesia consultation*. Australia New Zealand College of Anaesthetists, Melbourne. Available from http://www.anzca.edu.au/resources/professional-documents/professional-standards/ps7.html (accessed 13 January 2007).

Breen, K., Plueckhahn, V., Cordner, S. (1997). *Ethics, law and medical practice*. Allen & Unwin, St Leonards.

Cavell, R. (2007). Towards a better consent form. *Journal of Law and Medicine*, 14: 326–338.

Cox, C. (2000). A lesson in the age of litigation. *Nursing Standard*, 14: 61.

Kerridge, I., Lowe, M., McPhee, J. (1998). *Ethics and law for the health professions*. Social Science Press, Katoomba.

McLean, K. (2000). Victoria University of Wellington Law Review. Children and Competence to Consent: *Gillick* Guiding Medical Treatment in New Zealand. Available from http://www.austlii.edu.au/nz/journals/VUWLRev/2000/31.html (accessed 12 May 2009).

Murphy, E.K. (1997). Types of legal claims brought against perioperative nurses. *Association of Operating Room Nurses Journal*, 65: 972–973.

Murphy, E.K. (2000). Preparation of the patient for the procedure: Legal and ethical considerations. In: Phippen, M.L., Wells, M.P. *Patient care during operative and invasive procedures*. WB Saunders, Philadelphia, PA.

Potter, J. (2006). Rewriting the competency rules for children: Full recognition of the young person as rights-bearer. *Journal of Law and Medicine*, 14: 64–85.

Queensland Commission for Children and Young People and Child Guardian. (2007). Commission for Children and Young People and Child Guardian Amendment Bill 2007. Queensland Government. Available from http://www.austlii.edu.au/au/legis/qld/bill/cfcaypacgab2007601/ (accessed 12 May 2009).

Schroeter, K. (1997). Medical futility: Interpretation and ethical ramifications for the perioperative nurse. *Seminars on Perioperative Nursing*, 6: 138–141.

Shinn, L.J. (2001). *Yes, you can be sued. The nursing risk management series: An overview of risk management*. American Nurses Association. Silver Spring Available from http://www.nursingworld.org/mods/archive/mod310/cerm101.htm (accessed 13 January 2007).

Singapore Nurses Association. (2005). *Overview paper*. ICN Asia Workforce Forum. Available from http://www.icn.ch/Flash/sew_awf_overview05.swf (accessed 13 January 2007).

UNICEF (2007). *United Convention on the Rights of the Child, 1989*. Available on http://www.unicef.org/photoessays/30048.html (accessed 12 January 2007).

Index